Update Gastroenterology 2003

New developments in diagnosis and management of early and advanced GI malignancy

John Libbey Eurotext
127, avenue de la République
92120 Montrouge
Tél. : 33 (0) 1 46 73 06 60
e-mail : contact@john-libbey-eurotext.fr
http://www.john-libbey-eurotext.fr

John Libbey Eurotext Limited
42-46, High Street
Esher
Surrey
KT10 9QY
United Kingdom

© John Libbey Eurotext, 2003
ISBN : 2-7420-0497-1

Il est interdit de reproduire intégralement ou partiellement le présent ouvrage - loi du 11 mars 1957 - sans autorisation de l'éditeur ou du Centre Français du Copyright, 6 *bis*, rue Gabriel-Laumain, 75010 Paris.

Update Gastroenterology 2003

New developments in diagnosis and management of early and advanced GI malignancy

Edited by
G.N.J. Tytgat,
F. Penninckx

Combined EAGE, ISDS, EDS and EAES
Postgraduate Course 2003
Madrid, November 1-2

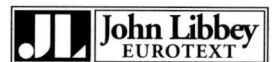

The publication of this book was made possible
thanks to the support from the NEGMA-GILD Laboratories.

Contents

Foreword
G.N.J. Tytgat IX

I – Upper GI malignancy

Indication for endoscopic mucosal resection or photodynamic therapy in superficial esophageal tumours
O. Pech, C. Ell 3

Indications for minimal invasive surgery in upper GI malignancy
A. Fingerhut 11

The role of induction chemotherapy in upper GI cancer
F. Lordick, J.R. Siewert 21

Extended vs limited resection for esophageal cancer: an individual approach
J.J.B. van Lanschot 35

II – Bilio-pancreatic malignancy

Critical appraisal of staging of bilio-pancreatic tumours
D.J. Gouma 41

Endoscopic and endosonographic approaches to biliopancreatic lesions
T. Rösch 55

Surgery for pancreatic cancer
N. Alexakis, J.P. Neoptolemos 63

Pancreatic and biliary tract carcinoma: any role for photodynamic therapy?
S.P. Pereira 79

III – General oncology

What should the clinician/surgeon know about molecular oncogenesis?
H.E. Blum, C. Arnold, O. Opitz, H. Usadel 95

Colitis-Associated Cancer - Time for New Strategies
F. Shanahan 107

Stress response after laparoscopic surgery
M. Buunen, M. Gholghesaei, R. Veldkamp, N.D. Bouvy, D.W. Meijer, H.J. Bonjer.... 113

To what extent will *Helicobacter pylori* eradication reduce gastric cancer?
A. Axon 131

Is antireflux surgery an effective prevention of malignant transformation in GERD?
L. Lundell... 141

Adenocarcinoma of the gastric cardia and gastro-esophageal junction
K.E.L. McColl.. 151

Familial cancer syndromes of the gastrointestinal tract and the role of surgery
G.O. Ceyhan, J. Kleeff, M.W. Büchler, H. Friess.. 161

Is the novel grading/staging system of neoplasia useful?
K. Geboes 175

Endoscopic mucosal resection for treatment of early gastric cancer. Indication and new technique, IT knife method
H. Ono 183

IV – Secondary liver tumours

Local ablative therapy for liver metastases
R. Lencioni, C. Franchini, L. Crocetti, D. Cioni 191

Interstitial laser coagulation: liver metastases
T.J. Vogl, R. Straub, K. Eichler, M. Mack.. 201

V – Lower GI malignancy

Critical appraisal of staging rectal cancer
R.G.H. Beets-Tan.. 219

Endoscopic management of early colorectal lesions
B. Saunders 227

Multi-modality treatment in advanced rectal tumours
L. Påhlman 233

The role of stenting as temporary and palliative treatment
M.C. Parker... 239

Rationale and techniques of intra-operative hyperthermic intraperitoneal chemotherapy in peritoneal surface malignancy
A.J. Witkamp, V.J. Verwaal, S. van Ruth, E. de Bree, F.A.N. Zoetmulder 247

List of contributors

Alexakis N., Department of Surgery, University of Liverpool, Royal Liverpool University Hospital, 5th floor UCD Building, Daulby St, Liverpool, L69 3GA, United Kingdom
Arnold C., Abteilung Innere Medizin II, Medizinische Universitatklinik, Freiburg, Germany.
Axon A., Department of Gastroenterology, Room 190A, Clarendon Wing, The General Infirmary at Leeds, Great George Street, Leeds, LS1 3EX, UK.
Beets-Tan R.G.H., Department of Radiology, University Hospital Maastricht, P.O. Box 5800, 6202 AZ Maastricht, The Netherlands.
Blum H.E., Abteilung Innere Medizin II, Medizinische Universitatklinik, Freiburg, Germany.
Bonjer H.J., Department of Surgery, Dr. Molewaterplein 40, 3015 GD, Rotterdam, The Netherlands.
Bouvy N.D., Department of Surgery, Dr. Molewaterplein 40, 3015 GD, Rotterdam, The Netherlands.
Büchler M.W., Department of General Surgery, University of Heidelberg, Im Neuenheimer Feld 110, D-69120 Heidelberg, Germany.
Buunen M., Department of Surgery, Dr. Molewaterplein 40, 3015 GD, Rotterdam, The Netherlands.
Ceyhan G.O., Department of General Surgery, University of Heidelberg, Im Neuenheimer Feld 110, D-69120 Heidelberg, Germany.
Cioni D., Division of Diagnostic and Interventional Radiology, Department of Oncology, Transplants, and Advanced Technologies in Medicine, University of Pisa; Via Roma 67, I-56125 Pisa, Italy.
Crocetti L., Division of Diagnostic and Interventional Radiology, Department of Oncology, Transplants, and Advanced Technologies in Medicine, University of Pisa; Via Roma 67, I-56125 Pisa, Italy.
De Bree E., Department of Surgical Oncology, The Netherlands Cancer Institute/Antoni van Leeuwenhock Hospital, Plesmanlaan 121, CX 1066 Amsterdam, The Netherlands.
Eichler K., University of Frankfurt/Main, Department of Diagnostic and Interventional Radiology, Theodor-Stern-Kai 7, 60590 Frankfurt am Main, Germany.
Ell C., Department of Medicine II, Wiesbaden Hospital, Ludwig-Erhard-Strasse 100, 65199 Wiesbaden, Germany.
Fingerhut A., Centre Hospitalier Intercommunal, 78303 Poissy Cedex, France.
Franchini C., Division of Diagnostic and Interventional Radiology, Department of Oncology, Transplants, and Advanced Technologies in Medicine, University of Pisa; Via Roma 67, I-56125 Pisa, Italy.
Friess H., Department of General Surgery, University of Heidelberg, Im Neuenheimer Feld 110, D-69120 Heidelberg, Germany.
Geboes K., Department of Pathology, K.U. Leuven, Minderbroederstraat 12, 3000 Leuven, Belgium.
Gholghesaei M., Department of Surgery, Dr. Molewaterplein 40, 3015 GD, Rotterdam, The Netherlands.
Gouma D.J., Academic Medisch Centrum/Universiteit van Amsterdam, afd. Chirurgie, Meibergdreef 9, 1105 AZ Amsterdam, The Netherlands.

Kleeff J., Department of General Surgery, University of Heidelberg, Im Neuenheimer Feld 110, D-69120 Heidelberg, Germany.
Lencioni R., Division of Diagnostic and Interventional Radiology, Department of Oncology, Transplants, and Advanced Technologies in Medicine, University of Pisa; Via Roma 67, I-56125 Pisa, Italy.
Lordick F., Department of Surgery, Klinikum rechts der Isar, Technical University of Munich, Ismaninger Str. 22, D-81675 Munich, Germany.
Lundell L., Department of Surgery, Huddinge University Hospital, Stockholm, Sweden.
McColl K.E.L., University Department of Medicine and Therapeutics, Western Infirmary, Glasgow, Scotland, United Kingdom.
Mack M., University of Frankfurt/Main, Department of Diagnostic and Interventional Radiology, Theodor-Stern-Kai 7, 60590 Frankfurt am Main, Germany.
Meijer D.W., Laboratory of Expimental Surgery, AMC University Hospital of Amsterdam, Amsterdam, The Netherlands.
Neoptolemos J.P., Department of Surgery, University of Liverpool, Royal Liverpool University Hospital, 5th floor UCD Building, Daulby St, Liverpool, L69 3GA, United Kingdom.
Ono H., Endoscopy and GI oncology division, Shizuoka Cancer Center Hospital, Japan.
Opitz O., Abteilung Innere Medizin II, Medizinische Universitatklinik, Freiburg, Germany.
Påhlman L., Dept. Surgery, Colorectal Unit, University Hospital, Uppsala, Sweden.
Parker M.C., Department of Surgery, Darent Valley Hospital, Dartford, United Kingdom.
Pech O., Department of Medicine II, Wiesbaden Hospital, Ludwig-Erhard-Strasse 100, 65199 Wiesbaden, Germany.
Pereira S.P., Institute of Hepatology and National Medical Laser Centre, University College London Campus, Royal Free & University College London Medical School, London WC1E 6HX.
Rösch T., Department of Internal Medicine II, Technical University of Munich, Germany.
Saunders B., Wolfson Unit for Endoscopy, St. Mark's Hospital, Harrow, Middlesex, HA1 3UJ, United Kingdom.
Shanahan F., Alimentary Pharmabiotic Centre, Department of Medicine, Cork University Hospital and University College Cork, National University of Ireland, Cork, Ireland.
Siewert J.R., Department of Surgery, Klinikum rechts der Isar, Technical University of Munich, Ismaninger Str. 22, D-81675 Munich, Germany.
Straub R., University of Frankfurt/Main, Department of Diagnostic and Interventional Radiology, Theodor-Stern-Kai 7, 60590 Frankfurt am Main, Germany.
Usadel H., Abteilung Innere Medizin II, Medizinische Universitatklinik, Freiburg, Germany.
Van Lanschot J.J.B., Department of Surgery, Academic Medical Center at the University of Amsterdam, Meibergdreef 9, 1105 AZ Amsterdam, The Netherlands.
Van Ruth S., Department of Surgical Oncology, The Netherlands Cancer Institute/Antoni van Leeuwenhock Hospital, Plesmanlaan 121, CX 1066 Amsterdam, The Netherlands.
Veldkamp R., Department of Surgery, Dr. Molewaterplein 40, 3015 GD, Rotterdam, The Netherlands.
Verwaal V.J., Department of Surgical Oncology, The Netherlands Cancer Institute/Antoni van Leeuwenhock Hospital, Plesmanlaan 121, CX 1066 Amsterdam, The Netherlands.
Vogl T.J., University of Frankfurt/Main, Department of Diagnostic and Interventional Radiology, Theodor-Stern-Kai 7, 60590 Frankfurt am Main, Germany.
Witkamp A.J., Department of Surgical Oncology, The Netherlands Cancer Institute/Antoni van Leeuwenhock Hospital, Plesmanlaan 121, CX 1066 Amsterdam, The Netherlands.
Zoetmulder F.A.N., Department of Surgical Oncology, The Netherlands Cancer Institute/Antoni van Leeuwenhock Hospital, Plesmanlaan 121, CX 1066 Amsterdam, The Netherlands.

Foreword

It gives me a great pleasure also on behalf of Prof. Penninckx to introduce this syllabus to you, the result of fruitful collaboration between the EAGE and all European surgical societies (EAES, EDS, ISDS).

It truly reflects the main mission of these European societies: to promote teaching and education by bringing the latest clinical and basic science innovations in the various disciplines. This postgraduate course is a perfect example of this mission. The course focuses on all aspects of early malignancy throughout the GI tract. We come full circle as diagnosis, endoscopic nonsurgical and surgical aspects are covered in depth. Whenever possible the clinical advice is evidence-based and critically analysed. A galaxy of world renown experts covers the various topics. Their scientific and educational qualities guarantee a teaching performance of highest standard. A major virtue of this course is the integration or the blending of the medical and surgical approaches. There can be no doubt that such "integrative approach" is beneficial for the patients with malignancy for whom we care. What will be presented during this course stresses once again that early detection is of paramount importance in order to improve the ultimate outcome and prognosis of GI malignancy.

The organising societies owe a great debt to Prof. Penninckx, and particularly to prof. Gouma, the surgical motor in the organisation, to Mrs. Ewa Jonsson, the EAGE congress organiser, and to Prof. Galmiche, so helpful in producing the syllabus. Last but no least all organising societies are immensely grateful to Negma-Gild, France, once again realising the publication of this postgraduate course through the capable hands of the John Libbey publishing house.

I can only hope that the collaboration between EAGE and soon EAGE/ESGE and all surgical societies may continue and flourish at the time of our annual UEGW for many years to come.

Prof. G.N.J. Tytgat
Co-chairman organising committee

I

Upper GI malignancy

Indication for endoscopic mucosal resection or photodynamic therapy in superficial esophageal tumours

Oliver Pech, Christian Ell

Department of Medicine II, Wiesbaden Hospital, Wiesbaden, Germany

Introduction

In the early 1990s, there was a sudden increase in the clinical importance of Barrett's esophagus. This was mainly due to the marked increase in the incidence of adenocarcinoma at the esophagogastric junction and a growing understanding of the pathophysiological connections between reflux disease, Barrett's metaplasia and adenocarcinoma. Endoscopic technology (above all high-resolution video endoscopy), the training of endoscopists, enthusiasm on the part of pathologists and gastroenterologists, and epidemiological conditions thus all contributed to the current "Barrett's boom" [1].

The risk of developing severe dysplasia or adenocarcinoma in comparison with the normal population is 30-125 times higher in traditional Barrett's esophagus, and the incidence is reported to be between one in 52 and one in 208 patient-years [2]. The risk of carcinoma appears to correlate with the severity of the reflux symptoms. A Swedish population-based case-control study for the first time demonstrated a direct connection between gastro-esophageal reflux and the development of esophageal adenocarcinoma [3].

Radical esophageal resection is still the standard treatment in patients with early esophageal malignancies; however, it is associated with high rates of mortality and morbidity. Even in specialized centres with highly selected groups of patients, the mortality in early neoplasias is more than 3%, and the morbidity is reported to be 20-50% [4-6]. In patients over the age of 70, the mortality increases to as high as 11% [7]. Therefore new therapeutic methods would be desirable.

Methods

Endoscopic resection

The "suck-and-cut" technique is used in the esophagus more frequently than strip biopsy, due to the anatomical conditions, and is also the technique favoured by our own group. With a simple strip biopsy, with or without mucosal injection, sufficiently large specimens can be obtained in the esophagus, particularly in flat neo-plastic lesions. A study by Tanabe *et al.* [8] demonstrated that endoscopic suck-and-cut mucosectomy in early gastric cancer is more effective than strip biopsy with regard to the largest diameter of the resected specimen, the rate of en-bloc resection, and the complication rate.

In the early 1990s, Inoue and co-workers developed the cap technique, thereby improving the effectiveness of ER in comparison with simple strip biopsy [9]. In the ER cap technique, a specially developed transparent plastic cap is attached to the end of the endoscope. After injection under the target lesion, the lesion is sucked into the cap and resected with a diathermy loop that has previously been loaded onto a specially designed groove on the lower edge of the cap. Since injecting underneath early carcinomas often makes it difficult to distinguish them, prior marking of the lesion – *e.g.*, using electrocautery – is recommended.

ER with a ligation device is another suction mucosectomy technique. In this method, the target lesion is sucked into the ligation cylinder, and a polyp is created by releasing a rubber band around it. The polyp is then resected at its base, either above or below the rubber band, using a diathermy loop. In this technique, the endoscope being used for resection has to be withdrawn again and reintroduced in order to remove the ligation cylinder and introduce the loop. Ligation devices available include, in addition to single-use devices, a reusable ligator [10], with which comparable results can be achieved at reduced cost.

A recently conducted study by our research group compared the two suction mucosectomy techniques – the cap technique and the ligation technique – in the resection of early esophageal neoplasias [11]. In this prospective study, 100 consecutive endoscopic mucosal resections were performed in 70 patients with early esophageal cancer. Fifty resections were carried out with the ligation device without prior injection, and 50 resections using the cap technique with prior submucosal injection with a diluted epinephrine-saline solution. The main criteria were the maximum diameter of the resected specimen, the resection area, and the complication rate. No significant differences were observed between the two groups with regard to the maximum diameter of the resected specimens and the resection area after 24 h. There was only a slight advantage for the ligation group in patients who had had prior treatment. One minor bleeding incident occurred in each group, but no severe complications were seen.

Photodynamic therapy

The principle of photodynamic therapy (PDT) is selective sensitisation of precancerous or malignant lesions using a systemically applicable photosensitiser with subsequent, endoscopically controlled, photochemically induced tissue ablation. While initially hematoporphyrin derivative (HPD), a photosensitiser with more side effects like posttherapeutic stenosis or prolonged photosensitivity of the skin over several weeks, was used in recent years 5-aminolevulinic acid-induced protoporphyrin IX (5-ALA-PpIX) has gained clinical application [12-14]. The main advantages of 5-ALA-PpIX are its only minimal phototoxic side effect and the well tolerated local reaction of the mucosa.

5-ALA, a naturally occurring precursor in the biosynthetic pathway for heme production, is administered orally and induces a relatively selective accumulation of PpIX in malignant tissue [15, 16]. Illumination with laser light of 635 nm wavelength generates cytotoxic oxygen species that in turn cause tissue destruction [14, 17].

PDT, as a local endoscopically guided treatment approach, is based on selective sensitisation of precancerous or malignant lesions and light-induced tissue destruction. The light sources now most often used are dye lasers in continuous-wave mode. Laser light with a defined wavelength is introduced into the gastrointestinal tract endoscopically via flexible optical fibres, and can be used for local irradiation of the sensitised dysplastic or malignant tissue. Photodynamic therapy exploits the phenomenon that light can activate photosensitised substances stored in the tissue, and can destroy the tissue by means of oxidation processes. In contrast to conventional high-energy lasers, the mode of action of PDT thus allows selective, nonthermal destruction of the target tissue while protecting the healthy surroundings as far as possible. To administer the light in tubular hollow organs such as the esophagus, cylindrical diffusers are used for circumferential light application [18]. Using the appropriate irradiation applicators, an area of up to 8 cm can be ablated in a single treatment session, depending on the laser energy used. The light doses applied range from 20 J to 300 J, depending on the photosensitizer used, with a power density of 100-400 – a fraction of the power applied using the Nd:YAG laser.

The advantage of PDT is that the ablation is homogeneous and extensive, allowing long segments of neoplasia to be completely treated in a few sessions. In comparison with other techniques, PDT requires the lowest number of sessions to achieve ablation of *e.g.* Barrett's epithelium. Side effects that have been observed involved phototoxic reactions in the skin, dysphagia and odynophagia, strictures and pleural effusion. However, these side effects mainly occurred with first-generation and second-generation photosensitizers [19]. PDT with 5-aminolevulinic acid, a new endogenous photosensitizer, has a reduced depth of penetration and thus a lower rate of stenosis [12]. In addition, the agent has faster decay kinetics in comparison with other photosensitizers, so that the risk of phototoxic effects in the skin is only present for a period of 36-48 hours [20]. This markedly improves the patients' quality of life, since they do not have to remain in darkened rooms for several weeks.

The advantages of EMR in comparison with all other local endoscopic treatment procedures are obvious. The histological preparation of the resection specimen provides information on the depth of invasion of the individual wall layers, and allows complete resection within healthy margins. The patient is still able to undergo surgical treatment even if submucosal invasion (associated with positive lymph nodes in 20-25% of patients) is not initially recognized at EMR. Therefore EMR should be used as the endoscopic treatment of choice, whenever possible.

Staging

An exact staging procedure, including chromoendoscopy, high resolution video endoscopy, magnification endoscopy and endoscopic ultrasound (EUS), is crucial before endoscopic therapy and influences the therapeutic concept.

In Barrett's esophagus chromoendoscopy with methylene blue and acetic acid should be performed. Methylene blue staining using a special spraying catheter has been found useful for characterising specialised columnar epithelium in Barrett's esophagus, with a sensitivity of ca. 90%. Methylene blue causes reversible staining of actively absorbant cells, particularly the goblet cells of the intestinal mucosa. Since the segment containing Barrett's epithelium may simultaneously include gastric epithelium (fundus), junctional epithelium (cardia) and intestinal epithelium, vital staining makes it easier to achieve precise biopsy identification of the specialised Barrett's epithelium [21]. In inhomogeneous or more weakly staining and unstained mucosal areas, dysplastic changes may be present, or there may be a focal adenocarcinoma [12, 22]. In combination with magnification endoscopes the detection of small malignancies could be improved decisively.

Iodine staining is successfully used in squamous cell neoplasias. Lugol's solution stains the intracellular glycogen content of squamous epithelium, which is reduced when there is tumour growth. Intestinal metaplasia and dysplastic or tumour-bearing segments do not take up the brown stain.

While endoscopy can delineate the intraluminal spread of the tumour, endosonography serves to assess the depth of tumour invasion into the surrounding area, including the lymph-node status. Endosonography is superior to computed tomography for classic tumour staging, as it allows depiction of the individual wall layers and can therefore precisely describe the extent of tumour spread into the surrounding area. Staining using endosonographic techniques is adapted to the TNM classification [23, 24]. The endoscopic ultrasound devices with a 360° sector with a frequency between 7.5 MHz and 12 MHz has a penetration depth of 10 cm and is used for the detection of paraesophageal lymph nodes. Small ultrasound probes with a frequency from 15 to 20 MHz are thin and can be introduced through pro-grade endoscopes, and have recently also made it possible to carry out fine diagnosis in the mucosal and submucosal areas. They are used for specialised description of early esophageal carcinoma with submucosal assessment (mucosal (uT1m) *versus* submucosal involvement (uT1sm)) [25-28]. Accuracy rates of up to 90% for T staging and up to 80% for lymph-node status have been reported when pre-therapeutic tumour staging is correctly conducted. Despite the very good sensitivity of 80% for lymph-node involvement, the specificity is still low at 40%; however, there is still a lack of reliable endosonographic criteria for lymph-node metastases. Incipient invasion of the submucosa also appears to be problematic, and cannot be detected with absolute certainty.

After the careful and extensive staging procedure the decision about the best therapeutic way can be made according the "Wiesbaden Concept":

Barrett's neoplasia

– In patients with detectable early Barrett's neoplasia ER should be performed.

– In patients with not detectable neoplasia and proof of histology by a second experienced pathologist, ALA-PDT should be used as the way of treatment.

Squamous cell neoplasia

– Due to the high sensitivity of Lugol's staining neo-plastic lesions are always detectable. Therefore only ER should be performed in patients with squamous cell neoplasia. PDT is only used as a supportive therapy to ablate large areas of cis.

Results

Patients with early Barrett's neoplasia treated by ER show excellent acute and short time follow-up results: ER was performed in a prospective study in 64 patients with high grade intraepithelial neoplasia and early Barrett's cancer. Complete remission was achieved in 97% of all low risk situations. No major complications occurred [29]. Intermediate results in 115 patients with early Barrett's neoplasia, in whom our "Wiesbaden concept" was used, showed a minor complication rate of 9.5% and a complete local remission rate of 98%. The calculated overall 3-year survival rate is 88% [30]. Just now we have also the long term survival of > 100 patients available, who were treated by ER only. 5-year survival is not different to the average survival rate of normal German people (unpublished data)

The results of ALA-PDT as primary treatment in patients with superficial neoplasia in Barrett's esophagus are also promising. 66 patients (mean age 61.4 ± 10.2 years) with high grade intraepithelial neoplasia (HGIN) (group A; n = 35) and early adenocarcinoma (group B; n = 31) were treated by PDT. Protoporphyrin IX induced by oral administration of 5-aminolevulinic acid was used as photosensitizer. A total of 82 ALA-PDT were performed. 34 of the 35 patients in group A (97%) and all patients in group B (100%) achieved a complete response during a mean follow-up period of 41.7 ± 18.4 months.

Endoscopic resection of esophageal squamous-cell neoplasia with curative intent seems to show similar results as patients with early Barrett's neoplasia. A total of 39 patients (mean age 61.4 ± 10.2 years) with early esophageal carcinoma (n = 29) and carcinoma *in situ* (Cis) (n = 10) fulfilled the criteria for local endoscopic therapy and were treated using endoscopic resection. Ten patients had carcinoma *in situ* (group A), 19 patients had mucosal cancer (group B) and 10 patients had submucosal cancer (group C). All patients in group C were inoperable or had refused surgery. Nine of the 10 patients in group A (90%), 19 of the 19 in group B (100%) and 8 of the 10 in group C (80%) achieved a complete response during a mean follow-up period of 29.7 ± 14.3 months. Tumour-related deaths occurred in three patients (one in group B, who was inoperable; two in group C, who refused surgery). Calculated 5-year survival was 90% in group A, 89% in group B and 0% in group C [31].

References

1. Pracht AT, MacDonald TA, Hopwood DA, Johnston DA. Increasing incidence of Barrett's esophagus: education enthusiasm or epidemiology? *Lancet* 1997; 350: 933.
2. Drewitz DJ, Sampliner RE, Garewal HS. The incidence of adenocarcinoma in Barrett's esophagus: a prospective study of 170 patients followed 4.8 years. *Am J Gastroenterol* 1997; 92: 212-5.
3. Lagergren J, Bergström R, Lindgren A, Nyren O. Symptomatic gastroesophageal reflux as a risk factor for esophageal adenocarcinoma. *N Engl J Med* 1999; 340: 825-31.
4. Hölscher AH, Bollschweiler E, Schneider PM, et al. Early adenocarcinoma in Barrett's esophagus. *Br J Surg* 1997; 84: 1470-3.
5. Nigro JJ, Hagen JA, DeMeester TR, et al. Occult esophageal adenocarcinoma: extent of disease and implications for effective therapy. *Ann Surg* 1999; 230: 433-40.
6. Rice TW, Falk GW, Achkar E, et al. Surgical management of high grade dysplasia in Barrett's esophagus. *Am J Gastroenterol* 1993; 88: 1832-6.
7. Thomas P, Doddoli C, Neville P, et al. Esophageal cancer resection in the elderly. *Eur J Cardiothorac Surg* 1996; 11: 941-6.
8. Tanabe S, Koizumi W, Kokutou M, et al. Usefulness of endoscopic aspiration mucosectomy as compared with strip biopsy for the treatment of gastric mucosal cancer. *Gastrointest Endosc* 1999; 50: 819-22.
9. Inoue H, Endo M. A new simplified technique of endoscopic esophageal mucosal resection using a cap-fitted panendoscope. *Surg Endosc* 1993; 6: 264-5.
10. Ell C, May A, Wurster H. The first reusable multiple-band ligator for endoscopic hemostasis of variceal bleeding and mucosal resection. *Endoscopy* 1999; 31: 738-40.
11. May A, Gossner L, Behrens A, Ell C. A prospective randomized trial of two different suck-and-cut mucosectomy techniques in 100 consecutive resections in patients with early cancer of the esophagus. *Gastrointest Endosc* 2003; 58: 167-75.
12. Gossner L, Stolte M, Sroka R, et al. Photodynamic ablation of high-grade dysplasia and early cancer in Barrett's esophagus by means of 5-aminolevulinic acid. *Gastroenterology* 1998; 114: 448-55.
13. Gossner L, May A, Sroka R, Stolte M, Hahn EG; Ell C. Photodynamic destruction of high grade dysplasia and early carcinoma of the esophagus after the oral administration of 5-aminolevulinic acid. *Cancer* 1999; 86 (10): 1921-8.
14. Regula J, MacRobert AJ, Gorchein A, et al. Photosensitization and photodynamic therapy of esophageal, duodenal and colorectal tumours using 5-aminolevulinic acid induced protoporphyrin IX – a pilot study. *Gut* 1995; 36: 67-75.
15. El-Far M, Ghonheim M, Ibraheim E. Biodistribution and selective *in vivo* tumour localization of endogenous porphyrins induced and stimulated by 5-aminolevulinic acid: a newly developed technique. *J Tumour Marker Oncol* 1990; 5: 27-34.
16. Bedwell J, MacRobert AJ, Phillips D, Bown SG. Fluorescence distribution and photodynamic effect of ALA-induced PpIX in the DMH rat colonic tumour model. *Br J Cancer* 1992; 65: 818-24.
17. Orenstein A, Kostenich G, Roitman L, et al. A comparative study of tissue distribution and photodynamic therapy selectivity of chlorine 6, Photofrin II and ALA-induced protoporphyrin IX in a colon carcinoma model. *Br J Cancer* 1996; 73 (8): 937-44.
18. Gossner L, Sroka R, Ell C. A new long-range through-the-scope balloon applicator for photodynamic therapy in the esophagus and cardia. *Endoscopy* 1999; 31: 370-6.
19. Overholt BF, Panjehpour M, Halberg DL. Photodynamic therapy for Barrett's esophagus with dysplasia and/or early stage carcinoma: Long-term results. *Gastrointest Endosc* 2003; 58: 183-8.
20. Kennedy JC, Pottier RH. Endogenous porphyrin IX, a clinically useful photosensitizer for photodynamic therapy. *J Photochemistry and Photobiology* 1992; 14: 275-92.
21. Canto MI, Setrakia S, Petras RE, et al. Methylene blue selectively stains intestinal metaplasia in Barrett's esophagus. *Gastrointestinal Endoscopy* 1996; 44 (1): 1-7.

22. Canto MI. Methylene blue staining and Barrett's esophagus. *Gastrointestinal Endoscopy* 1999; 49: S12-6.
23. Tio TL, Cohen P, Coene PPLO, Udding J, den Hartog Jager FCA, Tytgat GNJ. Endosonography and somputed tomography of esophageal carcinoma: Pre-operative classification compared to the new (1987) TNM system. *Gastroenterology* 1989; 96: 1478-86.
24. Tio TL, Coene PPLO, den Hartog Jager FCA, Tytgat GNJ. Preoperative TNM classification of esophageal carcinoma by endosonography. *Hepato-Gastroenterology* 1990; 37: 376-81.
25. Akahoshi K, Chijiwa Y, Hamada S, *et al.* Pre-treatment staging of endoscopically early gastric cancer with a 15 Mhz ultrasound catheter probe. *Gastointestinal Endoscopy* 1998; 48: 470-6.
26. Hünerbein M, Ghadimi BM, Haensch W, *et al.* Transendoscopic ultrasound of esophageal and gastric cancer using miniaturized ultrasound catheter probes. *Gastrointestinal Endoscopy* 1998; 48: 470-6.
27. Natsugoe S, Yoshinaka H, Morinage T, *et al.* Ultrasonographic detection of lymph-node metastases in superficial carcinoma of the esophagus. *Endoscopy* 1996; 28: 674-9.
28. Yanai H, Masahiro T, Karita M, Okita K. Diagnostic utility of 20-megahertz linear endoscopic ultrasonography in early gastric cancer. *Gastrointestinal Endoscopy* 1996; 44: 29-33.
29. Ell C, May A, Gossner L, Pech O, Seitz G, Stolte M. Endoscopic mucosal resection of early cancer and high-grade dysplasia in Barrett's esophagus. *Gastroenterology* 2000; 118: 670-7.
30. May A, Gossner L, Pech O, Vieth M, Stolte M, Ell C. Local endoscopic therapy for intraepithelial high-grade neoplasia and early adenocarcinoma in Barrett's esophagus: acute-phase and intermediate results of a new treatment approach. *Europ J Gastro Hep* 2002; 14: 1085-91.
31. Pech O, Gossner L, May A, Vieth M, Stolte M. Curative endoscopic resection of early squamous cell cancer and cancer *in situ*. *Am J Gastro* 2003 (accepted).

Indications for minimal invasive surgery in upper GI malignancy

Abe Fingerhut

Centre Hospitalier Intercommunal, 78303 Poissy Cedex, France

Presently, the main indications for minimal invasive surgery in upper gastrointestinal (GI) surgery are diagnosis and staging. The indications for resective surgery for upper GI malignancy are for the moment limited, but an expansion in certain settings can be foreseen. The theoretical advantages include the minimal invasive aspect of laparoscopic surgery, and whenever applicable, better vision to ensure adequate dissection. One hitherto under-emphasized advantage of the laparoscopic approach concerns the reduction of wound complications, seemingly greatly minimized by the laparoscopic approach (Duepree *et al.*, *J Am Coll Surg*, 2003). The limitations for diagnostic, staging, and therapeutic laparoscopy, on the other hand, have focused on missed lesions, incomplete vision, the (non)-radicality of resection, potential dissemination and port-site metastasis.

Diagnostic laparoscopy was introduced and developed in the 1970's (Christoffsen *et al.*, *Acta Pathologica*, 1970; Cushieri *et al.*, *Gut*, 1978), and has allowed these authors to confirm the diagnosis of cancer, to access the operability of tumour, and has proven useful for retrieval of material for diagnosis (Irving *et al.*, *Br J Surg*, 1978; Ishida *et al.*, *Endoscopy*, 1981). The role of laparoscopy for diagnosis, staging and eventually therapeutic purposes is still increasing (Shoup *et al.*, *Ann Surg Oncol*, 2002) and laparoscopy has been used for assessment of esophageal (Shandell *et al.*, *Br J Surg*, 1985), gastric (Shandell *et al.*, *Br J Surg*, 1985; Possik *et al.*, *Cancer*, 1986) and pancreatic (Freiss *et al.*, *J Am Coll Surg*, 1998; Warshaw *et al.*, *Am J Surg*, 1986; Irving *et al.*, *Br J Surg*, 1978; Cushieri, *Eur J Surg Oncol*, 1988; Pisters *et al.*, *Br J Surg*, 2001) carcinoma as well as to help detect hepatic metastasis (Possik *et al.*, *Cancer*, 1986). Laparoscopy should therefore represent another way of detecting extrapancreatic disease that cannot be found by standard pre-operative imaging. In some initial reports, up to one third of patients were found to have previously undetected disease through laparoscopic staging (Warshaw, *Am J Surg*, 1986; John, *Ann Surg*, 1995). Laparoscopy also plays an important role in the categorization of pancreatic carcinoma with respect to resectability.

Staging laparoscopy has been used both as a separate staging procedure (separate anaesthesia) and as part of a combined approach (Jiminez et al., Arch Surg, 2000; Fernanez del Castillo et al., Arch Surg, 1995), performed immediately before laparotomy under the same anaesthesia (Conlon et al., Ann Surg, 1996; Minnard et al., Ann Surg, 1998; Holzman et al., J Gastrointest Surg, 1997). In a recent review of the literature, Pisters et al. (Br J Surg, 2001) underscored that when state-of-the-art computerized tomography (CT) is available, the routine use of staging laparoscopy may not be easily justified. High quality CT has an accuracy of radiological prediction of resectability ranging from 75 to 89 per cent (Spitz et al., J Clin Oncol, 1997; Gloor et al., Cancer, 1997; Freiss et al., J Am Coll Surg, 1998; Holzman et al., J Gastrointest Surg, 1997; Rumstadt, J Gastrointest Surg, 1997). Laparoscopic detection of CT occult M1 disease or local tumour extension involving the mesenteric vessels or coeliac axis can be as high as 24 per cent (Jiminez et al., Arch Surg, 2000; Fernandez del Castillo, Arch Surg, 1995) but carries a false negative rate of 3 to 9 per cent (Jiminez et al., Arch Surg, 2000; John et al., Ann Surg, 1995).

As concerns the respectability, Santori et al. (Hepatogastroenterology, 1999) studied 14 patients with cancer of the pancreas. Laparoscopy reported that three of the 14 cases (21%) had metastatic disease and were therefore unresectable. Cuschieri (Eur J Surg Oncol, 1988) reviewed 73 patients who had undergone laparoscopy for pancreatic cancer. Forty-two were correctly staged as having inoperable disease. Peritoneal or omental deposits were only detected by laparoscopy. Underwood and Soper described laparoscopic surgery of the pancreas, including the laparoscopic management of pancreatic pseudocysts and pancreatic resection for islet cell tumours.

In the study from the Massachusetts General Hospital describing 125 patients with non-metastatic (localized and locally advanced) (M0) pancreatic cancer, as assessed by CT between 1994 and 1998 (Jiminez et al., Arch Surg, 2000), 30 patients (24%) had extrapancreatic disease and nine patients (7%) had positive cytological evidence of extrapancreatic disease. Conlon et al. (Memorial Hospital) (Ann Surg, 1996) evaluated 115 patients with suspected or proven pancreatic tumours believed to be resectable after CT.

In fact, it is not only laparoscopic imaging as such that is the determining factor. Intraoperative ultrasound is the principal adjunctive investigation measure and has proven to be crucial in several series (John et al., Ann Surg, 1995; Pietrabissa et al., World J Surg, 1999). However, laparoscopic sonography also has its limitations (Vollmer et al., Ann Surg, 2002).

Diagnostic laparoscopy at one time was thought to be useful as it could have avoided unnecessary laparotomy in up to 18% of cases (Neiveen Van Dijkum, Cancer, 1997). Currently however, laparoscopic staging may not improve outcome in patients with peripancreatic carcinoma compared to standard radiology staging. Laparoscopy and laparoscopic ultrasound were performed in 297 consecutive patients with peripancreatic carcinoma scheduled for surgery after radiological staging (Nieveen Van Dijkum, Ann Surg, 2003). Patients with pathology-proven unresectable tumours were randomly allocated to either surgical or endoscopic palliation. All others underwent laparotomy. Laparoscopic staging detected biopsy-proven unresectable disease in 39 patients (13%). At laparotomy, unresectable disease was found in another 72 patients, leading to a detection rate for laparoscopic staging of 35%. In all, 145 of the 197 patients classified as having "possibly resectable" disease after laparoscopic staging underwent resection (74%). Average survival in the group of 14 patients with biopsy-proven unresectable tumours randomly allocated to endoscopic palliation was 116 days, with a mean hospital-free survival of 94 days; those for the 13 patients allocated to surgical palliation were 192 days and 164 days respectively. These authors then concluded that because of the limited detection rate for unresectable metastatic disease and the likely absence of a large gain after switching from surgical to endoscopic palliation, laparoscopic staging should not be performed routinely in patients with peripancreatic carcinoma.

The team from Memorial Hospital in New York reported their experience of laparoscopy in the diagnosis of ampullary, bile duct and duodenal (periampullar) cancer (Brooks, *J Gastrointest Surg*, 2002). One hundred forty-four patients with radiologically resectable periampullary adenocarcinoma, seen between August 1993 and December 2000 underwent laparoscopy. Criteria for laparoscopic unresectability included histologically proved peritoneal or hepatic metastases, distant nodal involvement, arterial involvement, and local extension outside the resection field. Laparoscopy was thought to be adequate in 134 cases (93%) and identified 13 patients (10%) with unresectable disease. Of 121 patients with laparoscopic resectable disease, 111 (92%) went on to subsequent resection; by comparison, CT correctly predicted resectability in 82%. Laparoscopy spared 36% of unresectable patients a nontherapeutic laparotomy. The addition of diagnostic laparoscopy to dynamic CT scanning in this selected patient population identified an additional 10% of patients with unresectable disease. The authors went on to state that laparoscopy should be used in a selective manner for pre-operative staging of patients suspected of having non-pancreatic periampullary tumours.

Urbach et coll. (*Arch Surg*, 2002) studied the outcome of elderly patients undergoing laparoscopy for diagnostic purposes: of 122 individuals with pancreatic cancer, median survival was 4.8 months, compared with 5.3 months in a group of 791 patients who had conventional surgery. Compared with this latter group, patients who had laparoscopic surgery did not have an increased rate of death when the two groups were adjusted for age, sex, tumour size, grade, the presence of nodal and distant metastases at diagnosis and the use of radiation, chemotherapy, therapeutic endoscopic retrograde cholangiopancreatography or biliary and gastric bypass procedures. In conclusion, exposure to laparoscopic surgery did not adversely affect survival in this group of elderly patients.

The role of laparoscopy for the diagnosis of ascites has been advocated in several series (Inadomi, *Gastrointest Endosc Clin N Am*, 2001). Chu (*Gastrointest Endosc*, 1994) studied the role of laparoscopy in the diagnostic evaluation of ascites of unknown origin in 129 patients: peritoneal carcinomatosis was found in 78 (60.5%). Peritoneal biopsies in 76 of these cases revealed malignancy in 67 (adenocarcinoma 62, lymphoma 4, mesothelioma 1) and tuberculosis in 5; specimens were inadequate for diagnosis in 4. Overall, laparoscopy in combination with biopsy established the cause of ascites of unknown origin in 111 (86.0%) of 129 patients.

Laparoscopic lavage of the peritoneal cavity for detection of neo-plastic cells was thought to be an useful adjunct (Warshaw, *Am J Surg*, 1991). However, Nieveen Van Dijkum *et al.* (*Ann Surg*, 1998) among others have shown that the yield was very low (less than 2%).

As concerns the potential risk of dissemination, in a recent study from Memorial Hospital, of 1965 laparoscopic procedures performed between January 1993 and January 2001, clinical outcome and recurrences were noted for 1,650 in 1548 patients. Port site implantation occurred in 13 instances, *i.e.* 0.79% of all procedures (n = 1650). The median time to recurrence was 8.2 months. Compared with open surgery, incisional site recurrence was noted in 9 (0.86%) of 1,040 patients (difference not significant). The authors concluded that port site metastasis after laparoscopy for upper GI malignancy was uncommon, occurred most often in advanced disease, and did not seem to be different from open incision site recurrence.

What can be concluded from these reports? There probably is a role, although limited for laparoscopic exploration before undertaking major pancreatic resections for tumours. Diagnostic accuracy of digitalized imaging technologies is still increasing and should help define that subgroup which will benefit most from complementary laparoscopic investigation (Vollmer *et al.*, *Ann Surg*, 2002).

Minimal invasive techniques can be employed to treat foregut carcinoma either with palliative or curative intent.

Bilateral thoracic splanchnicectomy can be performed to alleviate pain from solar plexus involvement (Cuschieri JR, *Coll Surg Edinb*, 1994) In the case of unresectable malignant obstruction of the biliary tree, treatment should be directed toward rapid and safe relief of symptoms (jaundice) in such a manner that the patient remains symptom-free as long as he or she survives: laparoscopy can be used to diagnose and palliate obstructive jaundice (Farello *et al.*, *J Chir* (Paris), 1993; Fletcher and Jones, *Surg Endosc*, 1992; Shimi *et al.*, *Br J Surg*, 1992; Fingerhut and Cudeville, *Sem Laparosc Surg*, 1996). The operations performed include cholecystojejunostomy *(figure 1)*, choledochojejunostomy *(figure 2)* and/or gastrojejunostomy *(figure 3)*. Technical details may vary somewhat from one author to another but the essential steps are similar, as outlined herein (Fingerhut and Cudeville, *Sem Laparosc Surg*, 1996). The open access technique is used in all cases for creation of the carbopneumoperitoneum. A 10-12 mm trocar/cannula was inserted to introduce an end-viewing video connected optical device, just to the left of the midline, two finger breaths above the umbilicus. Three or four further trocars/cannulas are placed, as needed, along a semi circle centered on the target organ (Ferzli and Fingerhut). Care must be exercised to obtain adequate angles of attack to perform the anastomosis (cholecystojejunostomy, choledochojejunostomy, and/or gastrojejunostomy). If the gallbladder is to be used, one major point is the necessity of obtaining clear cholangioagrams through the gallbladder in order to confirm the patency of the cystic duct and make sure that its insertion into the common bile duct is at least 2 cm from the tumour (Shimi *et al.*, *Br J Surg*, 1992, Cushieri personal communication). Indeed the poor reputation of diversion using the gallbladder stems from either non patent cystic ducts or early obstruction of the cystic duct by ingrowing tumour (Cushieri, personal communication). Choledochoduodenostomy (Farello *et al.*, *J Chir*, Paris, 1993) or cholecystojejunostomy *(figure 2)* (Fingerhut and Cudeville, *Sem Laparosc Surg*, 1996; Fletcher and Jones, *Surg Endosc*, 1992; Shimi *et al.*, *Br J Surg*, 1992) can be performed either by hand or by mechanical (Fletcher and Jones, *Surg Endosc*, 1992; Shimi *et al.*, *Br J Surg*, 1992) sutures.

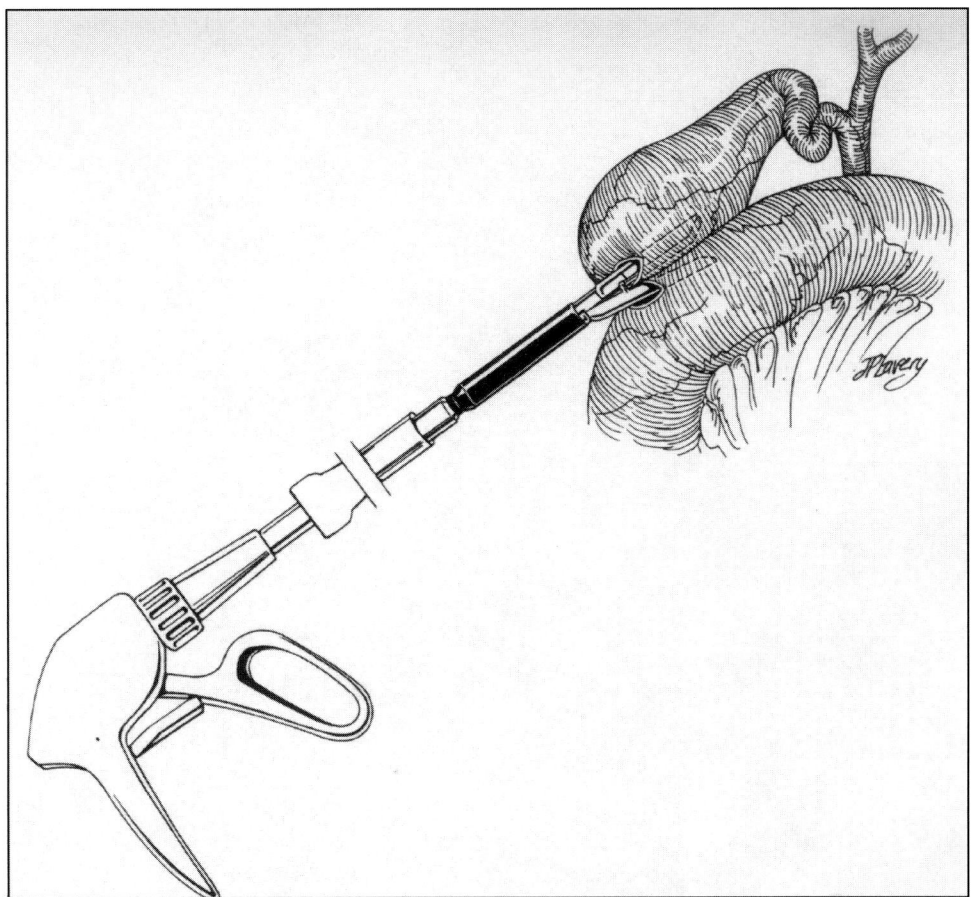

Figure 1. Laparoscopic cholecystojejunostomy.

While results of pancreatic resections have been published both for benign and malignant disease of the pancreas (Cuschieri, *Surg Endosc*, 2000), the indications and performances are limited to very few expert centers for the time being. The advantages are the same, but the time needed to perform these operations may counteract any of the traditional advantages of laparoscopic surgery.

The liver has also been the target of major technological and carcinological advances in the last few decades. Cryoablation of hepatic tumours has been performed for hepatic tumours, more and more often for primary as well as secondary tumours of the liver, and this can be performed laparoscopically (Lezoche *et al.*, *World J Surg*, 1998). New technologies and associated instruments allow performing resections with the least possible blood loss, a short resection time, and the need to interrupt the main vessels to the parenchyma as briefly as possible. Ischemia of the remaining parenchyma is therefore minimized, and untoward effects on the nearby structures due to ischemia, which must remain intact after resection, are avoided.

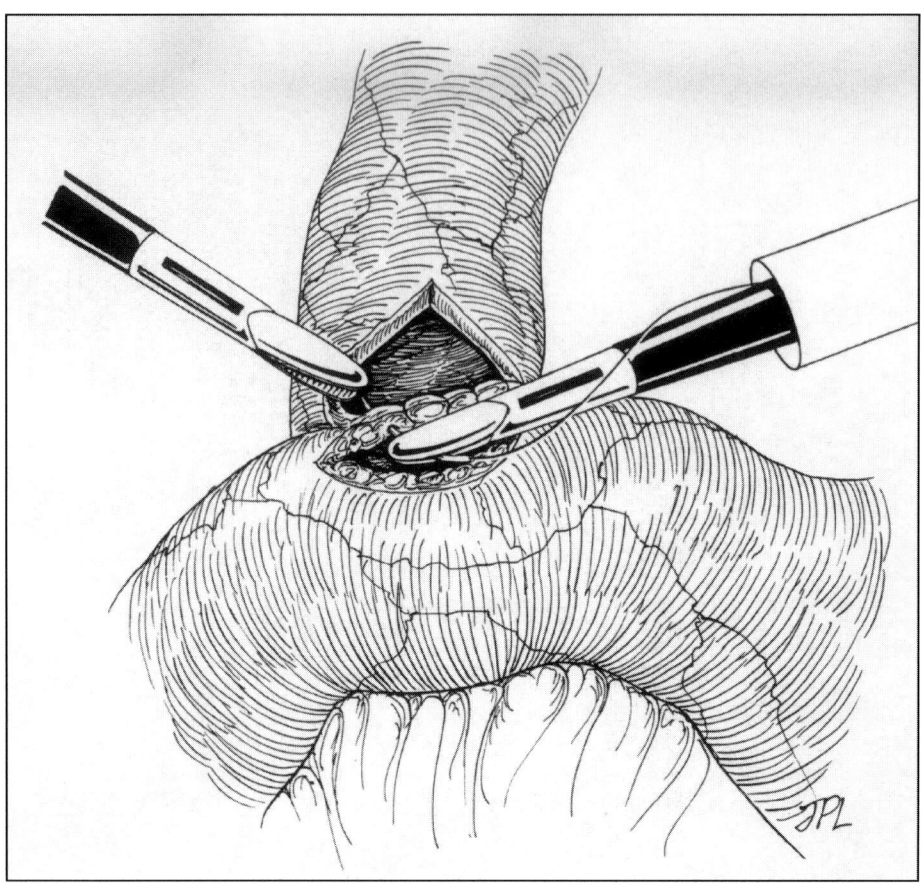

Figure 2. Laparoscopic choledochojejunostomy.

A variety of laparoscopic resectional techniques for liver tumours are currently available and this will certainly be developing in the next few years. As experience increases and technology progresses, larger resections, either laparoscopic or hand-assisted (Cuschieri, *Endscopy*, 2000), will be undertaken (Lesurtel, *J Am Coll Surg*, 2003). For the moment the domain of a few gifted surgeons around the globe, the short and long term benefits of such surgical feats, however, remain to be shown.

Laparoscopy may have a role as well in the pre-operative assessment of gastric (Ballesta Lopez *et al.*, *Surg Endosc*, 2002) and esophageal neoplasms.

Gastric stromal neoplasms are rare, accounting for < 2% of gastric tumours. Definite criteria for the malignant nature of such tumours are difficult to establish. Although laparoscopic resection for stromal tumours of the stomach has been shown to be feasible and seems reasonable because of apparently small risk of dissemination (Bouillot, *Gastroenterol Clin Biol*, 2003; Cuschieri, *Endoscopy*, 2000), there is still debate as to how to handle

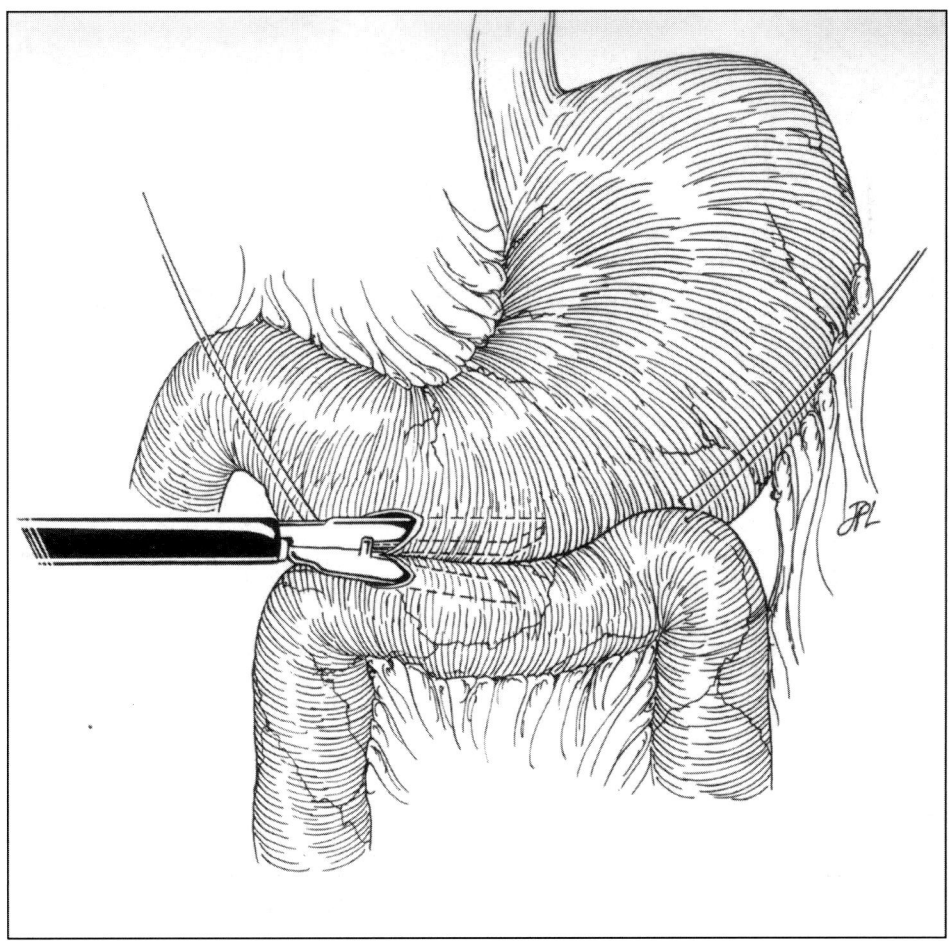

Figure 3. Laparoscopic gastrojejunostomy.

these tumours intraoperatively. Our technique (Yachouchy, *Surg Endosc*, 2002) consists of using the retrieval sac to apprehend the tumour and thus avoid operative dissemination of unsuspected malignancy. Further preventive measures include absence of manipulation of the tumour, elimination of direct contact with the abdominal wall, and avoidance of disruption of the mucosa.

Formal gastric resections have also been performed, whether with palliative or curative intent (Ballesta Lopez *et al.*, *Surg Endosc*, 2002; Noguchi, *Surg Oncol Clin N Am*, 2002). Experience is still limited but initial results seem promising, especially for early gastric carcinoma.

Although down-graded and then abandoned by some (Collard, *Ann Chir Gynaecol*, 1995), we have used the laparoscopic approach for patients with *in situ* carcinoma of the esophagus, notably those patients who have proven severe dysplasia in Barrett's esophagus on at least two successive endoscopic investigations. While theoretically advantageous (less large and debilitating incisions and ideally, better postoperative recovery), the operation is labor-intensive, takes a long time, and may induce hither to unknown complications in this fairly rare pathology (Collard, *Ann Chir Gynaecol*, 1995). Questions still remain as to whether associated adenolymphadectomy (as opposed to none), routine mediastinal clearance (as opposed to none), extrathoracic (as opposed to intrathoracic) anastomosis, use of whole stomach (as opposed to gastric tubes) can reduce postoperative complications and/or recurrence. Initial results for this technique show that postoperative respiratory failure may be related more to the duration of operation rather than the type of approach.

Currently we have treated 12 patients (age: 49-84). Nine were followed for 2 months to 5 years. One perioperative death occurred (84 yr old patient), two were lost to follow-up. Anastomotic leaks occurred in the neck in two patients. Hypothermic coagulopathy was noted in two patients. A low limb compression syndrome occurred in one patient, while four patients sustained pulmonary compromise. The median operative time was 5.2 (3.6-9) hours, with a median hospital stay of 11 (7-59) days. For those patients followed, there were two recurrences, noted at 1 and at 6 months which leads us to ask the question of whether these tumours were really intramucosal at the time of operation. In spite of these few but preoccupying complications, we are still pursuing this route for resection of *in situ* carcinoma and high grade dysplasia of the lower esophagus.

References

1. Ballesta Lopez C, Ruggiero R, Poves I, Bettonica C, Procaccini E. The contribution of laparoscopy to the treatment of gastric cancer. *Surg Endosc* 2002; 16: 616-9.
2. Bouillot JL, Bresler L, Fagniez PL, Samama G, Champault G, Parent Y. Laparoscopic resection of benign submucosal stomach tumours: a report of 65 cases. *Gastroenterologie Clin Biol* 2003; 27: 272-6.
3. Brooks AD, Mallis MJ, Brennan MF, Conlon KC. The value of laparoscopy in the management of ampullary, duodenal, and distal bile duct tumours. *J Gastrointest Surg* 2002; 6: 139-45.
4. Chu CM, Lin SM, Peng SM, Wu CS, Liaw YF. The role of laparoscopy in the evaluation of ascites of unknown origin. *Gastrointest Endosc* 1994; 40: 285-9.
5. Collard JM. Role of videoassisted surgery in the treatment of esophageal cancer. *Ann Chir Gynaecol* 1995; 84: 209-14.
6. Cuschieri A. Laparoscopy for pancreatic cancer: does it benefit the patient? *Eur J Surg Oncol* 1988; 14: 41-4.
7. Cuschieri A. Laparoscopic surgery of the pancreas. *J R Coll Surg Edinb* 1994; 39: 178-84.
8. Cushieri A. Minimally invasive surgery: hepatobiliary-pancreatic and foregut. *Endoscopy* 2000; 32: 331-44.
9. Cushieri A, Hall AW, Clark J. Value of laparoscopy in the diagnosis and management of pancreatic carcinoma. *Gut* 1978; 19: 672-7.
10. Cuschieri A. Laparoscopic hand-assisted surgery for hepatic and pancreatic disease. *Surg Endosc* 2000; 14: 991-6.

11. Conlon KC, Dougherty E, Klinistra DS, Coit DG, Turnbull AD, Brennan MF. The value of minimal access surgery in the staging of patients with potentially resectable peripancreatic malignancy. *Ann Surg* 1996; 223: 134-40.
12. Duepree HJ, Senagore AJ, Delaney CP, Fazio VW. Does means of access affect the incidence of small bowel obstruction and ventral hernia after bowel resection? Laparoscopy *versus* laparotomy. *J Am Coll Surg* 2003; 197: 177-81.
13. Farello GA, Cerofolini A, Bergamischi G, et al. L'anastomose cholédocho-duodénale par voie laparoscopique. *J Chir (Paris)* 1993; 130: 226-30.
14. Fernandez Del Castillo C, Rattner DW, Warshaw AL. Standards for pancreatic resection in the 1990s. *Arch Surg* 1995; 130: 295-300.
15. Ferzli GS, Fingerhut A. Trocar placement for laparoscopic abdominal procedures: a simple standardized method. (Submitted for publication.)
16. Fingerhut A, Cudeville C. Laparoscopic bypass for inoperable disease of the pancreas. *Sem Laparosc Surg* 1996; 3: 10-4.
17. Fletcher DR, Jones RM. Laparoscopic cholecystjejunostomy as palliation for obstructive jaundice in inoperable carcinoma of pancreas. *Surg Endosc* 1992; 6: 147-9.
18. Friess H, Kleeff J, Silva JC, Sadowski C, Baer HU, Buchler MW. The role of diagnostic laparoscopy in pancreatic and periampullary malignancies. *J Am Coll Surg* 1998; 186: 675-82.
19. Gloor B, Todd KE, Reber HA. Diagnostic workup of patients with suspected pancreatic carcinoma: the University of California-Los Angeles approach. *Cancer* 1997; 79: 1780-6.
20. Holzman MD, Reintgen KL, Tyler DS, Pappas TN. The role of laparoscopy in the management of suspected pancreatic and periampullary malignancies. *J Gastrointest Surg* 1997; 1: 236-44.
21. Inadomi JM, Kapur S, Kinkhabwala M, Cello JP. The laparoscopic evaluation of ascites. *Gastrointest Endosc Clin N Am* 2001; 11: 79-91.
22. Irving AD, Cushieri A. Laparoscopic assessment of the jaundiced patient: a review of 53 patients. *Br J Surg* 1978; 65: 678-80.
23. Ishida H, Furukawa F, Kuroda H, Kobayashi M, Tsuneoka K. Laparoscopic observation and biopsy of the pancreas. *Endoscopy* 1981; 13: 68-73.
24. Jimenez RE, Warshaw AL, Ratner DW, Willet CG, McGrath D, Fernandez-del-Castillo C. Impact of laparoscopic staging in the treatment of pancreatic cancer. *Arch Surg* 2000; 135: 409-15.
25. John TG, Greig JD, Carter DC, Garden OJ. Carcinoma of the pancreatic head and periampullary region. Tumour staging with laparoscopy and laparoscopic ultrasonography. *Ann Surg* 1995; 221: 156-64.
26. Lezoche E, Paganini AM, Feliciotti F, Guerrieri M, Lugnani F, Tamburini A. Ultrasound-guided laparoscopic cryoablation of hepatic tumours: preliminary report. *World J Surg* 1998; 22: 829-35.
27. Lesurtel M, Cherqui D, Laurent A, Tayar C, Fagniez PL. Laparoscopic *versus* open left lateral hepatic lobectomy: a case-control study. *J Am Coll Surg* 2003; 196: 236-42.
28. Minnard EA, Conlon KC, Hoos A, Dougherty EC, Hann LE, Brennan MF. Laparoscopic ultrasound enhances standard laparoscopy in the staging of pancreatic cancer. *Ann Surg* 1998; 228: 182-7.
29. Noguchi Y, Morinaga S, Yamamoto Y, Yoshikawa T. Is there a role for nontraditional resection of early gastric cancer? *Surg Oncol Clin N Am* 2002; 11: 387-403.
30. Pietrabissa A, Caramella D, Di Candio G, et al. Laparoscopy and laparoscopic ultrasonography for staging pancreatic cancer: critical appraisal. *World J Surg* 1999; 23: 998-1002.
31. Pisters PWT, Lee JE, Vauthey JN, Charnsangavej C, Evans DB. Laparoscopy in the staging of pancreatic cancer. *Br J Surg* 2001: 88; 325-37.
32. Possik RA, Franco EL, Pires DR, Wohnrath DR, Ferreira EB. Sensitivity, specificity and predictive value of laparoscopy for the staging of gastric cancer and for the detection of liver metastases. *Cancer* 1986; 58: 1-6.
33. Rumstadt B, Schwab M, Schuster K, Hagmuller E, Trede M. The role of laparoscopy in the preoperative staging of pancreatic carcinoma. *J Gastrointest Surg* 1997; 1: 245-50.

34. Santori E, Carlini M, Carboni F. Laparoscopic pancreatic surgery, indications, techniques, and preliminary results. *Hepatogastroenterology* 1999; 46: 1174-80.
35. Shandall A, Johnson C. Laparoscopy or scanning in esophageal and gastric carcinoma? *Br J Surg* 1985; 72: 449-51.
36. Shimi S, Banting S, Cushieri A. Laparoscopy in the management of pancreatic cancer: endoscopic cholecystojejunostomy for advanced disease. *Br J Surg* 1992; 79: 317-9.
37. Spitz FR, Abbruzzese JL, Lee JF, *et al.* Preoperative and postoperative chemoradiation strategies in patients treated with pancreaticoduodenectomy for adenocarcinoma of the pancreas. *J Clin Oncol* 1997; 15: 928-37.
38. Underwood RA, Soper NJ. Current status of laparoscopic surgery of the pancreas. *J Hepato Bil Pancreat Surg* 1999; 6: 154-64.
39. Vollmer CM, Drebin JA, Middelton WD, *et al.* Utility of staging laparoscopy in subsets of peripancreatic and biliary malignancies. *Ann Surg* 2002; 235: 1-7.
40. Warshaw A, Tepper JE, Shipley WU. Laparoscopy in the staging and planning of therapy for pancreatic cancer. *Am J Surg* 1986; 151: 76-80.
41. Warshaw AL. Implications of peritoneal cytology for staging of early pancreatic cancer. *Am J Surg* 1991; 161: 26-30.

The role of induction chemotherapy in upper GI cancer

Florian Lordick, Jörg Rüdiger Siewert

Department of Surgery, Klinikum rechts der Isar, Technical University of Munich, Ismaninger Str. 22, D – 81675 Munich, Germany

Although important advances in the surgical and non-surgical treatment of upper GI cancer have been achieved in the last two decades, prognosis remains poor. Three main reasons can be identified to explain this situation: firstly, in the western world where esophago-gastro-duodenoscopy is not yet part of screening programs, upper GI tumours are commonly diagnosed in advanced stages (Hundahl 1997). Secondly, lymphogenous and occult hematogenic spread is often present even in early stages (Siewert 2002). Thirdly, upper GI tumours are relatively insensitive to chemotherapy and radiation therapy. Therefore, cure cannot be achieved in metastatic disease or after incomplete (R1/R2) resection.

In high-volume centers, the quality and outcome of oncological surgery is far better than in less experienced institutions (Birkmeyer 2002). On the other hand, it is doubtful that these results can be significantly improved. At present, most groups seeking to further improve long-term outcome in localized upper GI cancer, try to combine chemotherapy or chemoradiation with surgical resection in neoadjuvant or adjuvant study concepts. The general impression is that adjuvant treatment after radical tumour resection in the upper GI tract is hampered by bad tolerance due to increased toxicity. Neoadjuvant treatment strategies, on the other hand, have proved to be feasible and well tolerated by patients in different phase II and phase III trials. Results of the recently presented MAGIC trial which showed that 88% of patients completed three cycles of pre-operative ECF chemotherapy whereas only 55% of patients were able to start post-operative chemotherapy and only 40% were able to receive all six planned perioperative ECF cycles (Allum 2003) have confirmed this experience. Pre-operative treatment strategies may, theoretically, be superior to post-operative therapy for two further reasons. First, neoadjuvant treatment potentially leads to downsizing of the tumour and therefore may improve the complete resectability rate which is the cornerstone of cure in oncological surgery. Secondly, neoadjuvant induction chemotherapy is the earliest way of tackling the systemic spread of cancer cells which in many cases is the cause of poor long-term prognosis. In the following, published data are reviewed regarding the role of neoadjuvant treatment in upper GI cancer.

Gastric cancer

Although its incidence in the western world has declined, cancer of the stomach still remains one of the most common human malignancies. Interestingly enough, a shift from distal to proximal tumours has been noted during the past two decades (Devesa 1998). The reasons for this shift are not yet clearly understood. There is an ongoing debate about the impact on survival of extended lymph node dissection after gastrectomy. Two adequately powered randomized studies have been published showing no significant 5-year survival difference between standard (D1) and extended (D2) lymphadenectomy (Bonencamp 1999, Cuschieri 1999). In the *Dutch Gastric Cancer Trial*, the 5-year survival rate was 45% for D1 and 47% for D2 resection. In the *British Medical Research Council Gastric Cancer Surgical Trial* the 5-year survival rate was 35% for D1 and 33% for D2 resection. In both studies, patients who underwent D2 resection experienced a far higher postoperative morbidity and mortality rate compared to patients who underwent D1 resection (4.0% *versus* 10.0% in the DGCT and 6.5 *versus* 13.0% in the MRC trial). On the other hand, highly experienced centers are able to perform extended (D2) lymphadenectomy with low morbidity and mortality rates (Siewert 1998). In a cohort of 1096 patients who had undergone extended (D2) lymphadenectomy, the 30-day-postoperative mortality rate was 5.0%. In stages T2N1 and T3N0 the German trial also showed significantly higher cure rates in the D2 group thus suggesting that there was a therapeutic benefit for subgroups at least. The fact that staging is more precise in patients who have undergone extended lymphadenectomy could constitute another advantage. Determining the extent of lymphadenectomy in gastric cancer surgery is, furthermore, of importance for combined modality treatment strategies as the discussion about the appropriate interpretation of the adjuvant chemoradiotherapy data delivered by the U.S. Intergroup study 0116 clearly showed (Macdonald 2001).

Another lesson that we have learned from the German Gastric Cancer Study is the high prognostic impact of the pT and the pN stage. Whereas patients with pT2N0 disease had a relatively good 5-year-survival of 66.5% after D2 lymphadenectomy, 5-year survival of patients with pT3N1 tumours was found to be only 21.2%. The ratio of invaded to removed lymph nodes was identified as the single most important independent prognostic factor ($p < 0.0001$) followed by the residual tumour (R) category ($p < 0.0001$), the pT category ($p < 0.0001$), post-surgical complications ($p < 0.0001$), and the presence of distant metastases ($p < 0.0001$).

We have learned that in locally advanced tumour stages (> T2, > N0), results after resection are unsatisfactory. Hence, there are strong arguments for administering induction chemotherapy before attempting resection. Patients with locally advanced tumours taken directly to laparotomy are frequently found to have such extensive disease that a R0 resection cannot be achieved. Moreover, the risk of local and distal failure is high after resection. Because clinical assessment of lymph node involvement is difficult with currently available pre-operative staging techniques, patients should be included in neoadjuvant treatment protocols and stratified according to the clinically assessed T stage. Metastatic disease should be excluded first. As peritoneal carcinomatosis usually cannot be detected by the routinely performed staging procedures, laparoscopy should be performed in any patient who is to undergo neoadjuvant treatment in order to achieve the most accurate information on pre-treatment tumour stage (Feussner 1999). Endoscopic ultrasound (EUS) has proved to be superior to other methods in the prediction of pathologically confirmed T stage with an accuracy of between 79-92% and a somewhat lower 50%-87% for the N stage (Rösch 1995a). The accuracy of EUS to predict R0 resectability has been evaluated as being 85% and 90%, respectively (Dittler 1995, Willis 2000). Consequently, before commencement of neoadjuvant treatment, staging procedures should include endoscopic ultrasound to define T stage, computed tomography to exclude distant metastases and laparoscopy to exclude peritoneal carcinomatosis. The value of positron emission tomography is limited in gastric cancer as its ability to detect tumours is reduced to 41-63% in non-intestinal type histology according to the Lauren classification (De Potter 2002, Stahl 2003). Owing to progress in investigational techniques, the accuracy of clinical staging has certainly improved. On the other hand, monitoring during neoadjuvant treatment and accurate response evaluation are still unsatisfactory. Clinical response evaluation criteria frequently used for metastatic disease have not been validated for localized upper GI tumours (Therasse 2000). EUS, although accurate in assessing T stage in patients who have not been pretreated, cannot be relied on in patients who have received neoadjuvant chemotherapy. Preoperative EUS after induction chemotherapy was found to be inaccurate, particularly in differentiating between T2 and T3 tumours (Kelsen 1996). The use of PET scan in assessing response during neoadjuvant chemotherapy in stomach cancer is very promising but certainly still in a preliminary phase and should be reproduced by other investigators (Ott 2002). In short, there is as yet no reliable morphological or functional surrogate parameter for response and for the true value of neoadjuvant chemotherapy in gastric cancer. Therefore, the goal of clinical studies must be to increase the rate of R0 resections and, more importantly, to lengthen disease-free and overall survival.

Although assessing tumour response is difficult, phase II studies of neoadjuvant chemotherapy have demonstrated that such treatments can be given with acceptable toxicity and without excessive postoperative morbidity and mortality *(table 1)*. Another lesson we have learned from the phase II trials is the fact that patients who respond to neoadjuvant chemotherapy have a markedly improved prognosis compared to clinical non-responders (Lowy 1999, Schuhmacher 2001). In the Munich trial, response to pre-operative chemotherapy proved to be a significant prognostic factor in univariate analysis using the log-rank test ($p = 0.008$, *figure 1*). Chemotherapy responders had a superior median survival of 45.0 months compared to 19.1 months for the whole study population (Schuhmacher 2001).

On the basis of the insights derived from the phase II studies one could hypothesize that patients with operable gastric cancer might benefit from neoadjuvant chemotherapy. However, until recently, no data from larger randomized studies were available. At the meeting of the American Society of Clinical Oncology 2003 in Chicago the first results from the UK Medical Research Council "MAGIC" trial were presented. In this multi-center trial 503 patients with stage II or greater esophagogastric cancer were randomized to receive surgery alone (S) or three cycles of pre-operative chemotherapy (ECF-schedule) followed by surgery followed by three post-operative ECF-cycles (CSC). A higher proportion of smaller tumours and of stage pT1 and pT2 tumours was found after induction chemotherapy suggesting a downsizing effect of induction chemotherapy and resulting in a higher proportion of potentially curative resections (79% *versus* 69%, $p = 0.018$, χ^2 test). Unfortunately, pathologically assessed data on the R classification are missing. Consequently we do not know how many resections deemed "curative" by the surgeon

Table I. Neoadjuvant chemotherapy for gastric cancer: results of phase II/small phase III studies

Study	Regimen	No. Patients	Resectable (R0)	Median Survival	2-Year Survival
Wilke 1989	EAP	34	10 (29%)	18 mo	26%
Ajani 1991	EAP	48	37 (77%)	16 mo	42%
Ajani 1995	EFP	25	18 (72%)	15 mo	44%
Alexander 1995	FU-LV-INF	22	18 (82%)	18 mo	52%
Kelsen 1996	CDDP-FU post-op. ip. CTX	56	34 (61%)	15 mo	40%
Crookes 1997	CDDP-FU post-op. ip. CTx	59	42 (71%)	> 4 yr	64%
Siewert 1997	CDDP-FU-LV	41	30 (73%)	NS	56%
Lowy 1999	CDDP-FU-INF	30	25 (83%)	18 mo	52%
Schuhmacher 2001	EAP	42	31 (74%)	19 mo	40%

CDDP = Cisplatinum; CTx = chemotherapy; EAP = Etoposide-Adriamycin-Cisplatinum; EFP = Etoposide-Fluorouracil-Cisplatin; FU = 5-Fluorouracil; ip. = intraperitoneal; LV = Leucovorin, NS = not specified.

later revealed residual microscopic disease (R1). After a median follow-up of 2.0 years progression-free survival was significantly prolonged in patients randomized to the CSC arm (log rank p-value = 0.002, hazard ratio = 0.7, 95% CI 0.56-0.88). For overall survival, the hazard ratio was 0.8 in favour of the peri-operative chemotherapy arm, but this difference had not yet reached significance (p=0.063). The 2-year survival rate was 48% for CSC *versus* 40% for surgery alone. The authors of the study conclude that perioperative chemotherapy improves progression-free survival and increases resectability in operable gastric cancer. Survival data are not yet mature. However, one can criticize the inclusion of patients with cancer of the distal esophagus in the study (11%). This might have blurred the results to a certain extent. More importantly, the assessment of the clinical stage lacks routinely performed endoscopic ultrasound and diagnostic laparoscopy. As a result, over- and understaging of patients randomized to the CSC group cannot be excluded thus leading to possible imbalances between the two study populations with regard to clinical stage and the number of prognostic factors. Last but not least, surgical quality control was weak in this study particularly regarding the extent of lymph node dissection and pathological assessment of the UICC R stage. In summary, the MAGIC trial is the first large randomized trial that strongly supports the efficacy of perioperative chemotherapy in gastric cancer. On the other hand, the trial leaves us with some unanswered questions. Therefore, the results of confirmatory studies like the EORTC 40954 trial with a more precise patient selection based on pretherapeutic EUS and laparoscopy and a sophisticated surgical quality control should be waited for before one draws definite conclusions regarding the impact of neoadjuvant chemotherapy on the surgical treatment and outcome of locally advanced gastric cancer.

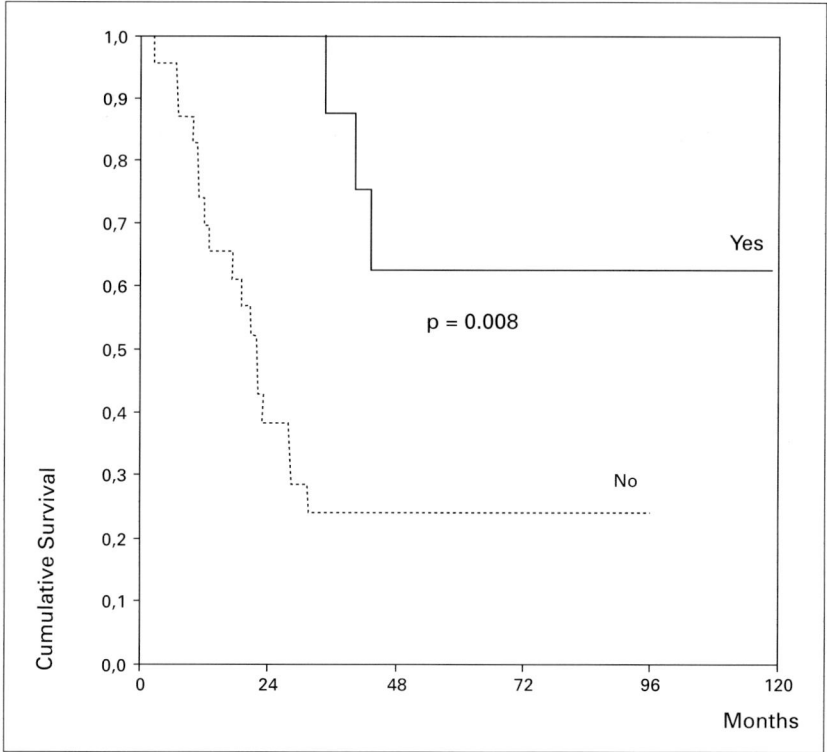

Figure 1. Graph illustrating cumulative survival after undergoing neoadjuvant chemotherapy and gastrectomy (R0 resection) in patients who achieved a complete endoscopic response (Yes) compared with patients who achieved less favorable endoscopic tumour reduction (No). From: Schuhmacher et al. Cancer 2001; 91: 918-27.

With the inclusion of new substances like oxaliplatin, the taxanes and irinotecan into the therapeutic arsenal, all of which have shown promising activity in the treatment of advanced upper GI cancer (Ajani 2002, Ajani 2003, Bouché 2003, Kollmannsberger 2000, Lordick 2003, Louvet 2001, Ridwelski 2001, Sumpter 2003), there is certainly a need for new, more active or at least better tolerated induction chemotherapy protocols to be tested in phase II (Newman 2002) and phase III trials.

Esophageal Cancer

While the incidence of esophageal squamous cell cancer is decreasing in the western world, there has been a rapid increase in the incidence rates of esophageal adenocarcinoma during the last decades with especially frequent occurrence among white males (Devesa 1998, Hesketh 1989, Siewert 2001, Wijnhoven 2002).

As in gastric cancer, locoregional staging is most reliably performed by means of endoscopic ultrasound (EUS). The accuracy for T staging is 84% (60%-90%) and for nodal staging 77% (50%-90%, Rösch 1995b). Barium swallow and computed tomography helps localize the tumour in relation to its neighbouring structures, particularly the tracheobronchial system. In proximal and mid-esophageal tumours, tracheo-bronchoscopy is recommended to rule out tumour infiltration which is equivalent to unresectability of the tumour and enhances the risk of esophago-tracheal fistula in case of radiation therapy. PET has been carefully evaluated in patients with esophageal cancer. Studies confirm that PET has good specificity (84%-100%) but limited sensitivity (38%-77%) for the detection of nodal and metastatic disease (Kim 2001, Kole 1998, Flamen 2000, Lerut 2000, Luketich 1999). A recently published decision analysis and cost-benefit analysis comparing the different staging modalities (EUS, CT, PET, thoracoscopy/laparoscopy) came to the conclusion that patients initially presenting with a diagnosis of esophageal cancer can be most effectively staged with PET scanning followed by EUS (Wallace 2002). Another obligatory prerequisite before esophagectomy or combined modality treatment in esophageal cancer is a sophisticated assessment of the physiological status of the patient (Bartels 1997).

Esophageal cancer is frequently diagnosed in locally advanced or metastatic stages. But even in earlier stages one must assume lymphatic spread due to the unique submucosal lymphatic drainage system of the esophagus. In stages T3/T4 virtually all patients show locoregional lymphatic spread (Rice 1997, Siewert 2001). As prognosis for patients with nodal metastases treated with surgery alone is very poor with a 5-year survival rate that rarely exceeds 20% (Eloubeidi 2001, Hölscher 1995, Rice 2001, Roder 1994), combined modality approaches have been investigated for the treatment of esophageal cancer.

Neoadjuvant chemoradiotherapy followed by resection has been the preferred investigational concept in the last decade. Unfortunately, most of the randomized studies have included squamous cell cancers together with adenocarcinomas although it has clearly been shown that the biology, clinical course and prognosis of both histologies is different (Siewert 2001, *figure 2*). Data indicate that in squamous cell carcinoma it is more difficult to achieve resection without residual tumour (*table 2*, Siewert 2002). Therefore, in the context of potentially curative treatment strategies, these two histological subtypes should be studied and treated as two different entities.

As *table 3* shows, all but one of the randomized studies assessing the value of neoadjuvant radiochemotherapy have yielded negative results. Admittedly, the interpretation of the results is difficult due to small sample sizes, inappropriate staging procedures, the inclusion of different histological types and tumour localizations, excessive postoperative mortalities in some of the studies and the use of meanwhile uncommon chemoradiotherapy schedules and techniques. Noteworthy is that, seen from the current perspective, the postoperative mortality rate was unacceptable in the earlier trials. Some of the studies suggest a better resectability rate (R0) after pre-operative chemoradiation (Law 1998, Nygaard 1992). Nonetheless, a significant survival benefit was noted in only one study (Walsh 1996). However, in this study the 3-year survival rate of patients randomized to the surgery alone arm was poorer than in any other randomized trial. Therefore, no definite conclusions can be drawn from the results of this study regarding the impact of neoadjuvant chemoradiation. It was hypothesized that the superior outcome of the combined modality treatment shown in the Walsh trial could be accounted for by the fact that only patients with

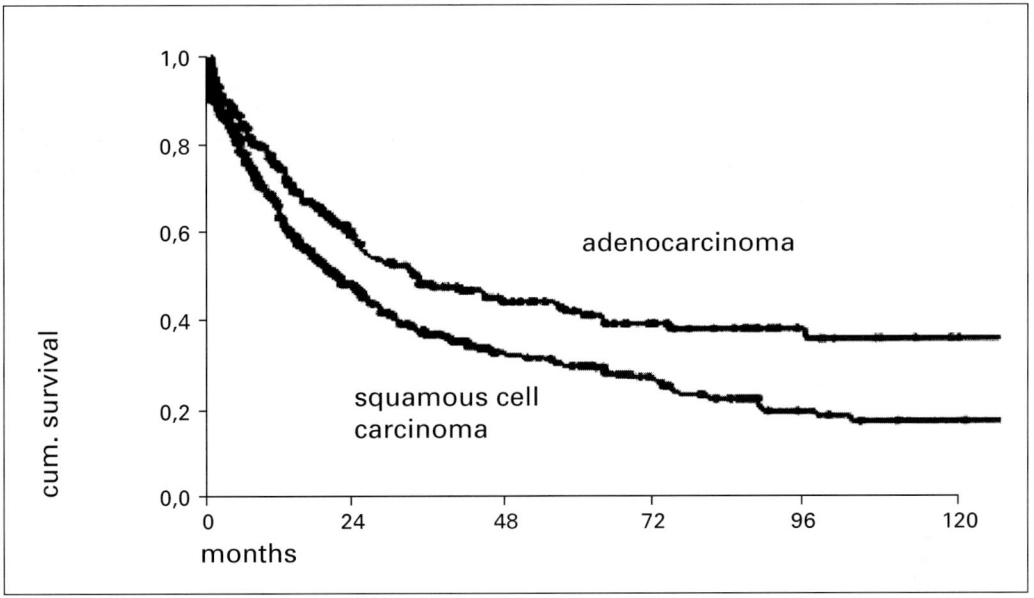

Figure 2. Overall 10-year survival curve of patients with resected adenocarcinoma (n = 407) *versus* patients with resected squamous cell carcinoma of the esophagus (n = 652). From: Siewert *et al. Ann Surg* 2001; 234: 360-9.

Table II. Rate of complete tumour resection (R0 by UICC definition) in squamous cell carcinoma and adenocarcinoma of the esophagus according to pathologic pT category

	SCC (%)	AC (%)
pT1		
Mucosa	100	100
Submucosa	91	100
PT2	84	84
PT3	70	68
PT4	48	59

AC = Adenocarcinoma of the esophagus, SCC = squamous cell carcinoma of the esophagus.
Data from the Department of Surgery, Klinikum rechst der Isar, Technical Universitiy of Munich.

adenocarcinoma were enrolled. On the other hand, the Australasian trial (Burmeister 2002) has shown improved recurrence-free survival (p = 0.03) for patients with squamous cell cancer, whereas for patients with adenocarcinoma an insignificant trend towards better recurrence-free survival was seen in the surgery alone arm. Certainly, this kind of subgroup analysis is not powerful enough for definite conclusions to be drawn, but on the other hand, the data suggest a possible benefit regarding the treatment sequence of chemoradiation followed by surgery for esophageal squamous cell carcinoma, provided that surgical quality and outcome is optimal.

Table III. Phase III trials to investigate the impact of neoadjuvant chemoradiation for potentially resectable esophageal carcinoma

Study	Protocol	Histology	n	R0 (%)	Mortality (%)	Median survival (mo)	Survival (%)	p value
Nygaard 1992	Surgery CDDP/BLM + 35Gy	SCC	41 47	37 55	13 24	7.5 7.5	3yr: 9 17	NS
Le Prise 1994	Surgery CDDP/5FU + 20Gy	SCC	45 41	84 85	7 8.5	10 10	3yr: 13.8 19.2	NS
Apinop 1994	Surgery CDDP/5FU + 40Gy	SCC	34 35	NA NA	15 14	7.4 9.7	5yr: 10 24	NS
Walsh 1996	Surgery CDDP/5FU + 40Gy	AC	55 58	NA NA	8 4	11 16	3yr: 6 32	0.01
Bosset 1997	Surgery CDDP + 37Gy	SCC	139 143	NA NA	4 12.3	18.6 18.9	5yr: 25 25	NS
Law 1998	Surgery CDDP/5FU + 40Gy	SCC	60 (tot)	42 80	0 0	26 27	NA NA	NS
Urba 2001	Surgery CDDP/VBL/5FU + 45Gy	SCC + AC	50 50	NA NA	2 7	17.6 16.9	3yr: 16 30	NS
Burmeister 2002	Surgery CDDP/5FU + 35Gy	SCC + AC	128 128	NA	4.6 (tot)	18.5 21.7	NA NA	NS

AC = Adenocarcinoma; BLM = Bleomycin; CDDP = Cisplatin; 5FU = 5-fluorouracil; NA = not available; NS = not significant, R0 = complete resection, SCC = squamous cell carcinoma, VBL = vinblastin.

As mentioned above, complete resection is a prerequisite for cure in esophageal cancer patients undergoing surgery but it is hard to achieve in squamous cell cancer, particularly if the tumour is topographically close to the tracheo-bronchial system. Most cisplatinum-based chemoradiation protocols show a considerable efficacy in squamous cell carcinoma with complete remission rates between 20-30% (Bosset 1997, Burmeister 2002, Urba 2001). Downsizing of the initial tumour is achieved in up to 50% of patients even in less effective treatment protocols (Brücher 2001). Therefore, some experienced surgeons restrict the indication for resection of locally ($\geq$ T3) advanced squamous cell carcinomas to tumours that have responded to induction chemoradiation and have shrunk in size. Indeed, non-responding tumours have a dismal prognosis with a 3-year survival rate of less than 20% unless R0 resection is achieved. If R0 resection is possible, the 3-year-survival rate was shown to be 35% even in patients who did not respond to neoadjuvant chemoradiaton (Stahl 2003b).

Although the activity of cisplatinum-based chemoradiation is relatively high, this therapy is demanding and leads to frequent toxicity-related dose reductions, delays and interruptions in administration. Therefore, there is a need for less toxic schedules with at least equivalent activity. One very promising approach is the combination of the platinum-derivate oxaliplatin with protracted-infusion fluorouracil and external beam radiation developed by the Roswell Park group. This protocol has led to a 38% pathologic complete response rate and an overall median survival of 25.3 months (Khushalani 2002).

Translational research has shown that tumour thymidylate synthase (TS) expression was down-regulated by oxaliplatin. Low TS levels at the end of treatment were independent indicators of favorable outcome (Leichman 2003). This result may suggest a possible advantage for a weekly oxaliplatinum schedule combined with 5-FU and radiation. At present, a similar weekly protocol is under phase I/II investigation at the Technical University of Munich.

Beyond neoadjuvant chemoradiation, induction chemotherapy without radiation has been investigated in potentially resectable esophageal cancer. Two adequately powered studies have been carried through and published. After the well performed US intergroup trial 0113 yielded negative results for three cycles of cisplatinum plus fluorouracil followed by surgery followed by two additional cycles of chemotherapy compared to surgery alone (Kelsen 1998), it came as a surprise that the UK MRC trial assessing a putatively similar treatment approach revealed a significant advantage for combined modality treatment in overall survival (16.8 months *versus* 13.3 months, hazard ratio = 0.79; 95% CI 0.67-0.93, p = 0.004; *figure 3*; MRC 2002). The conflicting results between the UK MRC and the US INT studies might be explained by the slightly different dosages and lengths of preoperative chemotherapy. The toxicity from the larger total doses of chemotherapy given in the US INT 0113 study may potentially diminish the survival benefit. Only 80% of patients in the US trial who received neoadjuvant chemotherapy proceeded to resection, whereas 92% of patients had surgery in the combined modality arm of the MRC trial. In previous randomized studies, patients who demonstrated a clinical response to induction chemotherapy fared better than non-responders. Indeed, the non-responders had worse survival than those who underwent immediate surgery (Ancona 2001, Law 1997, Roth 1988, Schlag 1992). Therefore, one can hypothesize that the longer duration of chemotherapy in the US Intergroup-0113, and the resulting delay in surgery were responsible for the detrimental effect on the clinical non-responders in the preoperative chemotherapy arm and may have contributed to the overall neutral effect of chemotherapy in the study (Chau 2003). In fact, even in the US INT 0113 trial clinical responders to chemotherapy had a better survival rate than non-responders (p = 0.002) and patients in the surgery alone group (p < 0.001, Kelsen 1999). This underlines the importance of a careful interpretation of the results of single studies as well as the rising need for reliable predictive markers and tools for early response evaluation during potentially curative combined modality therapies.

Response prediction

As we have learned, chemotherapy-responders have a markedly higher chance of cure after surgery compared to chemotherapy-non-responders (Kelsen 1999, Lowy 1999, Schuhmacher 2001). On the other hand, not all patients will benefit from neoadjuvant therapy and may instead lose time with inefficient therapy and suffer from substantial side effects. Thus, the crucial goal of clinical research in this context is to find reliable prognostic and predictive markers in order to customize treatment strategies for the individual patient.

One approach uses molecular biology to measure, on a qualitative or semi-quantitative basis, levels of individual target molecules or molecules associated with the mechanism of action of an individual agent that could predict the likelihood of response. There is preliminary evidence that the expression of tumour thymidylate synthase, thymidine phosphorylase, dipyrimidine dehydrogenase (all as markers for fluorouracil resistance) and of

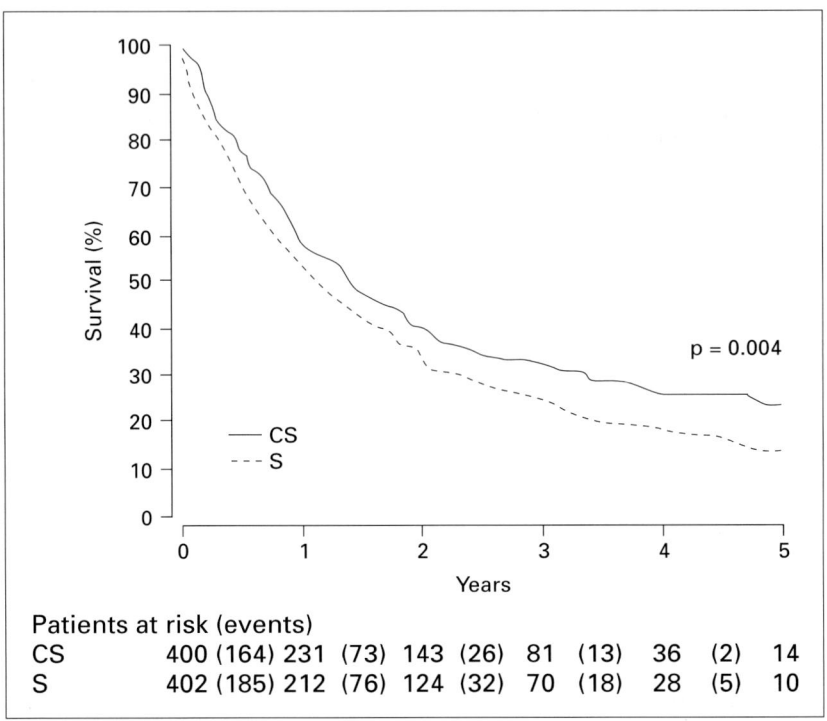

Figure 3. Kaplan-Meier curve showing survival of patients with resectable esophageal cancer randomized to either neoadjuvant chemotherapy followed by surgery (CS) or surgery alone (S). From: MRC Esophageal Cancer Working Party. *Lancet* 2002; 359: 1727-33.

the excision repair gene ERCC-1 helps predict response to chemotherapy containing 5-fluorouracil and cisplatin. (Alexander 1995, Boku 1998, Lenz 1995, Metzger 1998). Results on the impact of p53 expression are still very inconsistent. It must be emphasized that all these findings are not mature and cannot yet serve as a basis for clinical decision-making. However, the direction is clear and the time has come to implement promising molecular markers in prospective clinical trials as a stratification criterion.

An alternative approach is the early assessment of tumour glucose metabolism by means of FDG positron emission tomography during chemotherapy in order to predict response. Two studies have demonstrated that PET imaging may differentiate responding and non-responding tumours early in the course of neoadjuvant systemic chemotherapy (Ott 2002, Weber 2001). Based on these findings, the Munich group has started a prospective clinical study, the so-called MUNICON trial, in which neoadjuvant treatment in adenocarcinoma of the distal esophagus and esophago-gastric junction is monitored by means of PET imaging. According to the findings on day 14 of the first course of induction chemotherapy, patients receive three months of neoadjuvant therapy if there is metabolic response. If only minor metabolic changes are seen, patients undergo early tumour resection or, in the case of unresectable tumours, they are included in salvage protocols.

Presumably, the future will bring tailored treatment strategies based on the reliable specification of constitutional and tumour-related characteristics. Many believe that gene profiling will be a clue for technology in this context. A better understanding of individual tumour biology and prognosis may reduce over-and under-treatment which up to the present day has remained the main problem in all neoadjuvant and adjuvant treatment concepts.

References

1. Ajani JA, Baker J, Pisters PWT, et al. CPT-11 plus Cisplatin in patients with advanced, untreated gastric or gastroesophageal junction carcinoma. *Cancer* 2002; 94: 641-6.
2. Ajani JA, Van Cutsem, Moiseyenko V, et al. Docetaxel (D), cisplatin, 5-fluorouracil compare to cisplatin (C) and 5-fluorouracil (F) for chemotherapy-naive patients with metastatic or locally recurrent, unresectable gastric carcinoma (MGC): interim results of a randomized phase III trial (V325). *Proc Am Soc Clin Oncol* 2003; 999 (abstract).
3. Ajani JA, Ota DM, Jessup JM, et al. Resectable gastric carcinoma. An evaluation of preoperative and postoperative chemotherapy. *Cancer* 1991; 68: 1501-6.
4. Ajani JA, Roth JA, Putnam JB, et al. Feasibility of five courses of pre-operative chemotherapy in patients with resectable adenocarcinoma of the esophagus or gastro-esophageal junction. *Eur J Cancer* 1995; 31A: 665-70.
5. Alexander, HR, Grem JL, Hamilton M, et al. Thymidylate synthase protein expression association with response to neoadjuvant chemotherapy and resection for locally advanced gastric cancer and gastroesophageal adenocarcinoma. *Cancer J Sc Am* 1995; 1: 49-54.
6. Allum W, Cunningham D, Weeden S on behalf of the NCRI Upper GI Clinical Study Group. Perioperative chemotherapy in operable gastric and lower esophageal cancer. A randomised controlled trial (the MAGIC trial ISRCTN 93793971); *Proc Am Soc Clin Oncol* 2003, 998 (abstract).
7. Ancona E, Ruol A, Santi S, et al. Only pathologically complete response to neoadjuvant chemotherapy improves significantly the long-term survival of patients with resectable esophageal squamous cell carcinoma: Final report of a randomized controlled trial of preoperative chemotherapy *versus* surgery alone. *Cancer* 2001; 91: 2165-74.
8. Apinop C, Puttisak P, Preecha N. A prospective study of combined therapy in esophageal cancer. *Hepatogastroenterology* 1994; 41: 391-3.
9. Bartels H, Stein HJ, Siewert JR. Preoperative risk analysis and postoperative mortality of esophagectomy for resectable esophageal cancer. *Br J Surg* 1998; 85: 840-4.
10. Birkmeyer JD, Siewers AE, Finlayson EVA, et al. Hospital volume and surgical mortality in the United States. *N Engl J Med* 2002; 346: 1128-37.
11. Boku N, Chin K, Hosakawa K, et al. Biological markers as a predictor of response and prognosis of unresectable gastric cancer patients treated with 5-fluorouracil and cisplatinum. *Clin Cancer Res* 1998; 4: 1469-74.
12. Bonenkamp JJ, Hermans J, Sasako M, Van de Velde CJH for the Dutch Gastric Cancer Group. Extended lymph-node dissection for gastric cancer. *N Engl J Med* 1999; 340: 908-14.
13. Bosset JF, Gignoux M, Triboulet JP, et al. Chemoradiotherapy followed by surgery compared to surgery alone in squanous-cell cancer of the esophagus. *N Engl J Med* 1997; 337: 161-7.
14. Bouché O, Raoul JL, Giovanini M, et al. Randomized phase II trial of LV5FU2, LV5FU2-cisplatinum or LV5FU2-irinotecan in patients (pts) with metastatic gastric or cardial adenocarcinoma (MGA): final results of study FFCD 9803. *Proc Am Soc Clin Oncol* 2003; 1033 (abstract).
15. Brücher BL, Weber W, Bauer M, et al. Neoadjuvant therapy of esophageal squamous cell carcinoma: reponse evaluation by positron emission tomography. *Ann Surg* 2001; 233: 300-9.

16. Burmeister BH, Smithers BM, Fitzgerald L, et al. A randomized phase III trial of preoperative chemoradiation followed by surgery (CR-S) *versus* surgery alone (S) for localized resectable cancer of the esophagus. *Proc Am Soc Clin Oncol* 2002; 518 (abstract).
17. Chau I, Cunningham D. Perioperative chemotherapy for cancer of the esophagus and the esophagogastric junction. In: *Educational Book of the ASCO meeting* 2003: 429-40.
18. Cuschieri A, Weeden S, Fielding J, et al. for the Surgical Co-operative Group. Patient survival after D1 and D2 resections for gastric cancer: long-term results of the MRC randomized surgical trial – Surgical Co-operative Group. *Br J Cancer* 1999; 79: 1522-30.
19. De Potter T, Flamen P, van Cutsem E, et al. Whole-body PET with FDG for the diagnosis of recurrent gastric cancer. *Eur J Nucl Med* 2002; 29: 525-9.
20. Devesa SS, Blot WJ, Fraumeni JF. Changing pattern in the incidence of esophageal and gastric carcinoma in the United States. *Cancer* 1998; 83: 2049-53.
21. Dittler HJ. Assessment of resectability of gastrointestinal cancers by endoscopic ultrasonography. *Gastrointest Endosc Clin N Am* 1995; 3: 569-75.
22. Eloubeidi MA, Wallace MB, Hoffman BJ, et al. predictors of survival for esophageal cancer patients with and without celiac axis lymphadenpathy: Impact of staging endosonography. *Ann Thorac Surg* 2001; 72: 212-9.
23. Feussner H, Omote K, Fink U, Walker SJ, Siewert JR. Pretherapeutic laparoscopic staging in advanced gastric carcinoma. *Endoscopy* 1999; 31: 342-7.
24. Flamen P, Lerut A, Van Cutsem E. et al. Utility of positron emission tomography for the staging of patients with potentially operable esophageal carcinoma. *J Clin Oncol* 2000; 18: 3202-10.
25. Hesketh PJ, Clapp RW, Doos WG, Spechler SJ. The increasing frequency of adenocarcinoma of the esophagus. *Cancer* 1989; 64: 526-30.
26. Hölscher AH, Bollschweiler E, Bumm R, Bartels H, Höfler H, Siewert JR. Prognostic factors of resected adenocarcinoma of the esophagus. *Surgery* 1995; 118: 845-55.
27. Hundahl SA, Menck HR, Mansour EG, et al. The National Cancer Data Base report on gastric carcinoma. *Cancer* 1997; 80: 2333-41.
28. Kelsen DP, Ginsberg R, Pajak TF, et al. Chemotherapy followed by surgery compared to surgery alone for localized esophageal cancer. *N Engl J Med* 1998; 339: 1979-84.
29. Kelsen D, Karpeh M, Schwartz G, et al. Neoadjuvant therapy of high-risk gastric cancer: a phase II trial of pre-operative FAMTX and postoperative intraperitoneal fluorouracil-cisplatin plus intravenous fluorouracil. *J Clin Oncol* 1996; 15: 1818-28.
30. Kelsen D, Pajak T, Ginsberg R. Treatment of esophageal cancer. *N Engl J Med* 1999; 340: 1685-7.
31. Khushalani N, Leichman CG, Proulx G, et al. Oxaliplatin in combination with protracted-infusion fluorouracil and radiation: report of a clinical trial for patients with esophageal cancer. *J Clin Oncol* 2002; 20: 2844-50.
32. Kim K, Park SJ, Kim BT, et al. Evaluation of lymph node metastasis in squamous cell carcinoma of the esophagus with positron emission tomography. *Ann Thorac Surg* 2001; 71: 290-4.
33. Kole AC, Plukker JT, Nieweg OE, et al. Positron emission tomography for staging of esophageal and gastroesophageal malignancy. *Br J Cancer* 1998; 78: 521-7.
34. Kollmannsberger C, Qwuietzsch D, Haag C, et al. A phase II study of paclitaxel, weekly 24-hour continous infusion of 5-fluorouracil, folinic acid and cisplatin in patients with advanced gastric cancer. *Br J Canc* 2000; 83: 458-62.
35. Law S, Fok M, Chow S, et al. Preoperative chemotherapy *versus* surgical therapy alone for squamous cell carcinoma of the esophagus: A prospective randomized trial. *J Thorac Cardiovasc Surg* 1997; 114: 210-7.
36. Law S, Kwong DLW, Tung HM, et al. Preoperative chemoradiation for squamous cell esophageal cancer: a prospective randomized trial. *Can J Gastroenterol* 1998; 12 (Suppl B); A161 (abstract).

37. Lenz HJ, Leichman CG, Danenberg K, et al. Thymidylate synthase mRNA level in adenocarcinoma of the stomach. A predictor for primary tumour reponse and overall survival. *J Clin Oncol* 1995; 14: 176-82.
38. Le Prise E, Etienne PL, Meunier B, et al. A randomized study of chemotherapy, radiotherapy, and surgery *versus* surgery for localized squamous cell carcinoma of the esophagus. *Cancer* 1994; 73: 1779-84.
39. Lerut T, Flamen P, Ectors N, et al. Histopathologic validation of lymph node staging with FDG-PET scan in cancer of the esophagus and gastroesophageal junction: A prospective study based on primary surgery with extensive lymphadenectomy. *Ann Surg* 2000; 232: 743-52.
40. Lordick F, von Schilling C, Bernhard H, Hennig M, Bredenkamp R, Peschel C. Phase II trial of irinotecan and docetaxel in cisplatin-pretreated relapsed or refractory esophageal cancer. *Br J Canc* 2003 (in press).
41. Louvet C, André T, Lledo G, et al. Phase II study of oxaliplatin, fluorouracil, and folinic acid in locally advanced or metastatic gastric cancer patients. *J Clin Oncol* 2002; 23: 4543-8.
42. Lowy AM, Mansfield PF, Leach SD, et al. Response to neoadjuvant chemotherapy best predicts survival after curative resection for gastric cancer. *Ann Surg* 1999; 229: 303-8.
43. Luketich JD, Friedman DM, Weigel TL, et al. Evaluation of distant metastases in esophageal cancer: 100 consecutive positron emission tomography scans. *Ann Thorac Surg* 1999; 68: 1133-6.
44. Macdonald JS, Smalley SR, Benedetti J, et al. Chemoradiotherapy after surgery compared with surgery alone for adenocarcinoma of the stomach or gastroesophageal junction. *N Engl J Med* 2001; 345: 725-30.
45. Medical Research Council Esophageal Cancer Working Party. Surgical resection with or without preoperative chemotherapy in esophageal cancer: a randomised controlled trial. *Lancet* 2002; 359: 1727-33.
46. Metzger R, Leichman CG, Danenberg KD, et al. ERCC1 mRNA levels complement thymidylate synthase mRNA levels in predicting response and survival for gastric cancer patients receiving combination cisplatin and fluorouracil chemotherapy. *J Clin Oncol* 1998; 16: 309-16.
47. Newman E, Marcus SG, Potmesil M, et al. Neoadjuvant chemotherapy with CPT-11 and cisplatin downstages locally advanced gastric cancer. *J Gastrointest Surg* 2002; 6: 212-23.
48. Nygaard K, Hagen S, Hansen HS, et al. Pre-operative radiotherapy prolongs survival in operable esophageal carcinoma: a randomized, multicenter study of pre-operative radiotherapy and chemotherapy, the second Scandinavian trial in esophageal cancer. *World J Surg* 1992; 16: 1104-9.
49. Ott K, Weber WA, Becker K, Siewert JR, Schwaiger M, Fink U. Prediction of response to neoadjuvant chemotherapy in patients with gastric cancer by PET imaging. *Proc Am Soc Clin Oncol 2002*; 520 (abstract).
50. Rice TW, Adelstein DJ. Precise clinical staging allows treatment modification of patients with esophageal carcinoma. *Oncology (Huntington)* 1997; 11: 58-62.
51. Rice TW, Blackstone EH, Adelstein DJ, et al. N1 esophageal carcinoma: The importance of staging and downstaging. *J Thorac Cardiovasc Surg* 2001; 121: 454-64.
52. Ridwelski K, Gebauer T, Fahlke J, et al. Combination chemotherapy with docetaxel and cisplatin for locally advanced and metastatic gastric cancer. *Ann Oncol* 2001; 12: 47-51.
53. Roder JD, Busch R, Stein HJ, Fink U, Siewert JR. Ratio of invaded lymph nodes as a predictor of survival in squamous cell carcinoma of the esophagus. *Br J Surg* 1994; 81: 410-3.
54. Rösch T. Endosonographic staging of gastric cancer: a review of literature results. *Gastrointest Endosc Clin N Am* 1995; 5: 549-57.
55. Rösch T. Endosonographic staging of esophageal cancer: a review of literature results. *Gastrointest Endosc Clin N Am* 1995; 5: 537-47.
56. Roth JA, Pass HI, Flanagan MM, et al. Randomized trial of preoperative and postoperative adjuvant chemotherapy with cisplatin, vindesine and bleomycin for carcinoma of the esophagus. *J Thorac Cardiovas Surg* 1988; 96: 242-8.

57. Schlag PM for the CAO: Randomized trial for preoperative chemotherapy for squamous cell cancer of the esophagus. *Arch Surg* 1992; 127: 1446-50.
58. Schuhmacher CP, Fink U, Becker K, *et al.* Neoadjuvant therapy for patients with locally advanced gastric carcinoma with etoposide, doxorubicin, and cisplatinum. *Cancer* 2001; 91: 918-27.
59. Siewert JR, Böttcher K, Stein HJ, Roder JR and the German Gastric Carcinoma Study Group. Relevant prognostic factors in gastric cancer. *Ann Surg* 1998; 228: 449-61.
60. Siewert JR, Fink U, Sendler A, *et al.* Gastric cancer. *Curr Probl Surg* 1997; 34: 835-9.
61. Siewert JR, Stein HJ, Feith M, Bruecher BLDM, Bartels H, Fink U. Histologic tumour type is an independant prognostic parameter in esophageal cancer: Lessons from more than 1,000 consecutive resections at a single center in the Western world. *Ann Surg* 2001; 234: 360-9.
62. Siewert JR, Stein HJ, Sendler A, Molls M, Fink U. Esophageal Cancer: Clinical Management. In: Kelsen DP, Daly JM, Kern SE, Levin B and Tepper JE (ed.). *Gastrointestinal Oncology*. Lippincott Williams & Wilkins, Philadelphia 2002, 1st edition: 261-88.
63. Stahl A, Ott K, Weber WA, *et al.* PET imaging of locally advanced gastric carcinomas: correlation with endoscopic and histopathological findings. *Eur J Nucl Med Mol Imaging* 2003; 30: 288-95.
64. Stahl M, Wilke H, Walz MK, *et al.* Randomized phase III trial in locally advanced squamous cell carcinoma (SCC) of the esophagus: Chemoradiation with and without surgery. *Proc Am Soc Clin Oncol* 2003; 1001 (abstract).
65. Sumpter K, Harper-Wynne C, Cunningham D, *et al.* Randomised multicenter phase III study comparing capecitabine with fluorouracil and oxaliplatin with cisplatin in patients with advanced esophagogastric cancer receiving ECF: confirmation of dose escalation. *Proc Am Soc Clin Oncol* 2003; 1031 (abstract).
66. Therasse P, Arbuck SG, Eisenhauer EA, *et al.* New guidelines to evaluate the response to treatment in solid tumours. *J Nat Canc Inst* 2000; 92: 205-16.
67. Urba SG, Orringer MB, Turrisi A, Iannettoni M, Forastiere A, Strawderman M. Randomized trial of preoperative chemoradiation *versus* surgery alone in patients with locoregional esophageal carcinoma. *J Clin Oncol* 2001; 19: 305-13.
68. Wallace MB, Nietert PJ, Earle C, *et al.* An analysis of multiple staging management strategies for carcinoma of the esophagus: computed tomography, endoscopic ultrasound, positron emission tomography, and thoracoscopy/laparoscopy. *Ann Thorac Surg* 2002; 74: 1026-32.
69. Walsh TN, Noonan N, Hollywood D, *et al.* A comparison of multimodal therapy and surgery for esophageal adenocarcinoma. *N Engl J Med* 1996; 335: 1779-84.
70. Weber WA, Ott K, Becker K, *et al.* Prediction of response to preoperative chemotherapy in adenocarcinomas of the esophagogastric junction by metabiloc imaging. *J Clin Oncol* 2001; 19: 3058-65.
71. Wijnhoven BPL, Louwman MWJ, Tilanus HW, Coeberg JWW. Increased incidence of adenocarcinoma at the gastro-esophageal junction in Dutch males since the 1990s. *Eur J Gastroenterol Hepatol* 2002; 14: 115-22.
72. Wilke H, Preusser P, Fink U, *et al.* Preoperative chemotherapy in locally advanced and non-resectable gastric cancer: a phase II study with etoposide, doxorubicin and cisplatin. *J Clin Oncol* 1989; 7: 1318-26.
73. Willis S, Truong S, Gribnitz S, Fass J, Schumpelick V. Endoscopic ultrasonography on the preoperative staging of gastric cancer. Accuracy and impact on surgical therapy. *Surg Endosc* 2000; 14: 951-4.

Extended *vs* limited resection for esophageal cancer: an individual approach

J.J.B. van Lanschot

Department of Surgery, Academic Medical Center at the University of Amsterdam, The Netherlands

Introduction

More than half of the patients with a carcinoma of the esophagus or gastro-esophageal junction has incurable disease at the time of first presentation due to distant metastases and/or local ingrowth in surrounding organs. For these patients effective nonsurgical palliation (pertubation, brachytherapy) can be achieved for the relief of dysphasia as the predominant symptom. Operative resection is generally considered the treatment of first choice if cure is aimed at. The classical approach comprises a right-sided thoracotomy to mobilize the primary tumour with its immediately adjacent lymph nodes and a subsequent laparotomy for gastric tube reconstruction. This so-called Ivor-Lewis procedure was accompanied by substantial perioperative morbidity and even mortality [1]. Moreover, the majority of patients develops recurrent disease with a 5-year survival rate of about 20%, despite critical pre-operative selection. Various strategies have been explored to improve these disappointing results, including early detection (Barrett-surveillance), improved pre-operative selection (endosonography with fine needle aspiration, spiral CT-scanning, PET-scanning) and the addition of (neo-)adjuvant regimens (chemo- and/or radiotherapy). In the operative management two different and in fact opposite approaches have been developed. On the one hand the transhiatal approach has been developed to minimize the surgical trauma and thus to decrease perioperative morbidity and mortality. On the other hand more radical techniques have been applied to maximize long-term outcome.

The transhiatal approach to improve short term recovery

The transhiatal technique has been popularized, in which the tumour is mobilized from the abdomen via the widened hiatus. In this way a formal thoracotomy is prevented, which might decrease the incidence of (pulmonary) complications and thus result in a more favourable postoperative recovery without compromising long term outcome. This transhiatal technique is only feasible for tumours which are located distal to the carina. Several large volume centers, including the group by Orringer *et al.*, have published favourable short-term results with this transhiatal surgical approach [2, 3].

Extended esophagectomy to improve long term survival

Other groups have followed an opposite strategy, focussing on improved long-term survival rather than decreased early postoperative morbidity and mortality. Esophageal cancer is known for its early and scattered lymphatic dissemination. In order to decrease the risk of locoregional recurrence a more radical local excision of the primary tumour (including the azygos vein, the thoracic duct, the pleura and if necessary the pericardium) was combined with a more extensive lymph node dissection in the chest and abdomen (two fields) or even also in the neck (three fields). Several institutions have applied these supra-radical techniques and have claimed an improved long term survival [4, 5].

The recurrence pattern of the transhiatal resection

Different attempts have been undertaken to determine which surgical technique should be preferred under which circumstances. We performed a retrospective analysis of the pattern of recurrence after transhiatal esophagectomy [6]. Insight into the recurrence pattern might offer an indication of the possible advantages of a more extensive locoregional procedure. A group of 149 patients were followed for at least two years after potentially curative transhiatal resection. Recurrence was an early event after a median interval of 11 months; 51 patients (37%) developed locoregional recurrent disease. In 32 of these patients (23%) locoregional recurrence was the only detectable site of recurrent disease. This study indicates that at least theoretically a selective subgroup of about 20% might benefit from a more radical resection. Whether the potential advantage of improved long-term survival after extended resection outweighs the expected increase in perioperative morbidity and mortality, cannot be judged from these data.

Metaanalysis of transthoracic *versus* transhiatal resection

A metaanalysis was performed of the English literature published between 1990 and 1999 [7]. Fifty articles were identified, meeting predefined quality criteria. Transthoracic resections carried a higher risk of pulmonary complications, chylous leakage and wound infection. Anastomotic leakage and vocal cord paralysis were more frequent after transhiatal resection. In-hospital mortality was significantly higher after transthoracic resections: 9.2% *vs* 5.7% (RR = 1.60, 95%; CI = 1.89-1.35). There was no difference in three-year survival rates between transthoracic and transhiatal resections (25.0% *vs* 26.7%, RR = 0.94, 95%; CI = 0.83-1.07). When only the 24 comparative trials were considered, there was a statically significant difference in 5-year survival favouring transthoracic resection, but when all 50 studies were included, the 5-year survival rate was not significantly higher after transthoracic resection: 23.0% *vs* 21.7% (RR = 1.06, 95%; CI = 1.18-0.96).

However, this study could be criticized, because surgical approach (transhiatal *versus* transthoracic resection) was compared rather than extent of resection (Ivor-Lewis *versus* extensive lymphadenectomy). Moreover, only three randomized controlled trials were available with only small numbers of patients included (67, 39 and 32 patients respectively) [8-10]. For that reason we decided to perform a new randomized controlled trial.

Randomized comparison of transthoracic *versus* transhiatal resection

Between 1994 and 2000, 220 patients with a subcarinal adenocarcinoma of the esophagus were included in two Dutch large volume centers [11]. Perioperative morbidity was higher after transthoracic esophagectomy with 2-field lymphadenectomy, but there was no significant difference in in-hospital mortality (4% *vs* 2% after transhiatal resection; p = 0.45). Improved postoperative (esp. pulmonary) morbidity after transhiatal resection resulted in significantly shorter artificial ventilation (median 1 *vs* 2 days), ICU/MCU stay (median 2 *vs* 6 days), and hospital stay (median 15 *vs* 19 days). After a median follow-up of 4.7 years estimated overall 5-year survival was 29% after transhiatal resection and 39% after transthoracic resection. The estimated overall survival advantage was 10% (95% CI = − 3% + 23%). The power calculation of the study design was based on an estimated median overall survival of 14 months after transhiatal resection. However, this median survival appeared to be 21 months. For this reason, the nonsignificant 5-year survival advantage after transthoracic resection might probably be due to a type-II error.

How should (almost certain) short-term advantages of transhiatal resection be balanced against (probable) long-term survival advantages of transthoracic resection? Identification of subgroups that have relatively high long-term benefit helps translate the general outcome of the trial into individualized decision making [12]. Because we expected site-specific treatment effects, randomization was stratified according to the tumour site. Although we recognize the limitations of subgroup analysis, the long-term benefit of transthoracic esophagectomy is more substantial in patients with esophageal tumours (5-year survival advantage = 17%, 95% CI = − 3% to 37%) than in patients with junctional or cardiac tumours (5-year survival advantage = 1%) [13]. Based on this "best available evidence" we now consider transthoracic esophagectomy standard treatment for otherwise fit patients with potentially curable esophageal cancer, whereas transhiatal esophagectomy is the preferred approach in patients with junctional or cardiac cancer.

Implementation of individualization

Implementation of such individualized strategy should be done carefully and prudentially, because it requires sufficient experience with two totally different techniques. We and others have experienced, that the introduction of an operative technique which is new for a specific center has its learning curve. This might be all the more true in low volume hospitals [14].

References

1. Lewis I. The surgical treatment of carcinoma of the esophagus with special reference to a new operation for growths of the middle third. *Br J Surg* 1946; 34: 18-31.
2. Orringer MB, Marshall B, Iannettoni MD. Transhiatal esophagectomy: clinical experience and refinements. *Ann Surg* 1999; 230: 392-403.
3. Tilanus HW, Hop WCJ, Langenhorst BLAM, Lanschot JJB van. Esophagectomy with or without thoracotomy. *J Thorac Cardiovasc Surg* 1993; 105: 898-903.
4. Lerut I, Deleyn P, Coosemans W, Van Raemdonck D, Scheys I, LeSaffre E. Surgical strategies in esophageal carcinoma with emphasis on radical lymphadenectomy. *Ann Surg* 1992; 216: 583-90.
5. Altorki N, Kent M, Ferrara C, Port J. Three-field lymph node dissection for squamous cell and adenocarcinoma of the esophagus. *Ann Surg* 2002; 236: 177-83.
6. Hulscher JBF, Sandick JW van, Tijssen JGP, Obertop H, Lanschot JJB van. The recurrence pattern of esophageal carcinoma after transhiatal resection. *J Am Coll Surg* 2000; 191: 143-8.
7. Hulscher JBF, Tijssen JGP, Obertop H, Lanschot JJB van. Transthoracic *versus* transhiatal resection for carcinoma of the esophagus: a metaanalysis. *Ann Thorac Surg* 2001; 72: 306-13.
8. Goldminc M, Maddern G, LePrise E, Meunier B, Champion JP, Launois B. Esophagectomy by transhiatal approach or thoracotomy: a prospective randomized trial. *Br J Surg* 1993; 80: 367-70.
9. Chu KM, Law SY, Fok M, Wong J. A prospective randomized comparison of transhiatal and transthoracic resection for lower-third esophageal carcinoma. *Am J Surg* 1997; 174: 320-4.
10. Jacobi CA, Zieren HU, Müller M, Pichlmaier H. Surgical therapy of esophageal carcinoma: the influence of surgical approach and esophageal resection on cardiopulmonary function. *Eur J Cardiothorac Surg* 1997; 11: 32-7.
11. Hulscher JBF, Sandick JW van, Boer AGEM de, *et al*. Extended transthoracic resection compared with limited transhiatal resection for adenocarcinoma of the esophagus. *N Engl J Med* 2002; 347: 1662-9.
12. Kitajama M, Kitagawa Y. Surgical treatment of esophageal cancer; the advent of the era of individualization. *N Engl J Med* 2002; 347: 1705-9.
13. Lanschot JJB van, Tilanus HW, Obertop H. Surgical treatment of esophageal cancer. *N Engl J Med* 2003; 348: 1177-9 (letters).
14. Lanschot JJB van, Hulscher JBF, Buskens CJ, Tilanus HW, Kate FJW ten, Obertop H. Hospital volume and hospital mortality for esophagectomy. *Cancer* 2001; 91: 1574-8.

II

Bilio-pancreatic malignancy

New developments in diagnosis and management of early and advanced GI malignancy.
G.N. Tytgat, F. Penninckx, eds. John Libbey Eurotext, Paris © 2003, pp. 41-53.

Critical appraisal of staging of bilio-pancreatic tumours

D.J. Gouma

Academic Medical Center (AMC), Amsterdam, The Netherlands

Introduction

The incidence of pancreatic tumours is around 10/100.000 per year and the prognosis is dismal with a 5 year survival of only 4%. The poor prognosis is partly due to the late diagnosis and low curative resection rate. Surgical resection is the only potentially curative treatment, but the majority of patients are non surgical candidates due to advanced disease or significant co-morbidity. The clinical presentation, painless jaundice with a palpable gallbladder ("Courvoisier" sign) is typical in the majority of patients, however adequate staging of the disease is still more difficult.

Up to the early seventies in the last century the only diagnostic test was hypotonic duodenography and final staging was performed "durante operation".

Presently staging can be performed by many new modalities as ultrasound (US) + doppler, CT scan, MRI/MRCP (Magnetic Resonance Cholangio Pancreaticography), endoscopic ultrasound (EUS), ERCP or PTC with UDUS, Brush and fine needle biopsy and finally diagnostic laparoscopy.

The question remains which tests or combination of tests are necessary to establish the diagnosis as well as for accurate staging. Controversy exists about the following aspects of staging:

Should non-invasive tests be used first to evaluate metastases and/or local tumour ingrowth and if so, should CT scan or MRI be performed as primary test?

Is ERCP still indicated as a diagnostic procedure? Is pre-operative histology or cytology helpful? Should ERCP be used routinely to perform a pre-operative biliary drainage?

Finally should diagnostic laparoscopy be performed as final diagnostic procedure before explorative laparotomy?

These different aspects of staging bilio-pancreatic tumours will be discussed and finally a flow chart for diagnostic work-up and treatment is provided.

The first diagnostic procedure

During a consensus meeting in 1992 in The Netherlands it was already concluded that non invasive tests (CT scan) should preferably be performed before invasive procedures as ERCP. In a recent follow-up study we found that still in 30% of the patients ERCP and subsequent biliary drainage was performed before CT scan [1]. It is not clear whether the order was caused by waiting time for the CT scan or by the wish of the gastroenterologist to obtain the definitive diagnosis and pathological proof and to conduct a therapeutical intervention. Remarkably many patients (around 50%) did not undergo biliary drainage during ERCP, which is generally accepted to prevent biliary septic complications.

Because of the excellent quality of spiral CT and MRI/MRCP during the past years, it is questioned whether ERCP should be used or is anymore justified as a diagnostic procedure.

Data about the accuracy of CT scan and MRCP concerning detection of a pancreatic mass, showing the presence of livermetastases and local resectability are widely variable due to technical performance of these tests and patient selection. Based on randomized comparisons CT scan, MRI as well as endoscopy ultrasound (EUS) are comparable with an overall accuracy of more then 90% to demonstrate a pancreatic mass [2-6].

The specificity of the CT scan and MRI for evaluating liver metastases is respectively 82 and 92% and for local vascular extension around 60-70% for both procedures. For local extension EUS showed the same results. These different tests can be used as complementary procedures. In patients with more advanced disease the diagnostic accuracy of spiral CT and MRI is higher.

Considering the availability in general practice and cost-effectiveness, the spiral CT scan (preferably 2 mm slides) was selected as the first choice of test for non-invasive staging [6].

If ERCP is still used as a diagnostic procedure, intraductal ultrasound can be added to the procedure. A change in the diagnosis of the ERCP was made in around 25% however, pathology of the lesion is still mandatory if non surgical therapy is considered.

For proximal bile duct lesions the diagnosis and staging is more difficult. We found benign lesions in 15% of patients, who underwent a resection for so called "Klatskin tumours" [7]. Even during re-evaluation of the radiological tests most patients were categorized again as having suspected lesions.

Brush cytology and Fine Needle Aspiration (FNA)

Many studies have been performed analyzing Brush cytology and fine needle aspiration showing a relative low sensitivity and high specificity around 98-100% *(table I)*.

Table I. Diagnostic accuracy of Brush cytology and fine needle aspiration (FNA)

	n	sens	spec	ppv	npv
Grassbrenner	86	56%	91%	94%	43%
(proximal)	31	67%	88%	100	31%
Vandervoort	101	51%	100	100	47%
Stewart	406	60%	98%	98%	61%
Logrono	283	48%	98%	92%	76%
Farrell	24	57%	80%		
+dil./FNA	22	85%	100		
Foutch	772	52%	99%	99%	67%
Sturm					
– Cytology	312	36%	98%	98%	34%
– K-ras	312	42%	89%	92%	34%
– Combined	312	62%	89%	94%	44%

The combination of cytology and analysis of K-ras mutation did increase sensitivity but not overall accuracy [8].

It has been concluded that the positive predictive value is high but a negative sample does not exclude malignancy and for unsuspected strictures or predictive lesions exploration is still indicated.

Pre-operative biliary draining

Surgery in jaundiced patients carries an increased risk of postoperative complications. To avoid death and complications, pre-operative biliary drainage (PBD) has been proposed as a means of reversing the pathophysiologic disturbances seen in jaundiced patients. In 1935, Whipple already had performed a staged surgical approach with a preliminary bypass to reduce jaundice and improve hepatic function. Since then, numerous studies, randomized as well as retrospective, have compared the outcome of PBD with surgery without PBD.

Studies in experimental animals have shown benefit of PBD, especially after internal drainage when the enterohepatic circulation was restored. Arguments for internal biliary drainage as an improvement of liverfunction, improvement of nutritional status, reduction of endotoxemia, normalization of abnormal lipid spectrum, improvement of immune function, reduction of TNF/IL6 release and reduction of mortality [9-11].

Clinical studies have failed to show this benefit, and some studies even reported a deleterious effect. In two studies from our institution we did not find any difference in morbidity in patients who underwent pre-operative biliary drainage *versus* non drained patients. Recently deterious effects have been shown [12, 13], *(table II)*. PBD is mainly performed because of logistic problems, such as time needed for further staging and the expected waiting time for surgery.

Table II. Internal biliary drainage

Arguments in favor	Arguments against
• Improves liverfunction/hyperbilirubinemia	• Secondary inflammation bile duct
• Improves nutritional status	• Morbidity of drainage procedure
• Reduces endotoxemia	• Reduces endotoxemia
• Normalises abnormal lipid spectrum	• Increase:
• Improves immune function	– infected bile (stent clogging)
• Reduces TNF/IL-6 release	– wound infection
• Reduces mortality	– anastomotic leakage
	– intra abdominal sepsis

Despite the lack of a beneficial effect most jaundiced patients in many centres undergo surgery for tumours after pre-operative drainage. Therefore we performed recently a meta-analysis to examine the effectiveness of PBD in jaundiced patients with tumours, and to guide clinicians in their management of these patients [14]. The five level I randomized studies showed no difference in the overall death rate between patients who had PBD and those who had surgery without PBD. The overall complication rate, however, was significantly adversely affected by PBD compared with surgery without PBB *(figure 1)*.

At the 18 level II cohort studies there was no difference in the death rate between the two treatment modalities. The overall complications rate, however, was significantly adversely affected by PBD compared with surgery without PBD. If PBD had been without complications, then complications would be in favour of drainage based on level 1 studies, and no difference based on level 2 studies. Further, PBD was not able to reduce the length of postoperative hospital stay compared with surgery without PBD; instead, it prolonged the stay *(figure 2)*.

We concluded from this meta-analysis that pre-operative biliary drainage should not be performed routinely. The potential benefit of PBD in terms of postoperative rates of death and complications does not outweigh the disadvantage of the drainage procedure.

The indication for pre-operative biliary drainage is dependent on the time needed for extra diagnostic tests; probably the severity of jaundice (bilirubin levels > 300 µmol/1 l, logistics as waiting time for surgery or referral to centers, the use of pre-operative chemo-radiotherapy and last but not least the prevalence of the gastroenterologist [15]. Further randomized controlled trials with improved PBD techniques are necessary to analyze the potential benefit of this procedure.

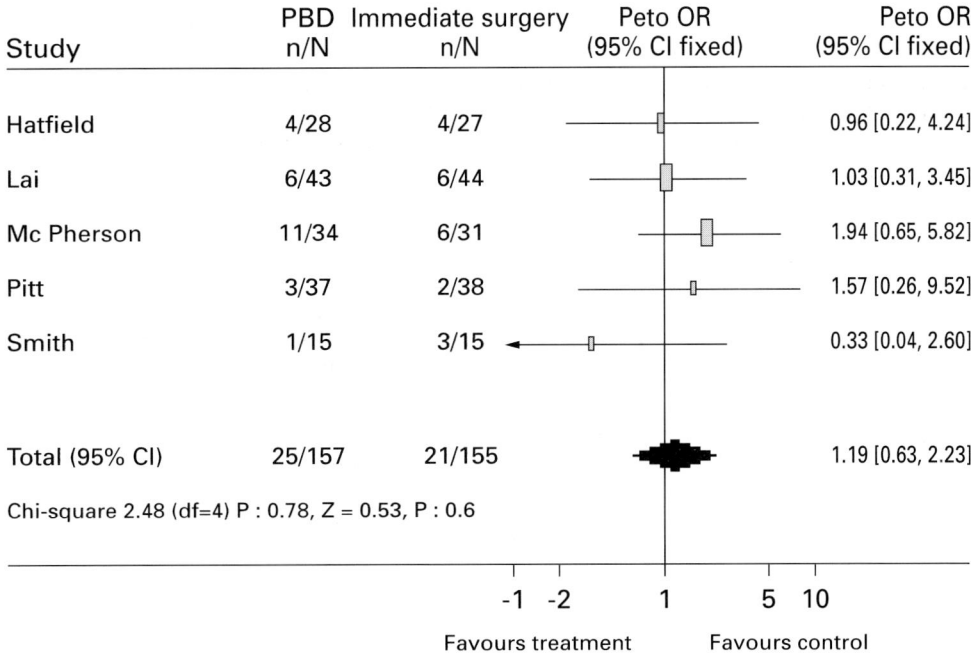

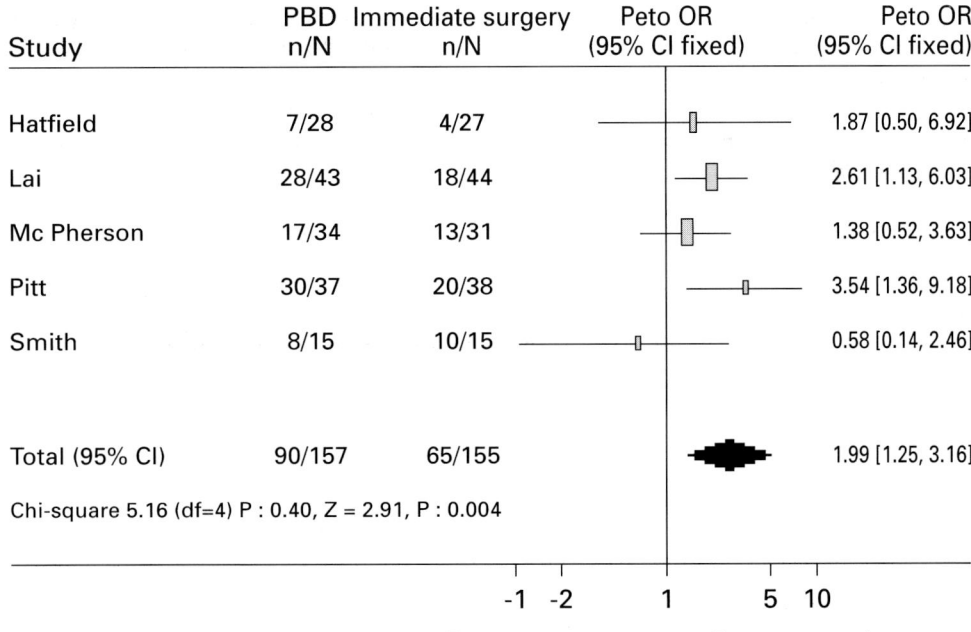

Figure 1. Preoperative biliary drainage meta-analysis 1966-2001, level I studies mortality and morbidity.

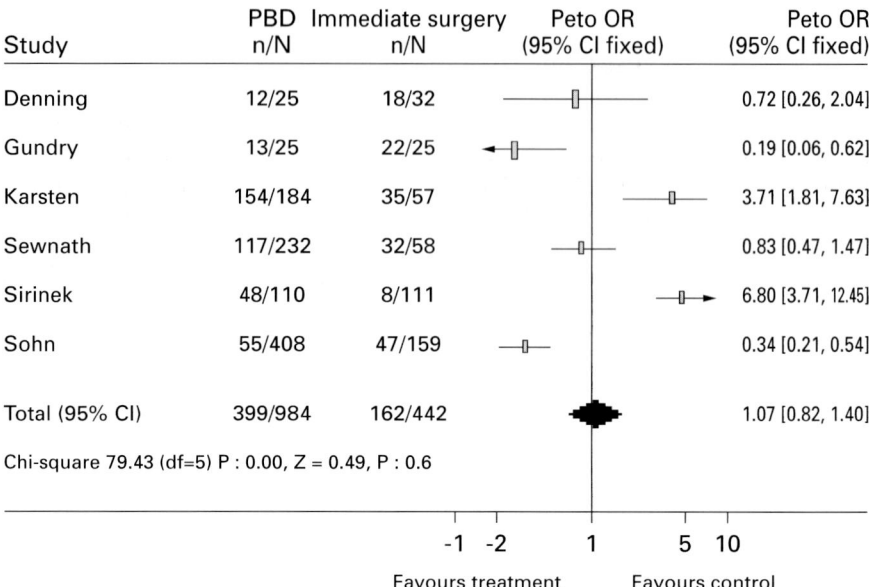
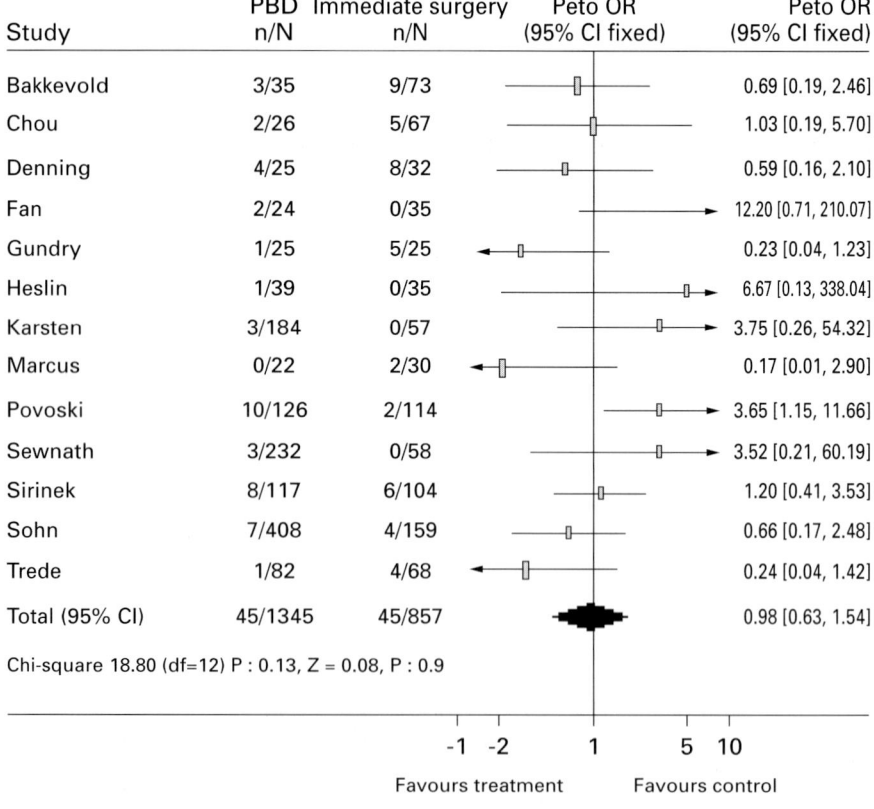

Figure 2. Overall mortality and morbidity level II studies.

Diagnostic laparoscopy

Diagnostic laparoscopy of peripancreatic malignancies has been reported to improve the assessment of tumour stage and to prevent unnecessary exploratory laparotomies. Laparoscopy enables the detection of small superficial metastases at the liver surface and the peritoneum that are easily missed with radiologic staging techniques and often first encountered during laparotomy. Diagnostic laparoscopy can be combined with laparoscopic ultrasound, which has been reported to be sensitive for the detection of small intrahepatic metastases and for the evaluation of enlarged lymph nodes and tumour ingrowth in vascular structures surrounding peripancreatic tumours.

As laparoscopy is the final staging procedure before surgery, the eventual benefits of laparoscopic staging apply to patients already selected for resection by radiologic imaging techniques.

The success rate of diagnostic laparoscopy is influenced by multiple factors. First of all it depends on the determination of the end-point for success of the procedure. This can be defined as new, additional finding (liver cysts) or a change in treatment strategy (bypass instead of resection) or the incidence of unnecessary laparotomy (detection metastases).

Secondly the success of laparoscopy depends also on tumour localization, the quality of pre-laparoscopy staging procedures, and at the timing in the staging process. Thirdly the success of diagnostic laparoscopy also depends on the indication for laparoscopy whether for selection for curative resection or for palliative radiotherapy or chemotherapy.

The first study in our institution to evaluate the additional value of diagnostic laparoscopy in patients with a pancreatic head carcinoma was performed between 1993 and 1994. The prelaparoscopic staging of 73 patients with potential resectable disease consisted of endoscopic retrograde cholangio-pancreatography (ERCP), abdominal ultrasound with Doppler examination and most (conventional) computed tomography (CT) in the referring hospital in the majority of the patients. Patients underwent diagnostic laparoscopy and 70 patients could be analysed. A change in tumour stage was found in 29 patients (41%). This resulted in a change in therapy in 14 patients (25%) and a laparotomy could be avoided in 17% [16]. In the same period, the additional value of diagnostic laparoscopy in patients with pancreatic head carcinoma varied widely in other studies between 18% and 55% with a mean of 39% [17-26], as shown in *table III*.

In recent years radiologic imaging techniques have been improved. New staging methods have been introduced, such as helical computed tomography, endoscopic ultrasonography, and intravascular ultrasonography, affecting patient selection for resection and increasing resectability rates. It is likely that the improved accuracy of radiologic staging techniques will also limit the additional value of laparoscopic staging.

In a recent review Pisters *et al.* stated that detection of occult metastatic disease should be less than 20% during laparoscopy because otherwise quality of prediagnostic imaging is not sufficient [27]. A number of recent studies from experienced centers in which the potential benefit of diagnostic laparoscopy in detection of metastases was evaluated during laparotomy after a high quality helical CT scan are in accordance with the reduced detection rate mentioned by Pisters and are summarized in *table IV*.

Table III. Results of diagnostic laparoscopy and detection of pathology proven metastases in pancreatic and periampullary carcinoma from the literature between 1991-1995

Author	Number of patients	Metastases	%
Bemelman [16]	70	12	17
Conlon [17]	108	39	39
Cushieri [18]	15	5	33
Cushieri [19]	51	16	18
Fernandez [20]	89	16	18
John [21]	40	14	35
Meduri [22]	56	31	55
Murugiah [23]	12	6	50
Pietrabissa [24]	21	9	43
Sand [25]	29	11	38
Warshaw [26]	57	17	30
Total	478	190	39

Table IV. Peritoneal and/or liver metastases detected during laparotomy after helical computed tomography (adapted from Pisters et al. BJS 2001; 88: 325-7)

Reference	patients considered resectable	Resection rate (%)	patients with metastases	maximum % prevented laparotomy*
Steinberg et al. [28]	32	75	4	13
Friess et al. [29]	159	75	16	10
Rumstadt et al. [30]	194	89	9	5
Holzman et al. [31]	23	78	1	4
Spitz et al. [32]	118	80	18	15
Sladinger et al. [33]	68	76	3	4

* Maximum percentage of patients who would have been spared laparotomy if laparoscopy had been performed with accuracy of 100%.

Laparoscopic staging and subsequent palliative treatment

Since evaluation of staging is incomplete without the assessment of the consequences for the treatment in terms of improvement of outcome, we decided to investigate the additional value of diagnostic laparoscopy after complete radiological staging as well as the outcome of patients with pathological proven unresectable carcinoma, who underwent palliative treatment by endoscopic stent placement or a surgical bypass procedure. In this study all patients with metastases at diagnostic laparoscopy were randomized for both palliative treatments. The primary end-point for the diagnostic part of the study was prevention of laparotomy and for the therapeutic part of this study hospital free survival after palliative treatment [34]. Diagnostic laparoscopy detected pathology proven metastases in 39/297 patients (13%). In another 13% of the patients unresectable disease was suspected but could not be proven with pathological examination.

The average hospital free survival in the endoscopically treated patients was 94 days compared to an average hospital free survival of 164 days after surgical palliative treatment *(figure 3)*. This study showed again a limited benefit of diagnostic laparoscopy (13%) in preventing laparotomy and more importantly no improved hospital free survival was found after subsequent non surgical palliation. Therefore diagnostic laparoscopy was abandoned as routine diagnostic procedure in patients with periampullary and pancreatic tumours in our institute.

During the past decade several studies have been performed to evaluate the potential benefit of diagnostic laparoscopy with pancreatic/periampullary tumours showing a decrease in the additional value in avoiding laparotomy from around 25% to 10%. The reduction of identifying metastases during laparoscopy is mainly caused by increasing quality of the radiological staging of the patients due to the CT scan and decreased thickness of the slices up to 2 mm as shown for our institution in *table V*. Therefore it can be concluded that there is no indication to perform diagnostic laparoscopy routinely in patients with pancreatic tumours. There might be an indication to perform laparoscopy in a well-defined selected group of patients with a high risk of advanced disease especially when good outcome in nonsurgical palliation can be expected.

Table V. The outcome of diagnostic laparoscopy at the AMC and change in radiological work-up of patients with periampullary tumours during 1993-2001

	year	radiological staging	prevented laparotomy
Introduction laparoscopy *BJS* [16]	93-94	Ultrasound	19%
Late laparotomy *Cancer* [35]	93-95	US conv. CT scan	15% (11%)
Randomized trial *Ann Surg* [19]	95-98	spiral CT scan 5 mm	13%
Implementation study (submitted) (stop laparoscopy)	99-01	spiral CT scan 2 mm	9.5%

CT scan findings and prognostic factors for survival

During the past years the accuracy of CT scan in staging pancreatic tumours has always been evaluated as sensitivity, specificity or positive productive value of resectability of the tumour or even more detailed resectability rate of microscopically radical resections.

It should be realized that resectability rate is also highly dependent on the surgical attitude in terms of acceptance or removal of the portal/mesenteric vein and/or acceptance of non-radical resections. Therefore we decided not to use the surgical resection itself as the reference standard for CT evaluation but the outcome in terms of survival of patients. In a recent study from our institution pre-operative CT scan findings/criteria were used as prognostic factors for survival in patients with pancreatic carcinoma.

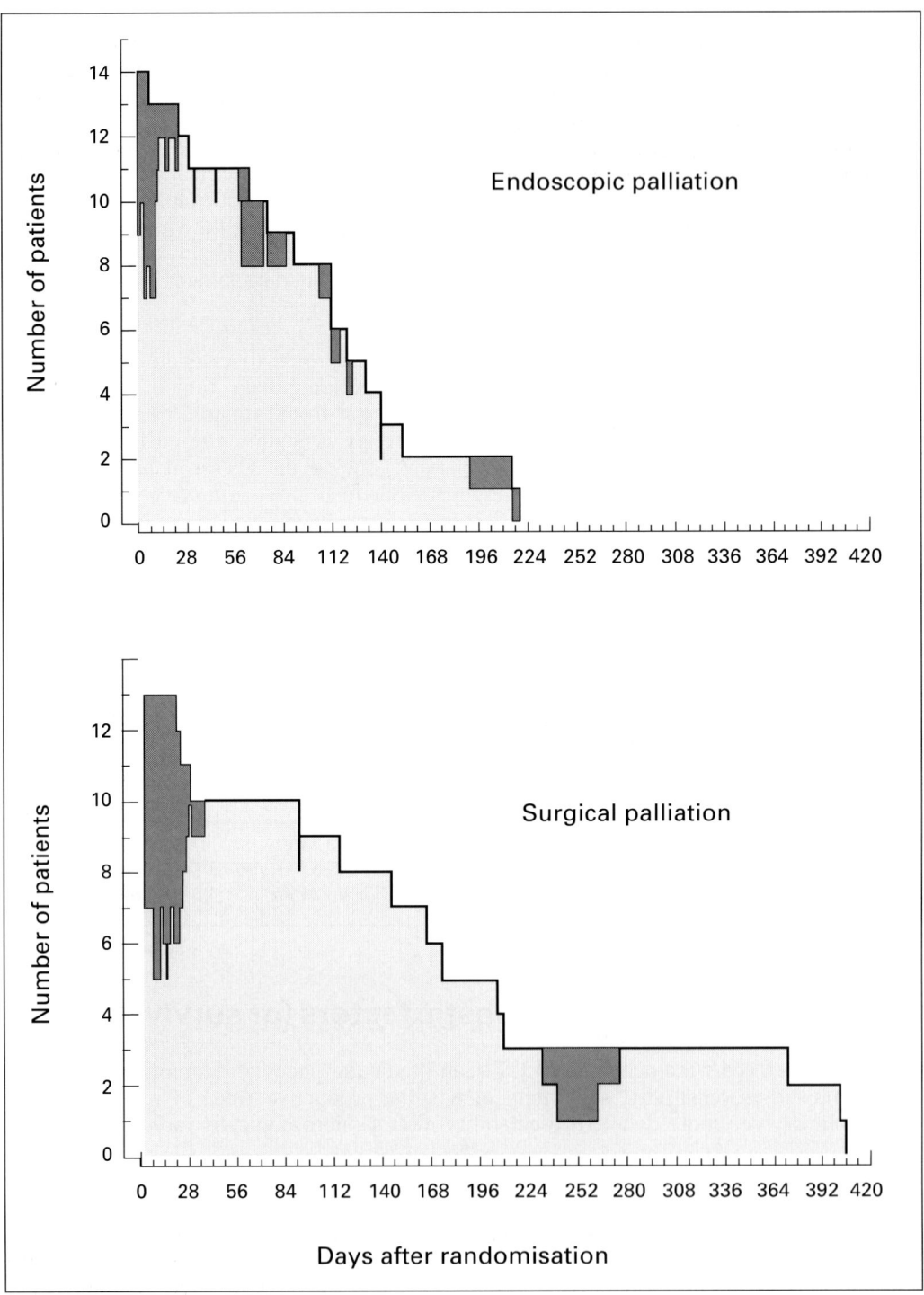

Figure 3. Endoscopic palliation.

In a consecutive group of 71 patients CT findings were directly correlated with survival after resection and bypass surgery. Median survival was 21 months for resectable tumours and 9.7 months after bypass surgery. In patients who underwent resection survival was limited (median 7-9 months) for patients with pre-operative CT scan signs of encasement of hepatic artery, mesenteric artery, venous involvement > 180 degrees, and fatty infiltration at the retroperitoneal resection plane.

It was concluded that CT findings might be useful to further select patients who should not undergo resection because of relative poor outcome.

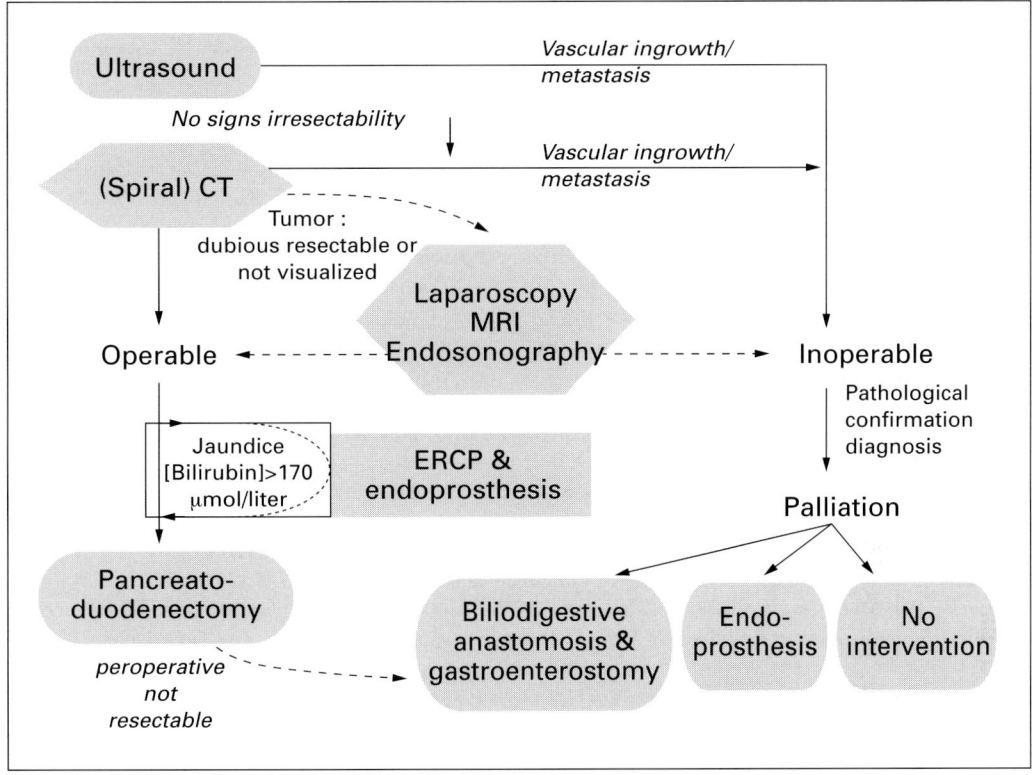

Figure 4. Flow chart for diagnosis work-up and treatment of periampullary and pancreatic carcinoma.

In summary

Spiral CT scan is currently the most important diagnostic tool for staging Brush cytology or fine needle aspiration have limited value. ERCP has minimal additional value for the diagnosis ERCP and pre-operative biliary drainage should not be used routinely. The additional value of laparoscopy is limited.

Considering the data as discussed above as well as recent data from the cost-effectiveness paper of Imaging Technologies for Assessing Resectability in Pancreatic Cancer [6] a flow chart for diagnostic work-up and treatment of pancreatic carcinoma is outlined in *figure 4*.

References

1. Tilleman EH, Benraadt J, Bossyt PM, Gouma DJ. Diagnostiek en behandeling van het pancreascarcinoom in de regio van het Integraal Kankercentrum Amsterdam in 1997. *Ned Tijdschr Geneeskd* 2001; 145 (28): 1358-62.
2. Freeny PC. Computed tomography in the diagnosis and staging of cholangiocarcinoma and pancreatic carcinoma. *Ann Oncol* 1999; 10 (4): 12-7.
3. Diehl SJ, Lehmann KJ, Sadick M, Lachman R, Georig M. Pancreatic cancer: value of dual-phase spiral CT in assessing resectability. *Radiology* 1998; 206: 373-8.
4. Sheridan MB, Ward J, Guthrie JA, *et al.* Dynamic contrast-enhanced MR imaging and dual-phase helical CT in the preoperative assessment of suspected pancreatic cancer: a comparative study with receiver operating characteristic analysis. *AJR Am J Roentgenol* 1999; 173 (3): 583-90.
5. Trede M, Rumstadt B, Wendl K, *et al.* Ultrafast magnetic resonance imaging improves the staging of pancreatic tumours. *Ann Surg* 1997; 226 (4): 393-405; discussion 405-7.
6. McMahon PM, Halpern EF, Fernandez-del Castillo C, Clark JW, Gazelle GS. Pancreatic cancer: cost-effectiveness of imaging technologies for assessing resectability. *Radiology* 2001; 221 (1): 93-106.
7. Gerhards MF, Vos P, Gulik TM van, Rauws EA, Bosma A, Gouma DJ. Incidence of benign lesions in patients resected for suspicious hilar obstruction. *Br J Surg* 2001; 88 (1): 48-51.
8. Sturm PD, Rauws EA, Hruban RH, *et al.* Clinical value of K-ras codon 12 analysis and endobiliary brush cytology for the diagnosis of malignant extrahepatic bile duct stenosis. *Clin Cancer Res* 1999; 5 (3): 629-35.
9. Gouma DJ, Coelho JC, Schlegel JF, Li YF, Moody FG. The effect of preoperative internal and external biliary drainage on mortality of jaundiced rats. *Arch Surg* 1987; 122 (6): 731-4.
10. Greve JW, Maessen JG, Tiebosch T, Buurman WA, Gouma DJ. Prevention of postoperative complications in jaundiced rats. Internal biliary drainage *versus* oral lactulose. *Ann Surg* 1990; 212 (2): 221-7.
11. Kimmings AN, van Deventer SJ, Obertop H, Rauws EA, Gouma DJ. Inflammatory and immunologic effects of obstructive jaundice: pathogenesis and treatment. *J Am Coll Surg* 1995; 181 (6): 567-81.
12. Sohn TA, Yeo CJ, Cameron JL, Pitt HA, Lillemoe KD. Do preoperative biliary stents increase postpancreaticoduodenectomy complications? *J Gastrointest Surg* 2000; 4 (3): 258-67; discussion 267-8.
13. Povoski SP, Karpeh MS Jr, Conlon KC, Blumgart LH, Brennan MF. Association of preoperative biliary drainage with postoperative outcome following pancreaticoduodenectomy. *Ann Surg* 1999; 230 (2): 131-42.
14. Sewnath ME, Karsten ThM, Prins MH, Rauws EJ, Obertop H, Gouma DJ. A meta-analysis on the efficacy of preoperative biliary drainage for tumours causing obstructive jaundice. *Ann Surg* 2002; 236 (1): 17-27 (review).
15. Isenberg G, Gouma DJ, Pisters PW. The on-going debate about perioperative biliary drainage in jaundiced patients undergoing pancreaticoduodenectomy. *Gastrointest Endosc* 2002; 56 (2): 310-5.
16. Bemelman WA, de Wit LT, van Delden OM, *et al.* Diagnostic laparoscopy combined with laparoscopic ultrasonography in staging of cancer of the pancreatic head region. *Br J Surg* 1995; 82: 820-4.

17. Conlon KC, Dougherty E, Klimstra DS, Coit DG, Turnbull AD, Brennan MF. The value of minimal access surgery in the staging of patients with potentially resectable peripancreatic malignancy. *Ann Surg* 1996; 223: 134-40.
18. Cuschieri A, Hall AW, Clark J. Value of laparoscopy in the diagnosis and management of pancreatic carcinoma. *Gut* 1978; 19: 672-7.
19. Cuschieri A. Laparoscopy for pancreatic cancer: does it benefit the patient? *Eur J Surg Oncol* 1988; 14: 41-4.
20. Fernandez-del CC, Rattner DW, Warshaw AL. Further experience with laparoscopy and peritoneal cytology in the staging of pancreatic cancer. *Br J Surg* 1995; 82: 1127-9.
21. John TG, Greig JD, Carter DC, Garden OJ. Carcinoma of the pancreatic head and periampullary region. Tumour staging with laparoscopy and laparoscopic ultrasonography. *Ann Surg* 1995; 221: 156-64.
22. Meduri F, Diana F, Merenda R, *et al*. Implication of laparoscopy and peritoneal cytology in the staging of early pancreatic cancer. *Zentralbl Pathol* 1994; 140: 243-6.
23. Murugiah M, Paterson-Brown S, Windsor JA, Miles WF, Garden OJ. Early experience of laparoscopic ultrasonography in the management of pancreatic carcinoma. *Surg Endosc* 1993; 7: 177-81.
24. Pietrabissa A, Di Candio G, Giulianotti PC, Mosca F. Exposure of the pancreas and staging of pancreatic cancer. *Laparoscopic Semin Laparosc Surg* 1996; 3: 3-9.
25. Sand J, Marnela K, Airo I, Nordback I. Staging of abdominal cancer by local anesthesia outpatient laparoscopy. *Hepatogastroenterology* 1996; 43: 1685-8.
26. Warshaw AL. Implications of peritoneal cytology for staging of early pancreatic cancer. *Am J Surg* 1991; 161: 26-9.
27. Pisters PW, Lee JE, Vauthey JN, Charnsangavej C, Evans DB. Laparoscopy in the staging of pancreatic cancer. *Br J Surg* 2001; 88 (3): 325-37.
28. Steinberg WM, Barkin J, Bradley EL, DeMagno E, Layer P. Controversies in clinical pancreatology. Workup of a patient with a mass in the head of the pancreas. *Pancreas* 1998; 17: 24-30.
29. Friess H, Kleeff J, Silva JC, Sadowski C, Baer HU, Büchler MW. The role of diagnostic laparoscopy in pancreatic and periampullary malignancies. *J Gastrointest Surg* 1998; 186: 675-82.
30. Rumstadt B, Schwab M, Schuster K, Hagmiller E, Trede M. The role of laparoscopy in the preoperative staging of pancreatic carcinoma. *J Gastrointest Surg* 1997; 1: 245-50.
31. Holzman MD, Reintgen KL, Tyler DS, Pappas TN. The role of laparoscopy in the management of suspected pancreatic and periampullary malignancies. *J Gastrointest Surg* 1997; 1: 236-44.
32. Spitz FR, Abbruzzese JL, Lee JE, *et al*. Preoperative and postoperative chemoradiation strategies in patients treated with pancreaticoduodenectomy for adenocarcinoma of the pancreas. *J Clin Oncol* 1997; 15: 928-37.
33. Saldinger PF, Reilly M, Reynolds K, *et al*. Is CT angiography sufficient for prediction of resectability of periampullary neoplasms? *J Gastrointest Surg* 2000; 4: 223-7.
34. Nieveen van Dijkum EJ, Romijn MG, Terwee CB, *et al*. Laparoscopic staging and subsequent palliation in patients with peripancreatic carcinoma. *Ann Surg* 2003; 237 (1): 66-73.
35. Van Dijkum EJ, de Wit LT, van Delden OM, *et al*. The efficacy of laparoscopic staging in patients with upper gastrointestinal tumours. *Cancer* 1997; 79 (7): 1315-9.

New developments in diagnosis and management of early and advanced GI malignancy.
G.N. Tytgat, F. Penninckx, eds. John Libbey Eurotext, Paris © 2003, pp. 55-61.

Endoscopic and endosonographic approaches to biliopancreatic lesions*

Thomas Rösch

Department of Internal Medicine II, Technical University of Munich, Germany

Endoscopic ultrasonography (EUS) is a technique which has been around for more than 20 years. In clinical practice, it is mainly used for diagnosis and staging of gastroenterological tumours, with some exceptions in the diagnosis of benign, non-neoplastic conditions (*e.g.* common bile duct stones). Some 10 years ago, linear EUS has been further developed for gaining tissue via EUS-guided fine needle aspiration (FNA) puncture [1], adding a substantial dimension to the diagnostic ability of EUS. Most recently, EUS has also been used to perform various therapeutic procedures [2]. In the following, the possibilities of these three areas shall be highlighted.

Technical factors

Echoendoscopes – with some recent exceptions – are oblique-viewing endoscopes which carry a rigid ultrasound transducer at their tip, which either generates a 360 degree round-view perpendicular to the shaft axis, or a linear image of variable width parallel to the endoscope axis. Radial scanners have been mechanical scanners, but recently electronic scanning – the principle of linear scanners – is being developed for radial scanning, too. EUS utilizes high ultrasound frequencies (5-20 MHz, 7.5 MHz being the most frequently used ultrasound frequency) which generate a high-resolution image in the near field with limited penetration depth, ranging from 1-2 to 5-6 cm, depending of the ultrasound frequency used. EUS is usually done with the patient in left lateral position, mostly under conscious sedation, and is associated with very low complication rates [3], with very few exceptions [4]. Details of the examination technique for the various organs in focus – GI

---

* Parts of that manuscript were taken from a recent Editorial in *Gut* (Rösch T: Endoscopic ultrasonography: Imaging and beyond. *Gut*; 2003, in press).

tract and immediate surroundings, mainly the pancreatobiliary tract – are described elsewhere [5, 6]. Miniprobes are a further development which mirror the miniaturization of the technique, they can be used intraductally in the biliary (and pancreatic duct) and are referred to below.

Linear echoendoscopes are necessary for the performance of EUS-guided FNA, since only with these instruments the course of the puncture needle can be followed. An average of 2-4 passes is necessary to obtain adequate tissue for cytologic smears, and the presence of an in-room cytopathologist seems to improve the yield [3]; some examiners try to obtain small core specimens for histopathologic analysis, but the relative yield and accuracy of cytologic and histologic analysis, as well as the best needle diameter (19 or 22 Gauge) are still unclear.

Endosonographic imaging in tumour diagnosis and staging

After primary suspicion diagnosis of pancreatobiliary tumours by ultrasound or CT, EUS is used for locoregional tumour staging. The use of EUS is limited to patients in whom surgery is considered, either primarily or (experimentally) after neo-adjuvant therapy, as EUS is not believed to be useful in inoperable patients or those with known unresectable disease or distant metastases. In contrast to equivocally good results in the GI tract for EUS staging, the situation in the pancreatobiliary tract is less clear-cut. EUS was repeatedly reported to be the most accurate method for diagnosing small cancers [7] but this was flawed by study designs with a very high disease prevalence, and has not consistently been confirmed by other papers [8]. The value of EUS in "screening" for pancreatic tumours in patients with only a vague suspicion is therefore not established. As with all other imaging tests including, most recently, PET [9], EUS is not useful for differentiating focal chronic pancreatitis from cancer [10], and its accuracy in locoregional staging is seen both enthusiastically [11-13] as well as more sceptically [14]. For pancreatic and biliary cancer staging, helical CT is probably at present the method of choice, merely due to its widespread existence – comparative studies between EUS and helical CT revealing greatly divergent results [15-17] – and EUS might be used as a second-line test in case of uncertainty on CT, or for additional information (FNA) or treatment (plexus neurolysis); these possibilities are discussed below.

In summary, in the year 2003, EUS may be used as a secondary step in cases with indeterminate CT and/or for FNA or treatment in pancreatic tumours. Recent studies showing less impressive results for EUS in GI and pancreatic cancer staging [14] have to be viewed in the perspective of a routine test usually doing less well under routine circumstances – a fact which is mostly not assessed with other imaging methods but probably applies to all of them.

Endosonographic imaging in benign pancreatobiliary disease

The diagnosis of common bile duct stones is another good indication for EUS as confirmed by a large number of pretty homogeneous studies from all over the world [18-21], yielding accuracy rate of well over 90%. Direct comparisons with MRCP showed EUS to be superior or equal [22]. EUS could therefore be used in patients with low or intermediate risk for common bile duct stones; a negative EUS examination has a very high negative predictive value [23]. The diagnosis of pancreatic endocrine tumours is another good indication for EUS, and other tests have repeatedly shown to be inferior to EUS [24].

Due to its good accuracy in detecting CBD dilatation, CBD stones, pancreatic tumours and – although disputed – chronic pancreatitis [25], EUS has been suggested as a primary tool in patients with a clinical suspicion of pancreatobiliary disease. However, data are mainly from tertiary referral centers which see preselected patients and some had a rather high rate of chronic pancreatitis cases [26]. Large and good outcome studies in patient populations with a low disease prevalence are still missing. The use of the echoendoscope as an endoscope for upper GI tract endoscopic screening including an endosonographic view on the pancreas is intriguing but has to be assessed properly. First data on patients with dyspepsia are appearing [27].

Diagnostic EUS with intraductal miniprobes

The intrabiliary use of MP has been published in a fair number of studies [28-30], but their real value in diagnosis of biliary strictures and staging of biliary tumours is still limited in clinical practice due to limited durability, costs, expertise and uncertain accuracy. New 3D miniprobes may fare much better, but evidence is largely missing for that statement.

Diagnostic EUS and outcome

A growing body of evidence deals with the impact of EUS on outcome and management [31-35], although it might be difficult to ascribe outcome in complex situations such as gastroenterologic tumours to one single imaging test. EUS predicition of advanced tumours has been linked to very poor prognosis in pancreatic cancer [58-63]. Calculations of cost-effectiveness in biliary pancreatitis [36] has mostly revealed encouraging results, but not all of the outcome studies showed huge differences induced by EUS; this however is not to be expected from a merely diagnostic tests, and it has to be mentioned, that outcome studies are usually avoided in the field of research dealing with GI imaging (endoscopy, radiology, nuclear medicine). A broader application of EUS in patients with abdominal pain/dyspepsia has therefore to be evaluated further.

Prior to the transluminal endoscopic drainage of pancreatic pseudocysts, EUS was shown to change management in almost 40% of cases [37]. EUS can diagnose intervening vessels, possibly preventing the blind transluminal approach, and it can guide the way to the best approach and non-bulging cysts. It is however not backed up by study data, whether in pseudocysts with clear bulging, the endoscopic drainage attempt should only be performed after EUS. It is nevertheless only logical that nowadays, cyst drainage can be performed under direct EUS-guidance (see below).

Endosonographic tissue acquisition

The addition of guided needle aspiration has clearly widened the spectrum of diagnostic EUS. Generally, specificity is close to 100% in all indications, but the diagnostic sensitivity somewhat depends on the indications [3, 38, 39], with the highest sensitivity being achieved in mediastinal tumours and lymph node metastases.

Pancreatic malignancy on the other hand, can be proven with a lower sensitivity, between 70 and 85%, and the influence on outcome is less clear: In irresectable tumours, EUS-FNA is necessary when radiochemotherapy regimens are applied, and can be performed in one step with staging and perhaps coeliac plexus blockade in case of severe pain. In resectable tumours, most would go straight to surgery and a negative FNA result would not change this approach; the minority opinion relies on the fact that resectable tumours may be of different histology than adenocarcinoma and then treated by limited surgery [40]. In pancreatic cystic lesions, the situation is less clear, and sensitivity of EUS imaging can be improved by FNA results, using cytology and tumour markers, but specificity may be negatively affected [41, 42].

Endosonographic therapy: current possibilities and future areas of research

A variety of therapeutic possibilities have either been partially explored or are evolving with some animal data presented. Transmural drainage of pancreatic and peripancreatic fluid collections under direct EUS guidance is one of the most logical applications of therapeutic use, and in a recent series of 35 cases, 20 of whom had infected cysts/abscesses, a 89% initial success rate with 3 recurrences was reported. Notably, almost all lesions (n = 32) lesions did not cause any bulging and would not have been amenable by conventional endoscopic drainage [43]. EUS may open the way to more aggressive therapy, such as direct endoscopic removal of pancreatic necroses [44]. EUS-guided coeliac plexus blockade has also been reported in a variety of studies on pancreatic cancer and chronic pancreatitis pain, with better results in cancer (78%) [45] than in chronic pancreatitis (55%) [46]; a small randomized study showed the EUS-guided technique to be superior to the CT-technique [47]. Other indications such as EUS-guided botulinum toxin injection, injection treatment for tumours, suprapapillary bile duct drainage and transgastric approach to the left biliary system have been reported in case reports, whereas other techniques such as creation of gastroenterostomy and antireflux techniques are still in the experimental stage [2,48]. Nevertheless, some of indications will remain and some new ones will evolve which will turn out to become clinically useful.

References

1. Fusaroli P, Caletti G. Endoscopic ultrasonography. *Endoscopy* 2003; 35 (2): 127-35.
2. Waxman I, Dye CE. Interventional endosonography. *Cancer J* 2002; 8 (Suppl. 1): S113-23.
3. Wiersema MJ, Vilmann P, Giovannini M, Chang KJ, Wiersema LM. Endosonography-guided fine-needle aspiration biopsy: diagnostic accuracy and complication assessment. *Gastroenterology* 1997; 112 (4): 1087-95.
4. Ryan AG, Zamvar V, Roberts SA. Iatrogenic candidal infection of a mediastinal foregut cyst following endoscopic ultrasound-guided fine-needle aspiration. *Endoscopy* 2002; 34 (10): 838-9.
5. Rösch T, Classen M. *Gastroenterologic Endosonograpy.* Thieme Stuttgart – New York 1992.
6. Rösch T, Will U, Chang K, Will U. *Longitudinal endosonography.* New York: Springer Heidelberg, 1992.
7. Rösch T, Lorenz R, Braig C, *et al.* Endoscopic ultrasound in pancreatic tumour diagnosis. *Gastrointest Endosc* 1991; 37 (3): 347-52.
8. Furukawa H, Okada S, Saisho H, *et al.* Clinicopathologic features of small pancreatic adenocarcinoma. A collective study. *Cancer* 1996; 78 (5): 986-90.
9. Sendler A, Avril N, Helmberger H, *et al.* Preoperative evaluation of pancreatic masses with positron emission tomography using 18F-fluorodeoxyglucose: diagnostic limitations. *World J Surg* 2000; 24 (9): 1121-9.
10. Rösch T, Schusdziarra V, Born P, *et al.* Modern imaging methods *versus* clinical assessment in the evaluation of hospital in-patients with suspected pancreatic disease. *Am J Gastroenterol* 2000; 95 (9): 2261-70.
11. Rösch T, Braig C, Gain T, *et al.* Staging of pancreatic and ampullary carcinoma by endoscopic ultrasonography. Comparison with conventional sonography, computed tomography, and angiography. *Gastroenterology* 1992; 102 (1): 188-99.
12. Ahmad NA, Lewis JD, Ginsberg GG, Rosato EF, Morris JB, Kochman ML. EUS in preoperative staging of pancreatic cancer. *Gastrointest Endosc* 2000; 52 (4): 463-8.
13. Gress FG, Hawes RH, Savides TJ, *et al.* Role of EUS in the preoperative staging of pancreatic cancer: a large single-center experience. *Gastrointest Endosc* 1999; 50 (6): 786-91.
14. Rösch T, Dittler HJ, Strobel K, *et al.* Endoscopic ultrasound criteria for vascular invasion in the staging of cancer of the head of the pancreas: a blind re-evaluation of videotapes. *Gastrointest Endosc* 2000; 52 (4): 469-77.
15. Mertz HR, Sechopoulos P, Delbeke D, Leach SD. EUS, PET, and CT scanning for evaluation of pancreatic adenocarcinoma. *Gastrointest Endosc* 2000; 52 (3): 367-71.
16. Tierney WM, Francis IR, Eckhauser F, Elta G, Nostrant TT, Scheiman JM. The accuracy of EUS and helical CT in the assessment of vascular invasion by peripapillary malignancy. *Gastrointest Endosc* 2001; 53 (2): 182-8.
17. Howard TJ, Chin AC, Streib EW, Kopecky KK, Wiebke EA. Value of helical computed tomography, angiography, and endoscopic ultrasound in determining resectability of periampullary carcinoma. *Am J Surg* 1997; 174 (3): 237-41.
18. Rösch T, Mayr P, Kassem MA. Endoscopic ultrasonography in acute biliary pancreatitis. *J Gastrointest Surg* 2001; 5 (3): 223-8.

19. Kohut M, Nowakowska-Dulawa E, Marek T, Kaczor R, Nowak A. Accuracy of linear endoscopic ultrasonography in the evaluation of patients with suspected common bile duct stones. *Endoscopy* 2002; 34 (4): 299-303.
20. Palazzo L, O'toole D. EUS in common bile duct stones. *Gastrointest Endosc* 2002; 56 (Suppl. 4): S49-57.
21. Berdah SV, Orsoni P, Bege T, Barthet M, Grimaud JC, Picaud R. Follow-up of selective endoscopic ultrasonography and/or endoscopic retrograde cholangiography prior to laparoscopic cholecystectomy: a prospective study of 300 patients. *Endoscopy* 2001; 33 (3): 216-20.
22. Fulcher AS. MRCP and ERCP in the diagnosis of common bile duct stones. *Gastrointest Endosc* 2002; 56 (Suppl. 6): S178-82.
23. Napoleon B, Dumortier J, Keriven-Souquet O, Pujol B, Ponchon T, Souquet J.C. Do normal findings at biliaryendoscopic ultrasonography obviate the need for endoscopic retrograde cholangiography in patients with suspicion of common bile duct stone? A prospective follow-up study of 238 patients. *Endoscopy* 2003; 25: 411-5.
24. Kahl S, Glasbrenner B, Leodolter A, Pross M, Schulz HU, Malfertheiner P. EUS in the diagnosis of early chronic pancreatitis: a prospective follow-up study. *Gastrointest Endosc* 2002; 55 (4): 507-11.
25. Coyle WJ, Pineau BC, Tarnasky PR, *et al.* Evaluation of unexplained acute and acute recurrent pancreatitis using endoscopic retrograde cholangiopancreatography, sphincter of Oddi manometry and endoscopic ultrasound. *Endoscopy* 2002; 34 (8): 617-23.
26. Sahai AV, Penman ID, Mishra G, *et al.* An assessment of the potential value of endoscopic ultrasound as a cost-minimizing tool in dyspeptic patients with persistent symptoms. *Endoscopy* 2001; 33 (8): 662-7.
27. Lee YT, Lai AC, Hui Y, *et al.* S in the management of uninvestigated dyspepsia. *Gastrointest Endosc* 2002; 56 (6): 842-8.
28. Domagk D, Poremba C, Dietl KH, *et al.* Endoscopic transpapillary biopsies and intraductal ultrasonography in the diagnostics of bile duct strictures: a prospective study. *Gut* 2002; 51 (2): 240-4.
29. Tamada K, Tomiyama T, Wada S, *et al.* Endoscopic transpapillary bile duct biopsy with the combination of intraductal ultrasonography in the diagnosis of biliary strictures. *Gut* 2002; 50 (3): 326-31.
30. Gress F, Chen YK, Sherman S, *et al.* Experience with a catheter-based ultrasound probe in the bile duct and pancreas. *Endoscopy* 1995; 27 (2): 178-84.
31. Fusaroli P, Caletti G. EUS and disease management. *Endoscopy* 2002; 34 (6): 492-4.
32. Ainsworth AP, Mortensen MB, Durup J, Wamberg PA. Clinical impact of endoscopic ultrasonography at a county hospital. *Endoscopy* 2002; 34 (6): 447-50.
33. Allescher HD, Rosch T, Willkomm G, Lorenz R, Meining A, Classen M. Performance, patient acceptance, appropriateness of indications and potential influence on outcome of EUS: a prospective study in 397 consecutive patients. *Gastrointest Endosc* 1999; 50 (6): 737-45.
34. Jafri IH, Saltzman JR, Colby JM, Krims PE. Evaluation of the clinical impact of endoscopic ultrasonography in gastrointestinal disease. *Gastrointest Endosc* 1996; 44 (4): 367-70.
35. Nickl NJ, Bhutani MS, Catalano M, *et al.* Clinical implications of endoscopic ultrasound: the American Endosonography Club Study. *Gastrointest Endosc* 1996; 44 (4): 371-7.
36. Buscail L, Pages P, Berthelemy P, Fourtanier G, Frexinos J, Escourrou J. Role of EUS in the management of pancreatic and ampullary carcinoma: a prospective study assessing resectability and prognosis. *Gastrointest Endosc* 1999; 50 (1): 34-40.
37. Fockens P, Johnson TG, van Dullemen HM, Huibregtse K, Tytgat GN. Endosonographic imaging of pancreatic pseudocysts before endoscopic transmural drainage. *Gastrointest Endosc* 1997; 46 (5): 412-6.
38. Giovannini M, Seitz JF, Monges G, Perrier H, Rabbia I. Fine-needle aspiration cytology guided by endoscopic ultrasonography: results in 141 patients. *Endoscopy* 1995; 27 (2): 171-7.
39. Williams DB, Sahai AV, Aabakken L, *et al.* Endoscopic ultrasound guided fine needle aspiration biopsy: a large single centre experience. *Gut* 1999; 44 (5): 720-6.

40. Fritscher-Ravens A, Brand L, Knofel WT, *et al.* Comparison of endoscopic ultrasound-guided fine needle aspiration for focal pancreatic lesions in patients with normal parenchyma and chronic pancreatitis. *Am J Gastroenterol* 2002; 97 (11): 2768-75.
41. Bounds BC, Brugge WR. EUS diagnosis of cystic lesions of the pancreas. *Int J Gastrointest Cancer* 2001; 30 (1-2): 27-31.
42. Hernandez LV, Mishra G, Forsmark C, *et al.* Role of endoscopic ultrasound (EUS) and EUS-guided fine needle aspiration in the diagnosis and treatment of cystic lesions of the pancreas. *Pancreas* 2002; 25 (3): 222-8.
43. Giovannini M, Pesenti C, Rolland AL, Moutardier V, Delpero JR. Endoscopic ultrasound-guided drainage of pancreatic pseudocysts or pancreatic abscesses using a therapeutic echo endoscope. *Endoscopy* 2001; 33 (6): 473-7.
44. Seifert H, Wehrmann T, Schmitt T, Zeuzem S, Caspary WF. Retroperitoneal endoscopic debridement for infected peripancreatic necrosis. *Lancet* 2000; 356 (9230): 653-5.
45. Gunaratnam NT, Sarma AV, Norton ID, Wiersema MJ. A prospective study of EUS-guided coeliac plexus neurolysis for pancreatic cancer pain. *Gastrointest Endosc* 2001; 54 (3): 316-24.
46. Gress F, Schmitt C, Sherman S, Ciaccia D, Ikenberry S, Lehman G. Endoscopic ultrasound-guided coeliac plexus block for managing abdominal pain associated with chronic pancreatitis: a prospective single center experience. *Am J Gastroenterol* 2001; 96 (2): 409-16.
47. Gress F, Schmitt C, Sherman S, Ikenberry S, Lehman G. A prospective randomized comparison of endoscopic ultrasound- and computed tomography-guided coeliac plexus block for managing chronic pancreatitis pain. *Am J Gastroenterol* 1999; 94 (4): 900-5.
48. Bhutani MS. Endoscopic ultrasonography (DDW report 2002). *Endoscopy* 2002; 34 (11): 888-9.

Surgery for pancreatic cancer

N. Alexakis, J.P. Neoptolemos

Department of Surgery, University of Liverpool, Royal Liverpool University Hospital, 5th floor UCD Building, Daulby St, Liverpool, L69 3GA, United Kingdom

Introduction

Pancreatic cancer (pancreatic ductal adenocarcinoma) is a devastating disease and represents an important health problem. It is the forth and sixth most common cancer death in the USA and UK respectively. The majority of patients present with advanced disease resulting in low resection rates especially outside of specialist centers. The late presentation is responsible in part for the overall median survival of less than 6 months and 5-year survival rate of 0.4 to 5.0% [1, 2]. For the 15-20% who undergoes pancreatic resection, the median survival is 10-18 months and the 5-year survival rate is 7-24%, but virtually all patients are dead within seven years of surgery [3].

Due to the poor 5-year survival, the incidence and mortality ratios are roughly equivalent, indeed the latest estimated figures from the IARC for the year 2000 demonstrate that there will be 217,000 new cases and 213,000 deaths from pancreatic cancer worldwide. The incidence of pancreatic cancer is rare before the age of forty-five and 80% of cases occur in the sixty to eighty year old age group [4]. With an increasingly elderly population, there can be no expectation of a marked reduction in incidence. Surgery offers the only possibility of cure, even thought any form of resectional surgery must be termed "potentially curative" [5]. The majority of pancreatic cancers affect the head of the pancreas and are removed by partial pancreatoduodenectomy. This was first successfully performed by Walter Kausch in Berlin in 1909 and later popularised by Allan O Whipple in 1935.

Nevertheless, there have been major improvements in operative mortality and morbidity in the past decade through the development of specialist units [6] and encouraging evidence of improved long-term survival with the use of adjuvant chemotherapy [7]. Our understanding of the disease has been also been improved but important aspects of pancreatic cancer biology remains poor [8].

Pathology

The most common exocrine pancreatic tumour is ductal adenocarcinoma which accounts for well over 90% of all tumours. They usually present at a stage when they are locally advanced, exhibit vascular invasion and lymph node metastases. Variants of ductal carcinomas and other malignant tumours of the pancreas are rare. In surgical resection series 80-90% of tumours are located in the head of the gland [9]. Lymph node metastases are common and are present at the time of surgery in 40-75% of primary tumours less than 2 cm in diameter [9]. Perineural infiltration and vascular invasion are both frequently seen in resection specimens.

Diagnosis, staging and assessment of resectability

In the majority of patients, the clinical diagnosis is fairly straightforward, although there are no positive clinical features which clearly identify a patient group with potentially curable disease. There are associated conditions, such as late onset diabetes mellitus or an unexplained attack of acute pancreatitis, which may point to an underlying cancer. Clinical features such as persistent back pain, marked and rapid weight loss, abdominal mass, ascites and supraclavicular lymphadenopathy usually indicate an unresectable tumour.

Initial investigation involves *abdominal ultrasonography* to identify a dilated extra hepatic main bile duct as well as perhaps the primary pancreatic tumour and if present large liver metastases. *ERCP* is important in the diagnosis of ampullary tumours by direct visualisation and biopsy. All other pancreatic tumours are detectable by ERCP only if they impinge on the pancreatic duct, so that small early cancers and those situated in the uncinate process, can be missed. The importance of ERCP is that it enables biliary stenting for symptomatic relief of jaundice. Brushings during ERCP have high specificity but lack sensitivity. In a contemporary series, positive cytology from sampling during ERCP was found in 87 (59.6%) of 147 patients with pancreatic cancer [10].

Contrast-enhanced *CT scanning*, particularly using multi-slice scanners with arterial and portal phases of contrast enhancement is the gold standard of staging and accurately predicts resectability in 80-90% of cases [11-13]. The assessment of local tumour extension with contiguous organ invasion, vascular involvement, hepatic metastases and lymph node metastases, correlate well with surgical findings in large tumours. CT is, however, much less accurate in identifying potentially resectable small tumours. Spiral computed tomography with multi-slice technology and 3-dimensional reconstruction may prove advantageous in the identification of small tumours and resectability [14]. Factors contraindicating resection include liver, peritoneal or other metastases, distant lymph node metastases, major venous encasement (> 2 cm in length, > 50% circumferential involvement), superior mesenteric, coeliac or hepatic artery encasement, as well as major co-morbidities. Factors that do not contraindicate resection include continuous invasion of the duodenum, stomach or colon, lymph node metastasis within the operative field, venous impingement or minimal invasion of the SMV-PV, gastro-duodenal artery encasement as well as the age of the patient. *Endosonography* (EUS) is highly sensitive in the detection of small tumours and invasion of major vascular structures [15]. EUS is superior to spiral computed tomography, MRI or PET scanning in the detection of small tumours and is being increasingly used [16, 17].

Laparoscopy, including *laparoscopic ultrasound*, can detect occult metastatic lesions in the liver and peritoneal cavity (in 10-15% of the cases), not identified by other imaging modalities [18-21], but the data are not entirely conclusive [22]. *Positron emission tomography* is an evolving technique that measures the metabolism in tumour cells – at the present time there is overlap with chronic pancreatitis but it does seem to be able to detect metastases not visible by other imaging modalities [23, 24].

Given the strong possibility of peritoneal tumour seeding there is no justification for transperitoneal biopsy in patients thought to have potentially resectable malignant tumours, even if they ultimately harbour benign disease [25]. Percutaneous FNA biopsy may be used to obtain a diagnosis in patients who are deemed inoperable on imaging and are selected for palliative treatment.

Pre-operative peritoneal cytology

There are a number of studies that suggest that patients with positive results from peritoneal washings have a poor outcome, even in the absence of macroscopic metastases [26, 27], but the results are not conclusive [28].

Pre-operative biliary drainage

There is no clear evidence that pre-operative endoscopic stenting is either of benefit or harmful in terms of surgical outcome. A study from Memorial Sloan-Kettering reported increased overall morbidity and mortality rates after resection with pre-operative biliary drainage [29]. Studies from other specialist units did not find any influence (only more wound infections in the stent group) [30-32]. If a stent is placed prior to surgery, this should be a plastic one and it should be placed endoscopically. Metal stents must be avoided in patients who are candidates for resection.

Standard *versus* pylorus preserving pancreatoduodenectomy

The majority of pancreatic resections for cancer are Kausch-Whipple (KW) resections of the head of the pancreas as this reflects the location of most cases of pancreatic cancer. Until recently there were no standardized descriptions of the Kausch-Whipple procedure or its pylorus preserving variant (PP-KW). This led to inconsistencies in both technique and pathological reporting that has hampered interpretation of data in reported series. These points were addressed at a pancreatic "workshop" and guidelines on surgery and pathological examination were drawn up and published [33, 34].

There are only two prospective randomized trials comparing the two techniques. The first, recruited a small number of patients (n = 31) and the major finding was more frequently delayed gastric emptying in the PP-KW group [35]. The second study randomized 77 patients (classic KW = 40, PP-KW = 37) [36] and reported a significantly higher morbidity in the classic KW group. The publication of two large trials from Holland and Switzerland are pending.

Large series have indicated that the pylorus preserving operation does not compromise long term survival figures compared to the standard Kausch-Whipple operation for carcinoma for head of the pancreas [37]. Opponents of the pylorus preserving operation point to the risk of recurrence in the resection margins and the limit in the lymphadenectomy to the nodes behind the stomach. These risks can be obviated by patient selection, so that the pylorus preserving operation is avoided in patients where there is proximal duodenal involvement or the tumour is close to the pylorus [38, 39] The advantages of pylorus preservation have not been conclusively established but may include a reduction in postgastrectomy complications, a reduction in enterogastric reflux and improved post operative nutritional status and weight gain compared to the standard operation [36, 37, 40, 41].

Reconstruction of the pancreatic-enteric anastomosis

A randomized trial of techniques in the Kausch-Whipple operation compared pancreatojejunostomy in 72 patients with pancreatogastrostomy in 73 patients for both benign and malignant peripancreatic disease [42]. The incidence of pancreatic anastomotic leak was 11% for the pancreatojejunostomy and 12% for the pancreatogastrostomy, with no perioperative mortality. In a retrospective study with 441 patients from Hanover-Germany, the leakage rates and the mortality due to leakage were significantly lower in the pancreatogastrostomy group in comparison with the pancreatojejunostomy group [43].

Major vein resection

Resection of the portal or superior mesenteric vein as a means of ensuring that resection with tumour-free margins becomes feasible is appropriate. This procedure does not increase operative morbidity or mortality [44] and long term outcome is not affected by the need for vein resection [45]. Resection in the presence of pre-operative detection of extensive portal vein encasement is rarely justified.

Complications after the Kausch-Whipple operation

A study from the University of Mainz-Germany found that intraoperative blood loss, pre-operative serum bilirubin, diameter of the pancreatic duct, and occurrence of complications were independent prognostic factors of mortality [46]. Many of the postoperative complications respond to medical treatment and radiological and endoscopic intervention. Complications that require reoperation are associated with a mortality of between 23% and 67% [47, 48].

Intraabdominal abscess

Intraabdominal abscess following pancreatic resection occurs in 1-12% of patients [49, 50]. The usual cause is anastomotic leak at the pancreatojejunostomy, the hepaticojejunostomy, the duodenojejunostomy, the gastrojejunostomy or the jejunojejunostomy and often herald as right sub-hepatic or left sub-diaphragmatic collections [51]. A contrast-enhanced CT scan is indicated whenever an intraabdominal collection is suspected. The preferred management of intraabdominal collections is CT-guided percutaneous drainage.

Haemorrhage

Postoperative haemorrhage occurs in 3-15% of patients following pancreatic resection [52]. Bleeding within the first 24 hours is usually due to insufficient intraoperative haemostasis or bleeding from an anastomosis. In the latter case management is conservative but immediate reoperation is usually required in the former cases [51]. Stress ulceration is rare and usually can be managed medically and/or endoscopically. Late haemorrhage (1-3 weeks following surgery) often has a more sinister underlying cause. It is commonly related to an anastomotic leak and secondary erosion of the retroperitoneal vasculature, with a mortality of 15-58% [53]. Another sinister cause is a pseudo-aneurysm. Investigations include CE-CT, endoscopy and selective angiography. If a bleeding point cannot be found endoscopically then selective embolisation of the source is undertaken providing that this can be identified by arteriography. Bleeding from a pancreatojejunostomy is particularly problematic with no clear evidence for the optimal re-interventional procedure. The choice lies between a completion total pancreatectomy and refashioning of the anastomosis after a limited resection of the jejunum and pancreas at the anastomosis [54].

Fistulae after pancreatoduodenectomy

The reported incidence of pancreatic fistula or leak ranges from 2% to 24% [46, 50, 55-62]. The mortality risk from a major pancreatic fistula is up to 28% and the cause of death is retroperitoneal sepsis and haemorrhage [46, 53, 59]. Several studies have reported risk factors for breakdown of the pancreatic anastomosis (a soft parenchymal texture of the pancreatic remnant, a small pancreatic duct size, ampullary carcinoma and the anastomotic technique) but other series have not found any parameter that predisposed to pancreatic leak [63, 57, 59, 61]. It is not clear which of the different anastomotic techniques produces optimal results [63-66]. Our unit now utilizes an end-to-side duct-to-mucosa technique (with an internal pancreatic stent) with an improvement of results. Adherence to a meticulous surgical technique may be more important than pancreatic texture.

Delayed gastric emptying

The incidence of delayed gastric emptying is 14% to 70% of patients after pancreatic resection [50, 54]. Yeo *et al.* have shown that delayed gastric emptying can be reduced by up to 37% following pancreatoduodenectomy with intravenous erythromycin [67]. Although delayed gastric emptying almost invariably resolves with conservative treatment operative correction is occasionally required. There are studies that suggest that pylorus preservation increases the risk of delayed gastric emptying [68]. There are many series that showed that delayed gastric emptying is related to the presence of intraabdominal complications, especially that of a pancreatic leak and also extended radical surgery [54].

The role of octreotide

The value of octreotide in the prevention and treatment of pancreatic fistulae and other complications following pancreatoduodenectomy is not clear. Interestingly all of the studies from Europe showed a benefit, whilst the studies from the USA have not. There are four randomized placebo-controlled trials from Europe (three multi-centre and one institutional). The group from Ulm [69] randomized 246 patients undergoing major elective pancreatic surgery of whom 200 underwent resection of the head of the pancreas, 31 underwent left resection and 15 had other procedures. The complication rate (including pancreatic fistula) was 32% in the octreotide group *vs* 55% in the placebo group ($p < 0.005$). The effect was more prominent in patients with peripancreatic tumours.

The Berne group randomized 247 patients undergoing major resection for chromic pancreatitis [70]. A total of 124 patients underwent resection of the head of the pancreas, 55 had a left resection, 61 had a pancreatojejunostomy and seven had other procedures. The postoperative complication rate in the octreotide group was 16.4% and in the placebo group 29.6% ($p < 0.007$). Similar results were reported from a multi-centre study from Italy [71] comprising 218 patients and from an institutional study with 75 patients from France [72].

The group from John Hopkins recruited 211 patients that had a pancreatoduodenectomy [73]. The pancreatic fistula rates were 9% in the control group and 11% in the octreotide group and the overall complication rates were 34% and 40% respectively. In study from the MD Anderson Cancer Center, 120 patients that underwent pancreatoduodenectomy for malignancy were randomized to either octreotide or placebo [74]. The rate of clinically significant pancreatic leak was 12% in the octreotide group and 6% in the control group ($p = 0.23$). The perioperative morbidity was 30% and 25% respectively. The latest trial from the USA, is a multi-centre, double-blind, placebo-controlled trial in 275 patients of whom 135 received vapreotide and 140 received placebo [75]. The procedures performed were: pancreatoduodenectomy ($n = 215$), distal pancreatectomy ($n = 52$) and central pancreatectomy ($n = 8$). There was no significant difference in the pancreas-anastomotic complication rates between the two groups (26.4% *vs* 30.4% respectively) nor does the overall complication rate (42% *vs* 40% respectively). A possible criticism is that 72 patients did not complete the study.

Standard *versus* extended lymphadenectomy

Two trials have addressed the role of extended lymphadenectomy. A multi-centre, randomized trial from Italy compared conventional pancreatoduodenectomy with and without extended lymph node resection: 40 patients were randomized to conventional resection and 41 patients were randomized to additional lymphadenectomy and retroperitoneal soft tissue clearance [76]. The conventional group had a median survival of 11.2 months with a 3-year survival rate of 10% and the radical group had a median survival of 16.7 months with a 3-year survival rate of 8% (no significant difference). Post-hoc subgroup analysis revealed a significantly longer survival rate in node positive patients after an extended rather than standard lymphadenectomy. It was claimed that radical surgery did not lead to an "up-staging" of lymph node status.

The Johns Hopkins group randomized 56 patients to a standard Kausch-Whipple and 58 patients to radical pancreatoduodenectomy. Perioperative morbidity and mortality were not significantly different between the two groups. The one year survival was 71% for the standard Kausch-Whipple group and 80% for the radical pancreatoduodenectomy group [77]. Updated results in 2002 showed 146 patients in the standard Kausch-Whipple arm and 148 in the extended pancreatoduodenectomy group [62]. Perioperative mortality was similar in the two groups but the overall complication rate was significantly higher in the extended pancreatoduodenectomy arm (43% *vs* 29%; p = 0.01). Radical pancreatoduodenectomy was not associated with a survival benefit (3-year survival of 38% *vs* 36% respectively). Thus there is no substantive evidence for the use of extended lymphadenectomy for pancreatic cancer.

Recurrence and survival after surgery for pancreatic cancer

The majority of patients will develop disease recurrence, which is usually at the resection site, the peritoneum and the liver (retroperitoneum 80%, liver 23-66%, peritoneum 27-62% and extra-abdominal sites 8-29%) [78, 79]. The majority of tumour recurrences occur within two years of surgery. Liver metastases frequently develop early following resection, indicating the presence of micrometastases at the time of surgery. Local recurrences by contrast tend to appear at a later stage. The reasons for recurrence following an apparently successful resection include residual retroperitoneal disease and an aggressive phenotype as shown by a very high frequency of perineural, lymphatic and vascular invasion and 5-year survival cannot be equated to cure [80].

Prognostic factors

Favourable independent prognostic factors are negative resection margins, well/moderately differentiated tumour, primary tumour diameter < 3 cm, and lymph node status [7, 81]. In a recent population-based study from Harvard Medical School-US, the strongest predictors of survival in multivariate analysis were tumour < 2 cm, negative lymph nodes, well differentiated histology, undergoing surgery in a teaching hospital, chemoradiation therapy, and higher socio-economic status [82]. The presence of favourable prognostic features however does not mean cure, as recurrence even if after five years is inevitable.

Volume-mortality relationship

The evidence base around specialist units has grown substantially and now clearly shows a reduced postoperative mortality that is a continuous effect, with no threshold, unaffected by case mix and only a possible single surgeon effect; reduced postoperative morbidity; reduced postoperative length of stay and cost; an increased resection rate; and probable increased long-term. A study conducted by the New York State Department of Public Health, demonstrated a clear correlation between caseload and surgical mortality. When surgeons performed less than nine resections annually, the mortality was 16%, compared to less than 5% for surgeons performing more than forty cases per year [83]. Similar relationships between hospital volume and mortality have been reported by other authors [84, 85]. A survey of 2.5 million complex surgical procedures in the US showed a large inverse relationship between the hospital volume and case mortality rates for pancreatic resection [86].

Other resections for pancreatic cancer

Total pancreaticoduodenectomy

This has no advantage in long-term survival compared to the Whipple's resection [87] and there are many nutritional and metabolic problems [88]. The procedure may be justified where there is diffuse involvement of the whole pancreas without evidence of distal spread [89].

Left pancreatectomy

A left resection is indicated for lesions in the body and tail of the pancreas. Pancreatic ductal carcinoma is seldom resectable in this location [90], but this procedure may be appropriate for other slow growing malignant tumours. Involvement of the splenic vein or artery is not in itself a contraindication to resection.

Adjuvant treatment

The best available level I evidence comes from the ESPAC-1 trial [7]. The European Study Group for Pancreatic Cancer (ESPAC) recruited 541 patients with pancreatic ductal adenocarcinoma. The ESPAC-1 trial assessed the roles of adjuvant chemoradiation (20 Gy in 10 daily fractions over 2 weeks with 500 mg/m^2 5FU i.v. bolus on the first three days and repeated after a planned break of 2 weeks) and chemotherapy (i.v. bolus 5FU, 425 mg/m^2 daily for 5 days, with folinic acid, 20 mg/m^2, monthly for six months). Clinicians could randomise patients into a 2 × 2 factorial design (observation, chemoradiation alone, chemotherapy alone or combination of the two) or into one of the main treatment comparisons (*i.e.* chemoradiation *versus* no chemoradiation or chemotherapy *versus* no chemotherapy. 285 patients were randomised to the 2 × 2 factorial design; an additional 68 patients were randomised to chemoradiation *versus* no chemoradiation and 188 patients were randomised to chemotherapy *versus* no chemotherapy. There was evidence of a survival benefit for adjuvant chemotherapy (median survival 19.7 months in 238 patients with chemotherapy *vs* 14.0 months in 235 patients without, p = 0.0005). With a median follow-up of the 227 (42%) patients still alive of 10 months (range 0-62, inter-quartile range 1-25 months) a nonsignificant beneficial effect of chemotherapy was observed in patients randomized in the 2 × 2 design to chemotherapy (n = 146; 17.4 months) *versus* no chemotherapy (n = 139; 15.9 months).

Palliative procedures for pancreatic cancer

Stent or surgical palliation for biliary obstruction?

The majority of patients with pancreatic cancer present with advanced disease that is not amenable to resection. The major symptom requiring intervention is obstructive jaundice. A number of randomized trials have compared operative bypass procedures with biliary stenting and shown that complications such as cholangitis and bile leaks are more common in bypass procedures, whilst recurrent jaundice is a feature of stenting (through stent occlusion or migration) [91, 92]. Around 20% of stented patients developed gastric outlet obstruction requiring further intervention [91]. No significant difference is seen in median survival or procedure related deaths. Self-expanding metal stents have greatly reduced the risk of obstruction and acute cholangitis [93]. Metal stents are very expensive compared to plastic stents and evidence supports the use of metal stents for patients with a good prognosis (primary < 3 cm) whilst plastic stents should be reserved for those with metastases and tumours > 3 cm in diameter [94].

Nevertheless there is still benefit for the patient with locally advanced disease only to undergo a surgical bypass as it may allow most of their remaining time to be spent at home without readmissions to treat recurrent jaundice. In a contemporary series of 56 patients using single loop biliary and gastric bypass only four needed subsequent biliary stenting and no reoperations were required before death [95]. For obstructive jaundice, most specialists construct a Roux-en-Y choledochojejunstomy. Biliary bypass should be constructed with the bile duct in preference to the gallbladder [96].

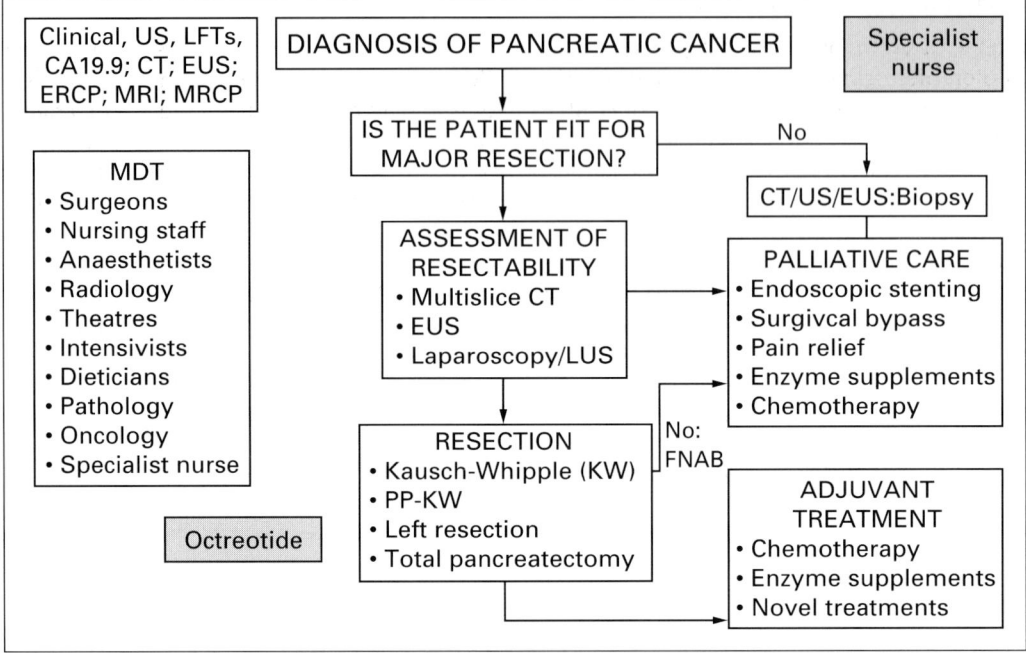

Figure 1. Examples of countries where intrahepatic cholangiocarcinoma is rising. ASMR, age standardised mortality rate. From Khan et al. [13], with permission from the *BMJ* Publishing Group.

The role of prophylactic gastrojejunostomy

A trial from Johns Hopkins randomized 87 patients who had unresectable disease of whom 44 underwent a gastrojejunostomy and 43 did not undergo a gastric bypass [97]. The mean survival in the gastrojejunostomy arm was 8.3 months and during that time none of the patients developed gastric outlet obstruction. The other group had similar survival (8.3 months), but eight (19%) out of 43 patients developed outlet obstruction requiring intervention. The deployment of expandable metallic stents endoscopically is an alternative approach [98]. The immediate success rate is 67%-87% with complications in up to 25% including perforation, fistula, and bleeding. Recurrent obstruction occurs in up to 23% due to stent migration or fracture.

The role of pancreatoduodenectomy in the palliation

The Johns Hopkins group retrospectively compared the outcomes of 64 patients undergoing pancreatoduodenectomy with gross or microscopic evidence of disease at the resection margins, with 62 patients with locally advanced disease that undergone surgical bypass [99]. Morbidity and mortality rates were similar. The overall actuarial survival in the pancreatoduodenectomy group was improved significantly ($p < 0.02$).

Procedures for pain relief

Pain is a common presenting feature and in patients with advanced disease and can be intolerable, providing a major therapeutic challenge despite advances in the formulation of opiates. Various factors are thought to produce pancreatic pain including increased parenchymal pressure secondary to ductal obstruction, neural infiltration, superimposed pancreatic inflammation and associated biliary stenosis. Randomized studies suggest a benefit from intraoperative neurolytic coeliac plexus block; using 5% phenol or 50% ethanol seems to produce effective palliation of pain in about 70% of patients [100, 101]. Percutaneous neurolytic coeliac plexus block guided by computed tomography shows reasonable results (with an overall success rate of 74%) in patients with cancers in the head of the pancreas but not in those with cancers in the body and tail of the pancreas [102]. Thoracoscopic division of the splanchnic nerves has also been described as an effective method [103]. Cancer in the head of the pancreas nearly always causes obstruction to the main pancreatic duct and consequent exocrine pancreatic failure. Pancreatic enzyme supplements given to patients with advanced pancreatic cancer enable them to enjoy a better quality of life and improved symptom score [104].

References

1. Bramhall SR, Allum WH, Jones AG, Allwood A, Cummins C, Neoptolemos JP. Treatment and survival in 13,560 patients with pancreatic cancer and incidence of the disease. An epidemiological study. *Br J Surg* 1995; 82: 111-5.
2. Warshaw A, Fernandez-del Castillo C. Pancreatic carcinoma. *N Engl J Med* 1992; 326: 455-65.
3. Nitecki SS, Sarr MG Colby TV, *et al.* Long-term survival after resection for ductal adenocarcinoma of the pancreas. Is it really improving? *Ann Surg* 1995; 221: 59-66.
4. Gourds L, Gold EB. Epidemiology of pancreatic cancer. *World J Surg* 1984; 8: 808-21.
5. Sener S, Fremgen A, Menck H, Winchester D. Pancreatic cancer: a report of treatment and survival trends for 100,313 patients diagnosed from 1985-1995, using the National Cancer database. *J Am Coll Surg* 1999; 189: 1-7.
6. Neoptolemos JP, Russell RC, Bramhall S, *et al.* Low mortality following resection for pancreatic and periampullary tumours in 1026 patients: UK survey of specialist pancreatic units. UK pancreatic cancer group. *Br J Surg* 1997; 84: 1370-76.
7. Neoptolemos JP, Dunn JA, Moffitt DD, *et al.* Adjuvant chemoradiotherapy and chemotherapy in resectable pancreatic cancer: a randomised controlled trial. *Lancet* 2001; 358: 1576-85.
8. Bardeesy N, CePinho R. Pancreatic cancer biology and genetics. *Nat Rev Cancer* 2002; 2: 897-909.
9. Solcia E CCKG. *Tumours of the pancreas*. Washington DC: Armed Forces Institute of Pathology, 1997.
10. Stewart CJ, Mills PR Carter R, *et al.* Brush cytology in the assessment of pancreatico-biliary strictures: a review of 406 cases. *J Clin Pathol* 2001; 54: 449-55.
11. McCarthy MJ, Evans J, Sagar G, Neoptolemos JP. Prediction of resectability of pancreatic malignancy by computed tomography. *Br J Surg* 1998; 85: 320-5.
12. Chong M, Freeny PC, Schmiedl UP. Pancreatic arterial anatomy. Depiction with dual phase helical CT. *Radiology* 1998; 208: 537-42.
13. Vedantham S, Lu DSK, Reber HA, *et al.* Small peripancreatic veins: improved assessment in pancreatic cancer patients using thin-section pancreatic phase helical CT. *Am J Roentgenol* 1998; 170: 377-83.

14. Novick SL, Fishman EK. Three-dimensional CT angiography of pancreatic carcinoma: role in staging extent of disease. *Am J Roentgenol* 1998; 170: 139-43.
15. Rosch T, Lightdale CJ, Botet JF, *et al.* Endosonographic localization of pancreatic endocrine tumours. *N Engl J Med* 1992; 326: 1721-26.
16. Howard TJ, Chin AC, Streib EW, *et al.* Value of helical computed tomography, angiography and endoscopic ultrasound in determining resectability of periampullary carcinoma. *Am J Surg* 1997; 174: 237-41.
17. Mertz HR, Sechopoulos P, Delbeke D, *et al.* EUS, PET and CT scanning for evaluation of pancreatic adenocarcinoma. *Gastrointest Endosc* 2000; 52: 367-71.
18. John TG, Greig JD, Carter DC, Garden OJ. Carcinoma of the pancreatic head and peri-ampullary region: tumour staging with laparoscopy and laparoscopic ultrasonography. *Ann Surg* 1995; 221: 136-46.
19. Henning R, Tempia-Caliera A, Hartel M, Buchler M, Friess H. Staging laparoscopy and its indications in pancreatic cancer patients. *Dig Surg* 2002; 19: 484-8.
20. Minnard EA, Conlon KC, Hoos A, *et al.* Laparoscopic ultrasound enhances standard laparoscopy in the staging of pancreatic cancer. *Ann Surg* 1998; 228: 182-7.
21. Callery M, Strasberg S, Doherty G, Soper N, Norton J. Staging laparoscopy with laparoscopic ultrasonography: optimizing resectability in hepatobiliary and pancreatic malignancy. *J Am Coll Surg* 1997; 185: 34-41.
22. Nieveen van Dijkum EJ, Romijn MG, Terwee CB, *et al.* Laparoscopic staging and subsequent palliation in patients with peripancreatic carcinoma. *Ann Surg* 2003; 237: 66-73.
23. Sendler A, Avril N, Helmberger H, *et al.* Pre-operative evaluation of pancreatic masses with positron emission tomography using 18F-fluorodeoxyglucose: diagnostic limitations. *World J Surg* 2000; 24: 1121-9.
24. Shreeve PD. Focal fluorine-18 fluorodeoxyglucose accumulation in inflammatory pancreatic disease. *Eur J Nucl Med* 1998; 25: 259-64.
25. Smith CD, Behrns KE, van Heerden JA, Sarr MG. Radical pancreatoduodenectomy for misdiagnosed pancreatic mass. *Br J Surg* 1994; 81: 585-9.
26. Makary M, Warshaw A, Centeno B, Willett C, Rattner D, Fernandez-del Castillo C. Implications of peritoneal cytology in pancreatic cancer management. *Arch Surg* 1998; 133: 361-5.
27. Merchant NB, Conlon KC, Saigo P, Dougherty E, Brennan MF. Positive peritoneal cytology predicts unresectability of pancreatic adenocarcinoma. *J Am Coll Surg* 1999; 188: 421-6.
28. Konishi M, Kinoshita T, Nakagohri T, Inoue K, Oda T, Takahashi S. Prognostic value of cytologic examination of peritoneal whashings in pancreatic cancer. *Arch Surg* 2002; 137: 475-80.
29. Povoski S, Karpeh M, Conlon K, Blumgard L, Brennan M. Association of preoperative biliary drainage with post operative outcome following pancreatoduodenectomy. *Ann Surg* 1999; 230: 131-42.
30. Sohn T, Yeo C, Cameron JL, Pitt H, Lillemoe K. Do preoperaive biliary stents incease post pancreaticoduodenectomy complications? *J Gastrointest Surg* 2000; 4: 258-68.
31. Pisters P, Hudec W, Hess K, *et al.* Effect of preoperative biliary decompresion on pancreaticoduodenectomy-associated morbidity in 300 consecutive patients. *Ann Surg* 2001; 234: 47-55.
32. Sewnath M, Birjmohun RS, Rauws E, Huibregtse K, Obertop H, Gouma D. The effect of preoperative biliary drainage on post operative complications after pancreaticoduodenectomy. *J Am Coll Surg* 2001; 192: 726-34.
33. Jones L, Russell C, Mosca F, *et al.* Standard Kausch-Whipple Pancreaticoduodenectomy. *Dig Surg* 1999; 16: 297-304.
34. Pedrazzoli S, Beger H, Obertop H, *et al.* A Surgical and pathological based classification of resection of pancreatic cancer: summary of an international workshop on surgical procedures in pancreatic cancer. *Dig Surg* 1999; 16: 337-45.

35. Lin PW, Lin YJ. Prospective randomized comparison between pylorus-preserving and standard pancreatoduodenectomy. *Br J Surg* 1999; 86: 603-7.
36. Seiler CA, Wagner M, Sadowski C, *et al.* Randomized prospective trial of pylorus-preserving *vs* Classic duodenopancreatectomy (Whipple procedure): initial clinical results. *J Gastrointest Surg* 2000; 4: 443-52.
37. Mosca F, Giulianotti PC, Balestracci T, *et al.* Long-term survival in pancreatic cancer: pyloruspreserving *versus* Whipple pancreatoduodenectomy. *Surgery* 1997; 122: 553-66.
38. Watanapa P, Williamson RCN. Resection of the pancreatic head with or without gastrectomy. *World J Surg* 1995; 19: 403-9.
39. Nakao A, Harada A, Nonami T, *et al.* Lymph node metastases in carcinoma of the head of the pancreas region. *Br J Surg* 1995; 82: 399-402.
40. Williamson RCN, Bliouras N, Cooper MJ, *et al.* Gastric emptying and enterogastric reflux after conservative and conventional pancreatoduodenectomy. *Surgery* 1993; 114: 975-79.
41. Zerbi A, Balzano G, Patuzzo R, *et al.* Comparison between pylorus-preserving and Whipple pancreatoduodenectomy. *Br J Surg* 1995; 82: 975-9.
42. Yeo CJ, Cameron JL, Maher MM, *et al.* A prospective randomized trial of pancreaticogastrostomy *versus* pancreaticojejunostomy after pancreaticoduodenectomy. *Ann Surg* 1995; 222: 580-8.
43. Schlitt H, Schmidt U, Simunec D, *et al.* Morbidity and mortality associated with pancreatogastrostomy and pancreatojejunostomy following partial pancreatoduodenectomy. *Br J Surg* 2002; 89: 1245-51.
44. Leach SD, Lee JE, Charnsangave JC, *et al.* Survival following pancreaticoduodenectomy with resection of the superior mesenteric-portal vein confluence for adenocarcinoma of the pancreatic head. *Br J Surg* 1998; 85: 611-7.
45. Sasson AR, Hoffman JP, Ross EA, *et al.* En bloc resection for locally advanced cancer of the pancreas: is it worthwhile? *J Gastrointest Surg* 2002; 6: 147-58.
46. Bottger T, Junginger T. Factors influencing morbidity and mortality after pancreaticoduodenectomy: critical analysis of 221 resections. *World J Surg* 1999; 23: 164-72.
47. Farley DR, Schwall G, Trede M. Completion pancreatectomy for complications after pancreatoduodenectomy. *Br J Surg* 1996; 83: 176-9.
48. Cunningham JD, Weyant MT, Levitt M, Brower ST, Aufses AH. Complications requiring reoperation following pancreatectomy. *Int J Pancreatol* 1998; 24: 23-9.
49. Bassi C, Falconi M, Salvia R, Mascetta G, Molinari E, Pederzoli P. Management of complications after pancreaticoduodenectomy in a high volume centre: results on 150 consecutive patients. *Dig Surg* 2001; 18: 453-7.
50. Yeo CJ, Cameron JL, Sohn T, *et al.* Six hundred and fifty consecutive pancreaticoduodenectomies in the 1990s. *Ann Surg* 1997; 226: 248-60.
51. Berberat PO, Friess H, Kleeff J, Uhl W, Bóchler MW. Prevention and Treatment of Complications in Pancreatic Cancer Surgery. *Dig Surg* 1999; 16: 327-36.
52. Rumstadt B, Schwab M, Korth P, Samman M, Trede M. Hemorrhage after pancreatoduodenectomy. *Ann Surg* 1998; 227: 236-41.
53. Van Berge Henegouwen MI, de Witt LT, van Guilk TM, Obertop H, Gouma DJ. Incidence, risk factors, and treatment of pancreatic leakage after a pancreatoduodenectomy: Drainage *versus* resection of pancreatic remnant. *J Am Coll Surg* 1997; 185: 12-24.
54. Halloran C, Ghaneh P, Bosonnet L, Hartley M, Sutton R, Neoptolemos JP. Complications of pancreatic cancer resection. *Dig Surg* 2002; 19: 138-46.
55. Bakkevold KE, Kambestd B. Morbidity and mortality after radical and palliative pancreatic cancer surgery. Risk factors influencing the short-term results. *Ann Surg* 1993; 217: 356-68.
56. Balcom JH 4th, Rattner DW, Warshaw AL, Chang Y, Fernandez-del Castillo C. Ten-year experience with 733 pancreatic resections: changing indications, older patients, and decreasing length of hospitalization. *Arch Surg* 2001; 136 (4): 391-8.

57. Bucher M, Friess H, Wagner M, Kulli C, Wagener V, Z'graggen K. Pancreatic fistula after pancreatic head resection. *Br J Surg* 2000; 87: 883-9.
58. Conlon KC, Labow D, Leung D, *et al.* Prospective randomized clinical trial of the value of intraperitoneal drainage after pancreatic resection. *Ann Surg* 2001; 234: 487-93.
59. Cullen JJ, Sarr MG, Ilstrup DM. Pancreatic anastomotic leak after pancreatcoduodenectomy: incidence, significance and management. *Am J Surg* 1994; 168: 295-8.
60. Trede M, Schwall G, Saeger HD. Survival after pancreatoduodenectomiy. 118 consecutive resections without an operative mortality. *Ann Surg* 1990; 211: 447-58.
61. Halloran CM, Ghaneh P, Bosonnet L, Hartley MN, Sutton R, Neoptolemos JP. Complications of pancreatic cancer resection. *Dig Surg* 2002; 19: 138-46.
62. Yeo C, Cameron JL, Lillemoe KD, *et al.* Pancreaticoduodenectomy with or without distal gastrectomy and extended retroperitoneal lymphadenectomy for periampullary adenocarcinoma, part 2. *Ann Surg* 2002; 236: 355-68.
63. Crist DW, Sitzmann JV, Cameron JL. Improved hospital morbidity, mortality and survival after the Whipple procedure. *Ann Surg* 1987; 206: 358-65.
64. Greene BS, Loubeau JM, Peoples JB, Elliott DW. Are pancreatic anastomoses improved by duct-to-mucosa sutures? *Am J Surg* 1991; 161: 45-9.
65. Marcus SG, Cohen H, Ranson JH. Optimal management of the pancreatic remnant after pancreaticoduodenectomy. *Ann Surg* 1995; 221: 635-45.
66. Williams JG, Bramhall SR, Neoptolemos JP. Purse-string pancreatico-jejunostomy following pancreatic resection. *Dig Surg* 1997; 14: 183-6.
67. Yeo CJ, Barry K, Sauter PK, *et al.* Erythromycin accelerates gastric emptying after pancreatoduodenectomy. *Ann Surg* 1993; 218: 229-38.
68. Van Berge Henegouwen MI, van Guilk TM, De Witt LT, *et al.* Delayed gastric emptying after standard pancreatoduodenectomy *versus* pylorus preserving pancreatoduodenectomy: An analysis of 200 consecutive patients. *J Am Coll Surg* 1997; 185: 373-9.
69. Buchler M, Friess H, Klempa I, *et al.* Role of octreotide in the prevention of postoperative complications following pancreatic resection. *Am J Surg* 1992; 163: 125-30.
70. Friess H, Beger Hépato-Gastro, Sulkowski U, *et al.* Randomized controlled multicentre study of the prevention of complications by octreotide in patients undergoing surgery for chronic pancreatitis. *Br J Surg* 1995; 82: 1270-3.
71. Montorsi M, Zago M, Mosca F, *et al.* Efficacy of octreotide in the prevention of pancreatic fistula after elective pancreatic resections: a prospective, controlled, randomized clinical trial. *Surgery* 1995; 117: 26-31.
72. Gouillat C, Chipponi J, Baulieux J, Partensky C, Saric J, Gayet B. Randomized controlled multicentre trial of somatostatin infusion after pancreaticoduodenectomy. *Br J Surg* 2001; 88: 1456-62.
73. Yeo CJ, Cameron JL, Lillemoe KD, *et al.* Does prophylactic octreotide decrease the rates of pancreatic fistula and other complications after pancreaticoduodenectomy? Results of a prospective randomized placebo-controlled trial. *Ann Surg* 2000; 232: 419-29.
74. Lowy AM, Lee JE, Pisters PW, *et al.* Prospective, randomized trial of octreotide to prevent pancreatic fistula afterpancreaticoduodenectomy for malignant disease. *Ann Surg* 1997; 226: 632-41.
75. Sarr MG for the Pancreatic Surgery Group. The potent somatostatin analogue Vapreotide does not decrease pancreas-specific complications after elective pancreatectomy: a prospective, multicentre, double-blinded, randomized, placebo-controlled trial. *J Am Coll Surg* 2003; 196: 556-65.
76. Pedrazzoli P, DiCarlo V, Dionigi R, *et al.* Standard *versus* extended lymphadenectomy associated with pancreaticoduodenectomy in the surgical treatment of adenocarcinoma of the head of the pancreas. Lymphadenectomy Study Group. *Ann Surg* 1998; 228: 508-17.
77. Yeo CJ, Cameron JL, Sohn TA, *et al.* Pancreaticoduodenectomy with or without extended retroperitoneal lymphadenectomy for periampullary adenocarcinoma: comparison of morbidity and mortality and short-term outcome. *Ann Surg* 1999; 229: 613-22.

78. Amikura K, Kobari M, et al. The time of occurrence of liver metastasis in carcinoma of the pancreas. *Int J Pancreatol* 1995; 17: 139-46.
79. Kayahara M, Nagakawa T, Ueno K, Ohta T, Takeda T, Miyazaki I. An evaluation of radical resection for pancreatic cancer based on the mode of recurrence as determined by autopsy and diagnostic imaging. *Cancer* 1993; 72: 2118-23.
80. Conlon KC, Klimstra D, Brennan M. Long-term survival aftre curative resection for pancreatic ductal adenocarcinoma. Clinicopahologic analysis of 5-year survivors. *Ann Surg* 1996; 223: 273-9.
81. Sohn TA, Yeo CJ, Cameron JL, et al. Resected adenocarcinoma of the pancreas 616 patients: results, outcomes and prognostic factors. *J Gastrointest Surg* 2000; 4: 567-79.
82. Lim J, Chien M, Earle C. Prognostic factors following curative resection for pancreatic adenocarcinoma. *Ann Surg* 2003; 237: 74-85.
83. Lieberman MD, Kilburn H, Lindsey M, Brennan MF. Relation of peri-operative deaths to hospital volume among patients undergoing pancreatic resection for malignancy. *Ann Surg* 1995; 222: 638-45.
84. Gouma DJ, van Geenen RC, van Gulik TM, et al. Rates of complications and death after pancreaticoduodenectomy: risk factors and the impact of hospital volume. *Ann Surg* 2000; 232: 786-95.
85. Birkmeyer JD, Warshaw AL, Finlayson SR, et al. Relationship between hospital volume and late survival after pancreaticoduodenectomy. *Surgery* 1999; 126: 178-83.
86. Birkmeyer JD, Siewers AE, Finlayson EV, et al. Hospital volume and surgical mortality in the United States. *N Engl J Med* 2002; 346: 1128-37.
87. Herter FP, Cooperman AM, Ahlborn TN, Antinori C. Surgical experience with pancreatic and periampullary cancer. *Ann Surg* 1982; 195: 274.
88. Andren-Sandberg A, Ihse I. Factors influencing survival after total pancreatectomy in patients with pancreatic cancer. *Ann Surg* 1983; 198: 605.
89. Launois B, Franci J, Bardaxoglou E, et al. Total pancreatectomy for ductal adenocarcinoma of the pancreas with special reference to resection of the portal vein and multicentric cancer. *World J Surg* 1993; 17: 122-7.
90. Johnson CD, Schwall G, Flechtenmacher J, Trede M. Resection for adenocarcinoma of the body and tail of the pancreas. *Br J Surg* 1993; 80: 1177-9.
91. Smith AC, Dowsett JF, Russell RCG, Hatfield ARW, Cotton PB. Randomised trial of endoscopic stenting *versus* surgical bypass in malignant low bile duct obstruction. *Lancet* 1994; 344: 1655-60.
92. Andersen JR, Sorensen SM, Kruse A, et al. Randomised trial of endoscopic endoprosthesis *versus* operative bypass in malignant obstructive jaundice. *Gut* 1989; 30: 1132-5.
93. Davids PH, Groen AK, Rauws EA, et al. Randomised trial of self-expanding metal stents *versus* polyethylene stents for distal malignant biliary obstruction. *Lancet* 1992; 340: 1488-92.
94. Prat F, Chapat O, Ducot B, et al. Predictive factors for survival of patients with inoperable malignant distal biliary strictures: a practical management guideline. *Gut* 1998; 42: 76-80.
95. Isla AM, Worthington T, Kakkar AK, Williamson RC. A continuing role for surgical bypass in the palliative treatment of pancreatic carcinoma. *Dig Surg* 2000; 17: 143-6.
96. Watanapa P, Williamson RCN. Surgical palliation for pancreatic cancer: developments during the past two decades. *Br J Surg* 1992; 79: 8-20.
97. Lillemoe KD, Cameron JL, Hardacre JM, et al. Is prophylactic gastrojejunostomy indicated for unresectable periampullary cancer? A prospective randomized trial. *Ann Surg* 1999; 230: 322-30.
98. Park KB, Do YS, Kang WK, et al. Malignant obstruction of gastric outlet and duodenum: palliation with flexible covered metallic stents. *Radiology* 2001; 219: 679-83.
99. Lillemoe KD, Cameron JL, Yeo CJ, et al. Pancreaticoduodenectomy. Does it have a role in the palliation of pancreatic cancer? *Ann Surg* 1996; 223: 718-25.
100. Lillemoe KD, Cameron JL, Kaufman HS, et al. Chemical splanchnicectomy in patients with unresectable pancreatic cancer. A prospective randomized trial. *Ann Surg* 1993; 217: 447-57.
101. Polati E, Finco G, Gottin L, et al. Prospective randomised double-blind trial of neurolytic coeliac plexus block in patients with pancreatic cancer. *Br J Surg* 1998; 85: 199-201.

102. Rykowski JJ, Hilgier M. Efficacy of neurolytic celiac plexus block in varying locations of pancreatic cancer: influence on pain relief. *Anesthesiology* 2000; 92: 347-54.
103. Ihse I, Zoucas E, Gyllstedt E, *et al.* Bilateral thoracoscopic splanchnicectomy: effects on pancreatic pain and function. *Ann Surg* 1999; 230: 785-90.
104. Bruno MJEB Haverkort, *et al.* Placebo controlled trial of enteric coated pancreatin microsphere treatment in patients with unresectable cancer of the pancreatic head region. *Gut* 1998; 42: 92-6.

Pancreatic and biliary tract carcinoma: any role for photodynamic therapy?

Stephen P. Pereira

Institute of Hepatology and National Medical Laser Centre, University College London Campus, Royal Free & University College London Medical School, London, England

Principles of photodynamic therapy

Photodynamic therapy (PDT) is a way of producing localised tissue necrosis with light (most conveniently from a low-power, red laser) after prior administration of a photosensitising agent, thereby initiating a localised nonthermal cytotoxic effect and tissue necrosis [1]. The cytotoxic intermediary is thought to be singlet oxygen. This moiety is highly cytotoxic, with a short lifetime (< 0.04 μs) and a short radius of action (< 0.02 μm) [2]. As the biological effect is photochemical, not thermal, there is little damage to connective tissues such as collagen and elastin, which helps to maintain the mechanical integrity of hollow organs like the gastrointestinal tract [3]. Furthermore, since the light used is non-ionising, PDT does not carry the cumulative toxicity associated with radiotherapy. Once a PDT-treated area has healed, it can be treated again if necessary. Much of the early interest in PDT centred around the selective retention of photosensitisers in malignant tissue compared with adjacent normal tissue as this raised the possibility of selective destruction of cancers. Although there is indeed some selectivity of uptake [4, 5], this is rarely enough to make selective tumour destruction feasible and there is essentially always some necrosis in adjacent normal tissue where normal and neo-plastic tissue meet. Nevertheless, if necrosis of normal tissue heals safely without loss of the mechanical integrity of the organ, PDT may have an important role to play in the local destruction of a range of cancers. Although most applications of PDT in gastroenterology to date have been on lesions of the luminal gut [6, 7], there is increasing interest in its use for the treatment of lesions of the biliary tract and pancreas.

Table 1. Selected clinical trials: PDT in the treatment of gastrointestinal and other malignant disease (from Hopper [2], with permission from Elsevier)

Tumour site	Photosensitiser	N	main results	Ref
Inoperable lung cancer	Porfimer sodium	100 patients	Mean endoluminal obstruction fell from 86% to 18%; improvement in FVC and FEV1; overall 2-year survival 19%; mean follow up 72 months; no treatment-related mortality	22
Early-stage lung cancer	Porfimer sodium	54 patients 64 tumours	50 (85%) of assessable carcinomas CR; median duration of CR 14 months; 5 recurrences within 18 months	21
SCC of lung	Porfimer sodium	21 patients 23 tumours	CR in 15 patients; duration of response longer than 1 year in 11 patients (mean follow-up 68 months); 5 pateints had recurrence after 12 months	23
Early SCC of esophagus	Temoporfin (14), HpD (9), porfimer sodium (8)	28 patients 31 tumours	CR of 84% in early cancers; 2 stenoses and 2 fistulas; mean follow-up 2 years	24
Early bronchial and esophageal cancers	Temoporfin	27 patients 40 tumours	83% of early cancers showed no recurrence after mean disease-free follow-up of 15.3 months; complications reduced with green light	29
Advanced esophageal cancer	Porfimer sodium vs Nd:YAG laser	218 patients	Improvement in dysphagia equivalent, but tumour response 32% with PDT and 20% after laser ablation; 9 vs 2 CR	25
Esophageal carcinoma	Porfimer sodium	77 patients	Minimal complications and no treatment-related mortality; length of palliation equal to, or better than other treatments	28
Inoperable esophageal cancer	Porfimer sodium	65 patients	Dysphagia relieved in all patients; 7 still alive after 2-30 months; mean survival 8 months; survival influenced by performance status	26
Early gastric cancer	Temoporfin	22 patients	CR in 80% of patients with intestinal cancer and 50% with diffuse Lauren's carcinoma; mean follow-up 12 and 20 months, respectively	27

CR = complete response; FVC = forced vital capacity; FEV1 = forced expiratory volume in 1 s; SCC = squamous-cell carcinoma; HpD = haematoporphyrin derivative.

Biliary tract carcinoma

Cholangiocarcinoma and cancer of the gall bladder are tumours of the biliary tract that are considered as one pathological entity (biliary tract carcinoma, BTC). Worldwide, BTC is the second most common primary liver cancer after hepatocellular carcinoma, accounting for 15% of all primary hepatic malignancies [8]. Overall, the incidence of BTC in Asia is 50 times higher than that in Europe, where it has been regarded as a rare tumour [8, 9]. However, recent epidemiological data from the UK, USA, Spain and Australia have shown a steady and steep rise in mortality rates from intrahepatic cholangiocarcinoma (but not gallbladder cancer or extrahepatic bile duct cancer) over the past 20 years, with smaller rises in France, Italy and Japanese men [9-12]. In the UK since the mid 1990s, more deaths have been coded annually as being due to this tumour than to hepatocellular carcinoma [12]. The cause of this rise is unknown and does not appear to be explained simply by improvements in diagnosis or changes in coding practice [12]. One hypothesis is that chronic and increasing exposure of biliary ductal epithelium to environmental chemical genotoxins in bile may play a role in the development of BTC [13].

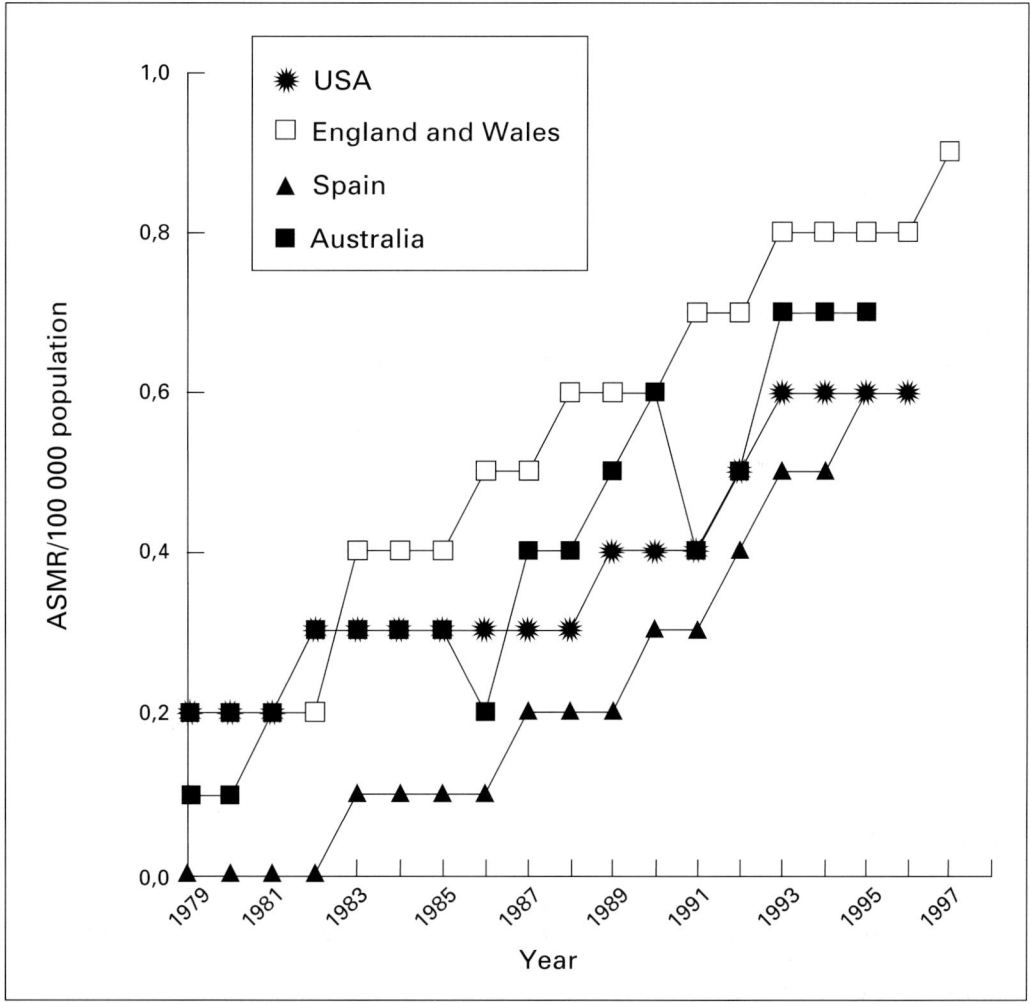

Figure 1. Examples of countries where intrahepatic cholangiocarcinoma is rising. ASMR, age standardised mortality rate. From Khan et al. [13], with permission from the BMJ Publishing Group.

BTC has a poor prognosis, with similar incidence and mortality rates and an overall five year survival of less than 5% [14]. Surgery is the only curative treatment for patients with BTC, but is appropriate in less than 20% of cases (Bismuth classification I-III [15]) and is associated with a 5-year survival of 9-30% in selected series [16-18].

Conversely, more than 80% of patients are diagnosed with proximal strictures involving both sides of the liver (Bismuth type III – stenosis of at least one second order branch or IV – bilobar involvement of second order branches), or have vascular involvement or metastases precluding resection [14]. Although most patients can be palliated promptly by endoscopic or percutaneous placement of one or more biliary stents [19], the prognosis remains poor, with complex hilar lesions having a median survival of less than six months [14, 20]. Since the cause of death in BTC after successful stenting is commonly due to recurrent biliary obstruction and intrabiliary sepsis, a key issue of palliative therapy is that of control of locally progressive disease. This is in contrast to upper gastrointestinal malignancies of the esophagus and pancreas, where metastatic disease is usually the primary factor in survival.

In theory, nonsurgical oncological approaches could have a beneficial impact on this disease. Uncontrolled studies suggest that intraluminal brachytherapy (iridium implants) [21-23], sometimes combined with external-beam radiotherapy [24-26], may prolong survival. However, the few controlled studies that have assessed this therapy have not found any significant clinical or survival advantage. In a retrospective comparison of endoscopic stenting alone with stenting and radiotherapy in 56 patients with irresectable cholangiocarcinoma from our Unit [27], there was a small survival advantage (11 *versus* 7 months) in those with Bismuth III/IV strictures given radiotherapy, but length of hospital stay and stent change requirements were also significantly increased. In the only prospective, randomised trial to date, reported as an abstract [28], preliminary survival figures in 21 patients with biliary stents randomised to observation alone or brachytherapy showed no advantage of brachytherapy over biliary drainage.

A systematic review of over 65 disparate studies of chemotherapy and/or radiation in BTC [20], and a recent UK consensus document on the diagnosis and treatment of cholangiocarcinoma [29], concluded that there was no strong evidence of survival benefit. To date, most studies have been small and have lacked a control group (level II evidence or less [30]) or sufficient power to test for differences in survival. A number of larger, multi-centre chemotherapy trials in BTC are currently underway, but at present there is no established treatment for advanced biliary cancer other than stenting and best supportive care.

Photodynamic therapy in BTC

Photofrin PDT

In 1991, McCaughan *et al* [31] reported on their experience with repeated PDT using dihematoporphyrin in a single patient with histologically proven adenocarcinoma of the common bile duct. The patient responded well to a total of seven PDT treatments performed through a percutaneous access, but after two years developed an unrelated endometrial carcinoma and died of pleural metastases after four years.

This case report stimulated preliminary studies in Germany of palliative endoscopic PDT for BTC. In two phase II studies of nine [32] and 23 patients [33] with histologically proven cholangiocarcinoma (Bismuth type III 2, Bismuth IV 30), endoscopic stenting plus PDT (repeated if there was evidence of tumour reduction or endoscopic biopsies of hilar strictures remained positive) resulted in an improvement in cholestasis, quality of life and survival compared with historical controls treated with stenting alone. Ortner *et al.* [32] demonstrated a median survival of 439 days in their study group, while Berr *et al.* [33] reported a median survival of 340 days and a six-month survival of 91% after diagnosis, compared with an expected survival of 50%. The 30-day mortality in the two studies was 0 and 4%, respectively. Similar findings were reported in a recent study from Bonn [34]. In 24 patients with histologically proven cholangiocarcinoma (Bismuth III 2, Bismuth IV 22) treated with a single course of PDT followed by metal stent insertion, the 30- and 60-day mortality was zero and the median survival post-PDT was approximately 300 days.

In the study by Ortner *et al.* [32], the mean change in the diameter of the bile duct at the area of greatest stenosis was 1.2 ± SD 1.0 mm before, to 5.9 ± 1.3 mm after PDT ($p < 0.001$), as a result of stricture dilatation by the endoprosthesis and/or tumour debulking by PDT. An apparent reduction in tumour mass was also seen in some intrahepatic ducts not directly illuminated with laser light. In the series by Berr *et al.* [33], 11 of the 23 patients presented with occlusion of either the left or right bile duct. The initial PDT reopened the occluded lobar duct in all of them, as well as an average of three segmental ducts. A potential explanation for these observations is that enough light to activate the photosensitiser reached affected areas by light propagation in the bile or through the hepatic parenchyma. Alternatively, PDT has been shown in animal models to induce a variety of immunologic responses that could potentially affect tumour growth in regions outside the treatment zone [35-37].

These phase II data have been supported by the results of a recent interim analysis of a multi-centre, randomised controlled trial of repeated PDT with stenting (mean 2.4 sessions) *versus* stenting alone for irresectable cholangiocarcinoma [38]. The trial was discontinued early by the monitoring committee after 39 patients had been randomised due to the marked survival advantage of the PDT group, with a median survival at the time of publication of 493 days compared with 98 days in the stent alone group ($p < 0.0001$). A further 31 patients with advanced disease (1 tumour stage III, 13 stage IVa, 17 stage IVb disease) who declined or had exclusion criteria for randomisation were also treated with PDT plus stenting, and had a median survival of 426 days.

In all of the above studies, the patients were photosensitised intravenously with the first generation photosensitiser, porfimer sodium (Photofrin®, Axcan Pharma Inc, Canada), followed by endoscopic illumination of the tumour with laser light at 630 nm. Adverse events related to PDT were minor (mainly cholangitis and photosensitivity). A UK phase II study using similar methodology is currently underway [39].

Technique

PDT for biliary cancer is performed either at the time of therapeutic ERCP or *via* a percutaneous transhepatic approach, or both. After diagnosis, patients undergo endoscopic and/or percutaneous drainage and insertion of endoprostheses into the right and left intrahepatic system. Following successful endoprosthesis placement and histological or cytological confirmation of cancer, patients receive porfimer sodium 2 mg/kg bodyweight, intravenously, 48 hours before laser activation. Patients remain in a darkened area of the ward for three days after injection, followed by readaptation to normal indoor light by day seven. If more intense exposure is necessary during this period, patients are advised to wear protective covering and sunglasses, and to avoid direct exposure to sunlight for at least a month after photosensitisation.

At 48 hours after photosensitisation, the endoprostheses are removed at repeat ERCP and intraluminal photoactivation is performed. In our Unit, this is done using a laser quartz fibre with cylindrical diffuser tip (20-50 mm length, 400 µm core diameter) with an x-ray marker on both sides of the diffuser – inserted either through a translucent endoscopic catheter introduced proximally above the strictures, or by placing the laser fibre directly across the stricture.

Photoactivation is performed at 630 nm using a light dose of 180 J/cm^2, which requires an irradiation time of approximately 10-12 minutes per treated biliary segment. All patients receive oxygen via a nasal catheter during the procedure as part of standard endoscopic practice, which in theory also optimises the PDT effect. Where tumour length exceeds the maximal diffuser length, overlap of treated fields is avoided by pulling the fibre back in controlled stages or using an opaque catheter to shield part of the fibre. After illumination of the first section of tumour length, the laser fibre is pulled back under radiological control using the markers viewed on the x-ray screen to the next segment of bile duct. In Bismuth IV strictures, a guidewire is inserted into the duct while treating one side, before repeating treatment on the other side. In the case of multiple intrahepatic strictures, second order branches that are accessible endoscopically and associated with obstructed liver segments are also treated. A new set of endoprostheses is inserted after completion of treatment.

Other photosensitisers

Foscan® (mTHPC: meso-tetrahydroxyphenyl chlorine; Biolitec Pharma Incorporated, Germany) is a second generation photosensitiser of the chlorine class with a more rapid elimination than porfimer sodium, and thus has the advantages of shorter treatment times and less prolonged skin photosensitivity. Photodynamic therapy with mTHPC has been used successfully to clear biliary metal stents blocked by malignant ingrowth [40]. The only major complications that occurred using this treatment were in patients whose tumours invaded large arteries, whereas infiltration of smaller vessels did not seem to contraindicate PDT.

Zoepf *et al.* [41] treated eight patients with non-resectable bile duct cancer with Photosan-3. After four weeks, there was a marked reduction in bile duct stenosis and bilirubin levels, with two infectious complications but no mortality. At the time of publication, the median survival was 119 days (range 52-443 days), with five patients still alive. A smaller study by the same group of four patients with bile duct cancer treated with 5-ALA revealed superficial fibrinoid necrosis at cholangioscopy performed 72 hours after treatment, but no significant reduction in bile duct stenoses [42].

Neo-adjuvant PDT before curative resection

After attempted curative resection of hilar bile duct carcinoma, there is an 80% probability of local recurrence and a five-year survival rate of approximately 20% [29]. Berr et al. [43] proposed that pre-operative local ablation of infiltrating tumour and dysplastic epithelium with PDT may increase the rate of cure after resection. A 72-year-old man underwent photofrin PDT to a Bismuth type II bile duct cancer, followed by surgical resection on day 23. Twenty-two hours after administration of porfimer sodium, biopsies from the adenocarcinoma exhibited 2.4-fold enrichment of porfimer-specific fluorescence as compared with the adjacent normal bile duct epithelium – similar findings to a previous pharmacokinetic study in human bile duct cancer which reported a mean ratio of fluorescence in tumour *versus* normal bile duct tissue of $2.3 \pm SD\ 1.2$ at 48 hours after photosensitisation with porfimer sodium [5]. In serial cross-sections of the surgical specimen, there was complete tumour necrosis with pigmentation of photodegraded porfimer to a depth of 4 mm, while in the outer layer of the wall (at 5-8 mm depth) viable cancer cell nests without degraded profimer were seen. Normal tissue suffered very little phototoxic damage, with no evidence of necrosis or inflammation within either the connective and muscular tissue in the treated tumour or the bile duct mucosa and muscular layer at the tumour-free resection margin. None of the 20 lymph nodes removed contained metastatic tumour. Eighteen months after surgery, neither tumour recurrence nor stricture formation was found at the pretreated bilioenteric anastomosis.

In a subsequent series of seven patients with advanced proximal bile duct cancer treated with neo-adjuvant PDT by the same group [44], R0 resection was achieved in all patients. Tumour recurred in two patients six and nine months after surgery, with a one-year recurrence-free survival of 83%. The authors concluded that neo-adjuvant PDT of localised bile duct cancer of porfimer sodium is safe and needs to be evaluated prospectively to determine whether it reduces the rate of local disease recurrence after potentially curative resection. If selective tumour phototoxicity to a depth of 8-10 mm wall thickness could be achieved with technical improvements, PDT may also have a role as a potentially curative procedure in some patients.

PDT for ampullary carcinoma

PDT has also been used with palliative intent in patients with carcinoma of the ampulla of Vater unsuitable for pancreaticoduodenectomy. In a series from The Royal London Hospital [45], 10 patients were treated endoscopically with PDT after haematoporphyrin derivative had been given intravenously 48 hours beforehand. The tumours were treated by three or four light applications at each session, and treatment repeated up to five times (median 2) at three to six month intervals. The sole complication was moderate skin photosensitivity in three patients, with no evidence of significant damage to the duodenum. In three of the four patients with small tumours confined to the ampulla but who were unfit for surgery, endoscopic biopsies post-PDT were negative for malignancy and endoscopic stents were no longer required for 8-12 months, by which time macroscopic tumour had recurred. In all three patients with local spread < 3 cm in diameter, there was an appreciable response with reduced tumour bulk but macroscopic tumour remained, while only one of three patients with advanced disease had a temporary reduction in tumour size. The authors concluded that PDT causes safe and effective tumour destruction in patients with ampullary carcinoma with periods of clinical remission for tumours confined to the ampulla, and with refinements in technique may prove curative for small tumours.

Pancreatic adenocarcinoma

Worldwide, adenocarcinoma of the pancreas is one of the top 10 leading causes of cancer death, and ranks fourth as a cause of cancer death in the UK and USA [46, 47]. In series from specialised centres, over 10% may be resectable at presentation [48], but in larger population-based studies the number undergoing resection with curative intent may be as low as 3% [49]. Even after resection, median survival is only 10-20 months and no more than 5-20% of resected patients survive five years [50]. Options available for the treatment of inoperable patients are largely limited to chemotherapy, radiotherapy, or some combination of the two. Gemcitabine is probably the most useful single agent for symptomatic relief although no agent has been shown to have a convincing benefit on survival [51]. Overall, the long term prognosis of the disease is poor with a one-year survival rate of no more than 10%. For non-metastatic disease, median survival is 6-10 months although for those with metastatic disease at presentation, median survival is only 3-6 months [52]. Given these dismal results, a minimally invasive treatment capable of local destruction of tumour tissue with low morbidity may have a place in the treatment of this disease.

PDT in pancreatic cancer: animal studies

In contrast to biliary tract carcinoma, PDT of the pancreas has been less well studied in humans, partly because of concerns related to the many vital structures in the vicinity of the pancreas that could be vulnerable to local insults, and the theoretical risks of pancreatitis, fistulation and inappropriate release of pancreatic secretions. However, a great deal of experimental work has been undertaken, mainly on hamsters, to study PDT effects on the pancreas and surrounding tissues as well as on tumours transplanted into the pancreas. This has been done with a range of photosensitisers including porfimer sodium [53], aluminium disulphonated phthalocyanine (AlS_2Pc) [54, 55], pheophorbide A [56], 5-aminolevulinic acid (ALA) [57, 58] and mTHPC [4, 59], with broadly similar results. In general, there was necrosis in normal pancreas and stomach, which healed without serious adverse effects. The tissue that was most vulnerable with all photosensitisers was the duodenum, with sealed duodenal perforations and late duodenal stenosis seen in some animals. In the aorta, there was endothelial and medial smooth muscle cell necrosis but this did not lead to any thrombotic events or weakening of the arterial wall.

Studies of treatment of chemically-induced pancreatic cancers transplanted into the hamster pancreas showed that it was possible to achieve tumour necrosis, with the only significant complication again being duodenal damage (sealed perforation or stenosis) when the site treated was close to the duodenal wall [54, 56, 58, 53]. Unlike tumours in the luminal gut, some selectivity of tumour necrosis was found relative to the effect in

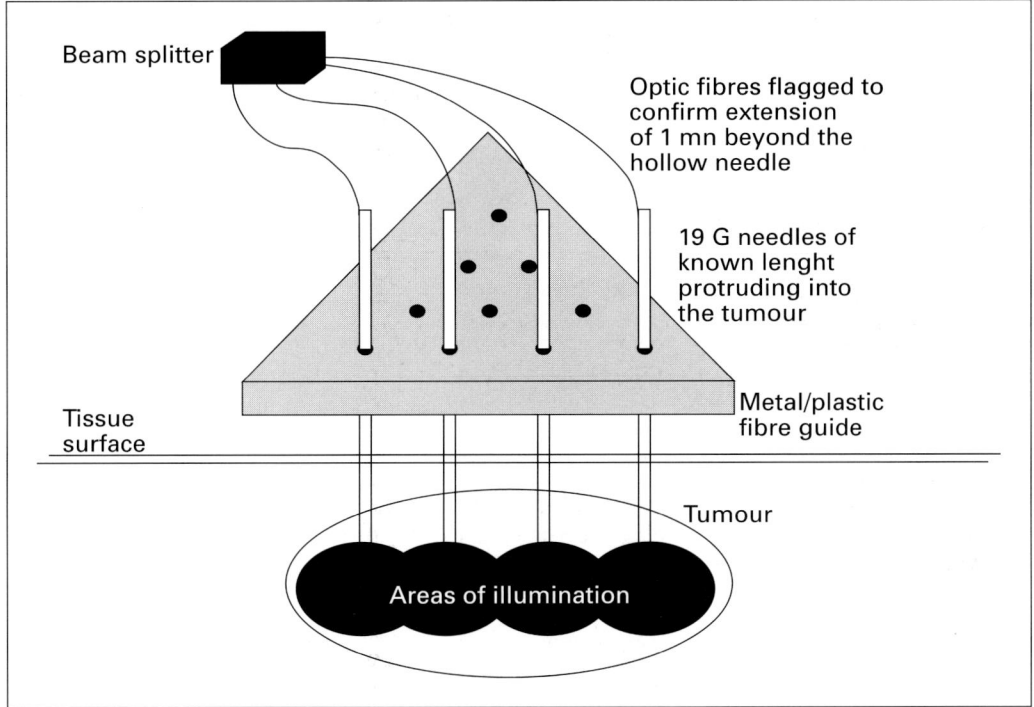

Figure 2. Placement of light delivery fibres in interstitial application of PDT. (From Hopper [2], with permission from Elsevier.)

the surrounding normal pancreas [4]. This was noted using $A1S_2Pc$, even though the selectivity of uptake in these tumours was only 2-3:1. It was suggested that this might be due to the presence of glutathione or some other substance in normal pancreatic secretions, not present in the tumour, that absorbed singlet oxygen. Another important result was found in a randomised, controlled study on implanted pancreatic cancers in hamsters using PDT with ALA. Tumour necrosis up to 8 mm deep was achieved and there was a significant increase in the survival time of treated animals compared with untreated controls [58].

PDT in pancreatic cancer: clinical studies

The lack of serious complications in these animal studies (apart from the duodenal effects which were thought to be a consequence of the very thin wall of the hamster duodenum) led to our Unit conducting a pilot clinical trial of PDT in pancreatic cancer, published in 2002 [60]. The photosensitiser used was mTHPC, as the experimental work had shown that this gave the largest zone of necrosis around each treatment site (up to 12 mm in diameter), and also because this drug requires the lowest light doses and therefore the shortest treatment times.

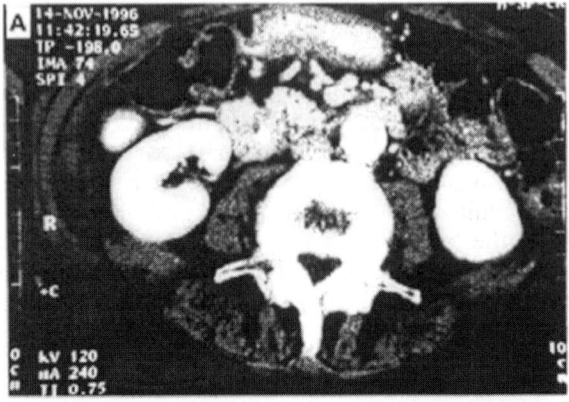

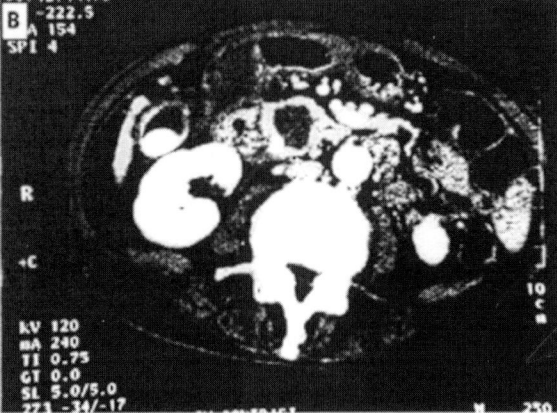

Figure 3. Contrast enhanced computerised tomography scans of a patient: (A) prior to mTHPC PDT, showing a 2.5 cm carcinoma in the head of the pancreas, and (B) four days after PDT, showing a large new area of non-enhancement. This patient had a biliary stent in place at the time of treatment. Technically, this tumour was thought to be operable but the general condition of the patient was considered to be too poor. From Bown et al. [60], with permission from the BMJ Publishing Group.

Technique

With the aims of assessing technical feasibility, safety and efficacy, 16 patients with locally advanced cancers in the head of the pancreas were treated with mTHPC *via* percutaneous needles placed under CT guidance. The documented maximum tumour diameter prior to PDT was 2.5-6.0 cm (median 4.0) and tumour volume was 3-63 cm^3 (median 27). The patients received mTHPC 0.15 mg/kg bodyweight, intravenously, 72 hours before laser activation. Patients remained in a darkened area of the ward for the first 24 hours, with the level of light kept below 100 lux (equivalent to a single 60 W bulb). On each subsequent day the permitted light exposure was increased by 100 lux so that by day three low level indoor lighting was acceptable and by seven days normal indoor lighting was safe.

Treatment was undertaken three days after photosensitisation under subdued lighting conditions. After prophylactic antibiotics and intravenous sedation, the anterior abdominal wall was infiltrated with local anaesthetic. Up to six 19 G needles were inserted into the deepest part of the tumour by the radiologist with their tips separated by about 1.5 cm using a combination of ultrasound and CT guidance, the number being determined by the size and position of the tumour.

The light source used was a diode laser delivering red light at 652 nm. Using a beam splitter, the light was divided equally between up to four 0.4 mm core diameter optical fibres. When all of the needles had been confirmed as correctly sited in the tumour, a fibre was passed down to the tip of each needle to leave 3 mm of bare fibre in direct contact with the tumour during delivery of the therapeutic light. In patients requiring six needles, the last two sites were illuminated after the first four rather than concurrently. Prior to use, the system was calibrated to deliver 100 mW at the tip of each fibre. This power setting was used to minimise photocoagulation of blood around the fibre tips which can reduce the amount of light delivered to the target site. After delivery of the planned light dose at the initial sites, the needles and fibres were pulled back under CT control in approximately 1 cm steps as required to cover the entire tumour and the same light dose delivered at each position. The light dose delivered at each site was kept at 20 J for each patient.

Results

On contrast-enhanced CT scans taken a few days after PDT, all patients had a new non-enhancing area in the pancreas (up to 6.5 cm diameter) consistent with tumour necrosis, which was confirmed on biopsy in the first patient. The median volume of necrosis produced by PDT was 36 cm^3 (range, 9.0 to 60.0 cm^3).

Transient procedure-related pain requiring opiate analgesia was the most common side effect. Ten patients experienced a temporary paralytic ileus but most were drinking normally by 48 hours and none developed pancreatitis. There was no treatment-related mortality, but two patients with gastroduodenal artery involvement had haemodynamically significant bleeds requiring transfusion and/or embolisation. Two others with major duodenal wall involvement developed significant PDT-induced duodenal stenosis requiring enteral stent placement. The treatment shrank the area of viable tumour, and tumour did not regrow at the site of PDT necrosis but often regrew from the edges of the treated areas. In 14 cases, the late stages of the disease were dominated by local tumour invasion and lymphadenopathy. In two patients, multiple liver metastases were detected soon after PDT and their subsequent clinical course was dominated by this development. Median survival for all patients from the time of diagnosis was 12.5 months (range 6-34 months). Seven of the 16 (44%) patients were alive one year after PDT, nine (56%) were alive one year after diagnosis and two patients survived two years.

These preliminary results suggest that the technique is feasible and safe for local debulking of pancreatic cancer. The survival values compare favourably with the median survival of 6-10 months from diagnosis in patients with non-metastatic locally advanced disease reported in other series [52]. However, randomised controlled studies will be required to assess the true influence of PDT on survival, and its potential additional role to palliative chemotherapy in the management of this disease. Technical aspects of future studies will be to match the distribution of laser effects to the extent of diseased tissue being treated, and ideally to extend the treated area beyond the tumour margins identified on pretreatment scans. The use of modified selection criteria, such as excluding patients with tumour encasement of a major artery or the duodenum, would also be expected to reduce the risk of major complications and allow treated areas to heal safely.

References

1. Dougherty TJ, Gomer CJ, Henderson BW, et al. Photodynamic therapy. *J Natl Cancer Inst* 1998; 90: 889-905.
2. Hopper C. Photodynamic therapy: a clinical reality in the treatment of cancer. *Lancet Oncol* 2000; 1: 212-9.
3. Barr H, Tralau CJ, Boulos PB, MacRobert AJ, Tilly R, Bown SG. The contrasting mechanisms of colonic collagen damage between photodynamic therapy and thermal injury. *Photochem Photobiol* 1987; 46: 795-800.
4. Mikvy P, Messman H, MacRobert AJ, et al. Photodynamic therapy of a transplanted pancreatic cancer model using meta-tetrahydroxyphenylchlorin (mTHPC). *Br J Cancer* 1997; 76: 713-8.
5. Pahernik SA, Dellian M, Berr F, Tannapfel A, Wittekind C, Goetz AE. Distribution and pharmacokinetics of Photofrin in human bile duct cancer. *J Photochem Photobiol B* 1998; 47: 58-62.
6. Ell C, Gossner L, May A, et al. Photodynamic ablation of early cancers of the stomach by means of mTHPC and laser irradiation: preliminary clinical experience. *Gut* 1998; 43: 345-9.
7. Sibille A, Lambert R, Souquet JC, Sabben G, Descos F. Long-term survival after photodynamic therapy for esophageal cancer. *Gastroenterology* 1995; 108: 337-44.
8. Nakanuma Y, Hoso M, Terada T. Clinical and pathologic features of cholangiocarcinoma. In: Okuda K, Tabor E, eds. *Liver cancer*. New York: Churchill Livingstone, 1997: 279-90.
9. Khan SA, Taylor-Robinson SD, Toledano MB, Beck A, Elliott P, Thomas HC. Changing international trends in mortality rates for liver, biliary and pancreatic tumours. *J Hepatol* 2002; 37: 806-13.
10. Nair S, Shiv Kumar K, Thuluvath PJ, Shivakumar KS, Shiva Kumar K. Mortality from hepatocellular and biliary cancers: changing epidemiological trends. *Am J Gastroenterol* 2002; 97: 167-71.
11. Patel T. Increasing incidence and mortality of primary intrahepatic cholangiocarcinoma in the United States. *Hepatology* 2001; 33: 1353-7.
12. Taylor-Robinson SD, Toledano MB, Arora S, et al. Increase in mortality rates from intrahepatic cholangiocarcinoma in England and Wales 1968-1998. *Gut* 2001; 48: 816-20.
13. Khan SA, Carmichael PL, Taylor-Robinson SD, Habib N, Thomas HC. DNA adducts, detected by 32P postlabelling, in human cholangiocarcinoma. *Gut* 2003; 52: 586-91.
14. de Groen PC, Gores GJ, LaRusso NF, Gunderson LL, Nagorney DM: Biliary tract cancers. *N Engl J Med* 1999; 341: 1368-78.
15. Bismuth H, Nakache R, Diamond T. Management strategies in resection for hilar cholangiocarcinoma. *Ann Surg* 1992; 215: 31-8.
16. Henson DE, Albores-Saavedra J, Corle D. Carcinoma of the extrahepatic bile ducts. Histologic types, stage of disease, grade, and survival rates. *Cancer* 1992; 70: 1498-501.
17. Madariaga JR, Iwatsuki S, Todo S, Lee RG, Irish W, Starzl TE. Liver resection for hilar and peripheral cholangiocarcinomas: a study of 62 cases. *Ann Surg* 1998; 227: 70-9.
18. Reding R, Buard JL, Lebeau G, Launois B. Surgical management of 552 carcinomas of the extrahepatic bile ducts (gallbladder and periampullary tumours excluded). Results of the French Surgical Association Survey. *Ann Surg* 1991; 213: 236-41.
19. Polydorou AA, Cairns SR, Dowsett JF, et al. Palliation of proximal malignant biliary obstruction by endoscopic endoprosthesis insertion. *Gut* 1991; 32: 685-9.
20. Hejna M, Pruckmayer M, Raderer M. The role of chemotherapy and radiation in the management of biliary cancer: a review of the literature. *Eur J Cancer* 1998; 34: 977-86.
21. Ede RJ, Williams SJ, Hatfield AR, McIntyre S, Mair G. Endoscopic management of inoperable cholangiocarcinoma using iridium-192. *Br J Surg* 1989; 76: 867-9.
22. Karani J, Fletcher M, Brinkley D, Dawson JL, Williams R, Nunnerley H. Internal biliary drainage and local radiotherapy with iridium-192 wire in treatment of hilar cholangiocarcinoma. *Clin Radiol* 1985; 36: 603-6.

23. Levitt MD, Laurence BH, Cameron F, Klemp PF. Transpapillary iridium-192 wire in the treatment of malignant bile duct obstruction. *Gut* 1988; 29: 149-52.
24. Foo ML, Gunderson LL, Bender CE, Buskirk SJ. External radiation therapy and transcatheter iridium in the treatment of extrahepatic bile duct carcinoma. *Int J Radiat Oncol Biol Phys* 1997; 39: 929-35.
25. Kuvshinoff BW, Armstrong JG, Fong Y, et al. Palliation of irresectable hilar cholangiocarcinoma with biliary drainage and radiotherapy. *Br J Surg* 1995; 82: 1522-5.
26. Vallis KA, Benjamin IS, Munro AJ, et al. External beam and intraluminal radiotherapy for locally advanced bile duct cancer: role and tolerability. *Radiother Oncol* 1996; 41: 61-6.
27. Bowling TE, Galbraith SM, Hatfield AR, Solano J, Spittle MF. A retrospective comparison of endoscopic stenting alone with stenting and radiotherapy in non-resectable cholangiocarcinoma. *Gut* 1996; 39: 852-5.
28. Ricci E, Mortilla MG, Conigliaro R, Sassatelli R, Palmieri T, D'Abbiero A. Endoscopic drainage and HDR brachytherapy in palliation of obstructive pancreatic and bile duct cancers: a prospective randomized study. *Ital J Gastroenterol Hepatol* 1998; 30: A88.
29. Khan SA, Davidson BR, Goldin R, et al. Guidelines for the diagnosis and treatment of cholangiocarcinoma: consensus document. *Gut* 2002; 51 (Suppl. VI): vi1-vi9.
30. Phillips B, Ball C, Sackett D, et al. http://cebm.jr2.ox.ac.uk/docs/levels.html Oxford Centre for Evidence-based Medicine, 2001.
31. McCaughan JS Jr., Mertens BF, Cho C, Barabash RD, Payton HW. Photodynamic therapy to treat tumours of the extrahepatic biliary ducts: a case report. *Arch Surg* 1991; 126: 111-3.
32. Ortner MA, Liebetruth J, Schreiber S, et al. Photodynamic therapy of nonresectable cholangiocarcinoma. *Gastroenterology* 1998; 114: 536-42.
33. Berr F, Wiedmann M, Tannapfel A, et al. Photodynamic therapy for advanced bile duct cancer: evidence for improved palliation and extended survival. *Hepatology* 2000; 31: 291-8.
34. Dumoulin FL, Gerhardt T, Fuchs S, et al. Phase II study of photodynamic therapy and metal stent as palliative treatment for nonresectable hilar cholangiocarcinoma. *Gastrointest Endosc* 2003; 57: 860-7.
35. Korbelik M, Krosl G. Enhanced macrophage cytotoxicity against tumour cells treated with photodynamic therapy. *Photochem Photobiol* 1994; 60: 497-502.
36. Wong Kee Song LM, Wang KK, Zinsmeister AR. Mono-L-aspartyl chlorin e6 (NPe6) and hematoporphyrin derivative (HpD) in photodynamic therapy administered to a human cholangiocarcinoma model. *Cancer* 1998; 82: 421-7.
37. Wong M, Wang KK, Alexander GL, Gutta K. Chlorin E6 and hematoporphyrin derivate (HPD) on photodynamic therapy of a human cholangiocarcinoma model. *Gastroenterology* 1996; 110: A595.
38. Ortner MA, Berr F, Liebetruth J, et al. Photodynamic therapy of non-resectable cholangiocarcinoma: a randomized prospective study – first results. *Gastrointest Endosc* 2001; 53: A3321.
39. Cancer Research UK. Biliary tree (gallbladder and bile duct). *http://www.cancerhelp.org.uk/trials/trials/default.asp*. 2003.
40. Rogowska AZ, Whitelaw DE, Hatfield AR, Ripley AM, Buonaccorsi G, Bown SG. Photodynamic therapy for recanalisation of occluded biliary metal stents. *Gastroenterology* 1999; 116: G0123.
41. Zoepf T, Jakobs R, Arnold JC, Apel D, Rosenbaum A, Riemann JF. Photodynamic therapy for palliation of nonresectable bile duct cancer-preliminary results with a new diode laser system. *Am J Gastroenterol* 2001; 96: 2093-7.
42. Zoepf T, Jakobs R, Rosenbaum A, Apel D, Arnold JC, Riemann JF. Photodynamic therapy with 5-aminolevulinic acid is not effective in bile duct cancer. *Gastrointest Endosc* 2001; 54: 763-6.
43. Berr F, Tannapfel A, Lamesch P, et al. Neoadjuvant photodynamic therapy before curative resection of proximal bile duct carcinoma. *J Hepatol* 2000; 32: 352-7.
44. Wiedmann M, Caca K, Berr F, et al. Neoadjuvant photodynamic therapy as a new approach to treating hilar cholangiocarcinoma: a phase II pilot study. *Cancer* 2003; 97: 2783-90.

45. Abulafi AM, Allardice JT, Williams NS, van Someren N, Swain CP, Ainley C. Photodynamic therapy for malignant tumours of the ampulla of Vater. *Gut* 1995; 36: 853-6.
46. Jemal A, Thomas A, Murray T, Thun M. Cancer statistics, 2002. *CA Cancer J Clin* 2002; 52: 23-47.
47. Parkin DM, Pisani P, Ferlay J. Global cancer statistics. *CA Cancer J Clin* 1999; 49: 33-64, 1.
48. Warshaw AL, Fernandez-del Castillo C. Pancreatic carcinoma. *N Engl J Med* 1992; 326: 455-65.
49. Bramhall SR, Neoptolemos JP. Advances in diagnosis and treatment of pancreatic cancer. *Gastroenterologist* 1995; 3: 301-10.
50. Stojadinovic A, Brooks A, Hoos A, Jaques DP, Conlon KC, Brennan MF. An evidence-based approach to the surgical management of resectable pancreatic adenocarcinoma. *J Am Coll Surg* 2003; 196: 954-64.
51. Burris HA 3rd, Moore MJ, Andersen J, *et al*. Improvements in survival and clinical benefit with gemcitabine as first-line therapy for patients with advanced pancreas cancer: a randomized trial. *J Clin Oncol* 1997; 15: 2403-13.
52. Hawes RH, Xiong Q, Waxman I, Chang KJ, Evans DB, Abbruzzese JL. A multispecialty approach to the diagnosis and management of pancreatic cancer. *Am J Gastroenterol* 2000; 95: 17-31.
53. Schroder T, Chen IW, Sperling M, Bell RH Jr., Brackett K, Joffe SN. Hematoporphyrin derivative uptake and photodynamic therapy in pancreatic carcinoma. *J Surg Oncol* 1988; 38: 4-9.
54. Chatlani PT, Nuutinen PJ, Toda N, *et al*. Selective necrosis in hamster pancreatic tumours using photodynamic therapy with phthalocyanine photosensitization. *Br J Surg* 1992; 79: 786-90.
55. Nuutinen PJ, Chatlani PT, Bedwell J, MacRobert AJ, Phillips D, Bown SG. Distribution and photodynamic effect of disulphonated aluminium phthalocyanine in the pancreas and adjacent tissues in the Syrian golden hamster. *Br J Cancer* 1991; 64: 1108-15.
56. Evrard S, Keller P, Hajri A, *et al*. Experimental pancreatic cancer in the rat treated by photodynamic therapy. *Br J Surg* 1994; 81: 1185-9.
57. Ravi B, Regula J, Buonaccorsi GA, MacRobert AJ, Loh CS, Bown SG. Sensitization and photodynamic therapy of normal pancreas, duodenum and bile ducts in the hamster using 5-aminolevulinic acid. *Lasers Med Sci* 1996; 11: 11-21.
58. Regula J, Ravi B, Bedwell J, MacRobert AJ, Bown SG. Photodynamic therapy using 5-aminolevulinic acid for experimental pancreatic cancer-prolonged animal survival. *Br J Cancer* 1994; 70: 248-54.
59. Mlkvy P, Messmann H, Pauer M, *et al*. Distribution and photodynamic effects of meso-tetrahydroxyphenylchlorin (mTHPC) in the pancreas and adjacent tissues in the Syrian golden hamster. *Br J Cancer* 1996; 73: 1473-9.
60. Bown SG, Rogowska AZ, Whitelaw DE, *et al*. Photodynamic therapy for cancer of the pancreas. *Gut* 2002; 50: 549-57.

III

General oncology

What should the clinician/surgeon know about molecular oncogenesis?

Hubert E. Blum, Christian Arnold, Oliver Opitz, Henning Usadel

Department of Medicine II, University of Freiburg, Germany

Abstract

Gastrointestinal malignancies, especially cancer of the esophagus, stomach, colon, rectum and pancreas as well as hepatocellular carcinoma and cancer of the biliary system are among the most frequent cancers in Western countries. In recent years, basic science oriented biomedical research has identified tumour-specific alterations in gene sequences and expression levels as well as in protein structure and function in these cancers, increasingly yielding tumour- and patient-specific expression profiles. As hallmarks of a given cancer these molecular markers can be useful to identify individuals at risk to develop a cancer, to detect pre-malignant lesions or cancer, to assess prognosis and monitor disease progression as well as to predict response to treatment. Thus, molecular markers of cancer are becoming increasingly relevant for patient care and will eventually be an integral part of clinical medicine. For the clinician/surgeon, therefore, a basic understanding of molecular oncogenesis and of the principle and clinical relevance of molecular markers are essential to implement strategies to prevent, diagnose and treat different types of cancer.

Introduction

With the sequencing and analysis of the human genome [1, 2] molecular biology, recombinant DNA technology, genomics and proteomics increasingly contribute to the diagnosis, therapy and prevention of human diseases [3]. Genetically, human diseases can be classified into three major categories:

(i) Hereditary monogenetic diseases that are caused by a single gene defect and that are inherited by the classical Mendelian rules. There are more than 4,000 monogenetic diseases described. For an increasing number of these diseases the molecular basis has been identified.

(ii) Acquired monogenetic diseases such as infections as well as some malignancies which are associated with genetic alterations that are acquired and frequently accumulated during life-time.

(iii) Complex genetic diseases which are associated with mutations of several genes, only some of which have been identified to date. Several common human diseases belong to this category, such as most malignancies, diseases of the cardiovascular system, hypertension, arthritis, diabetes and others.

Molecular methods allow the early and specific detection of known infectious, inherited and malignant diseases affecting the gastrointestinal (GI) tract. Such analyses increasingly lead to a better understanding of the molecular basis of inherited and malignant diseases which in turn have an increasing impact on patient management, including the presymptomatic identification of patients at risk, the correct staging of the disease, the choice of treatment and the follow-up of patients undergoing therapy. For GI tumours, the identification of individuals at risk and the early diagnosis are of critical importance since a large proportion can be prevented or cured by surgical removal before metastasis has occurred. With increasing understanding of the genetic basis of GI tumours it will become feasible to identify tumour-specific molecular markers for prevention, (early) diagnosis and staging, prognosis and selection of the appropriate therapeutic strategy. Molecular biology, therefore, has become an integral part not only of basic research in GI oncology but increasingly also of clinical gastroenterology.

While major advances in the understanding of the molecular pathogenesis have been made in recent years for all GI tumours, including esophageal cancer [4], hepatocellular carcinoma [5] and the relatively rare gastrointestinal stromal tumours [6, 7], the most frequent and best studied GI tumour is colorectal carcinoma (CRC). In the following we will, therefore, focus on CRCs and review our current understanding of their molecular pathogenesis and the significance of molecular markers for CRC prevention, diagnosis and patient management.

CRC – Molecular Pathogenesis

All cancers are caused by genetic and/or epigenetic alterations that enable cancer cells to provide their own growth signals, ignore growth inhibitory signals, avoid apoptosis, replicate indefinitely, sustain angiogenesis and proliferate in nonphysiologic locations [8]. In addition, the pathogenesis of CRC involves environmental factors which may interact with genetic and/or epigenetic alterations in the promotion of tumour development. Dietary factors, *e.g*, low fiber and high fat content, may promote CRC development by altering intestinal bacterial flora, slowing gastrointestinal transit time and increasing recycling of bile acids.

Genetic and epigenetic alterations

Genetic alterations range from point mutations to chromosomal alterations; epigenetic alterations are nonmutational phenomena (DNA methylation and histone modification) that modify gene expression *(table I)*. Genetic targets of mutations are oncogenes, tumour suppressor genes and mismatch repair genes.

Table I. Genetic and Epigenetic Alterations in Cancer

Genetic Alterations
Mutations
  Point mutations (missense, nonsense)
  Insertions
  Deletions
Chromosomal changes
  Rearrangements
  Deletions (loss of heterozygosity, LOH)
  Duplications
  Amplifications

Epigenetic Alterations
  DNA methylation
  Histone modification, *e.g*, acetylation

There is an increasing understanding of the genetic basis of hereditary and sporadic (non-hereditary) CRC [9-16]. The data suggest that CRC results from the aggregate effect of multiple sequential genetic alterations ("multistep carcinogenesis", *figure 1*) which may be inherited (germ-line mutations) or acquired (somatic mutations). Colon cancer cells contain a very large number of mutations. Approximately 20% of all chromosomal arm pairs in DNA from normal colon show a loss of one arm (loss of heterozygosity, LOH) in tumour DNA [16] and perhaps 100,000 microsatellite mutations are found in individual CRCs with microsatellite instability [17]. Mutations occur randomly in the genome, with certain types of mutations more common at specific genetic sequences (*e.g*, insertions/deletions more common at repetitive sequences, chromosomal rearrangements more common at complementary sites). Since < 2% of the genome encode for a gene, many mutations will not affect the expression of a gene. Thus, DNA from CRCs contains a large number of mutations, only some of which are involved in multistep carcinogenesis and essential for tumour formation. Mutations providing a growth advantage will result in the expansion of this cell clone; mutations affecting critical structural or functional proteins will result in a clonal collapse; mutations not affecting cell viability will be found as part of the signature mutations of the tumour cell.

The correction of mutations by the proof-reading subunit of DNA polymerase, DNA mismatch repair (MMR), base excision repair and nucleotide excision repair is central for the accurate replication of DNA. When there is damaged DNA, cell cycle proteins prevent the cells from dividing. If the damage is not repaired, the cell enters apoptosis.

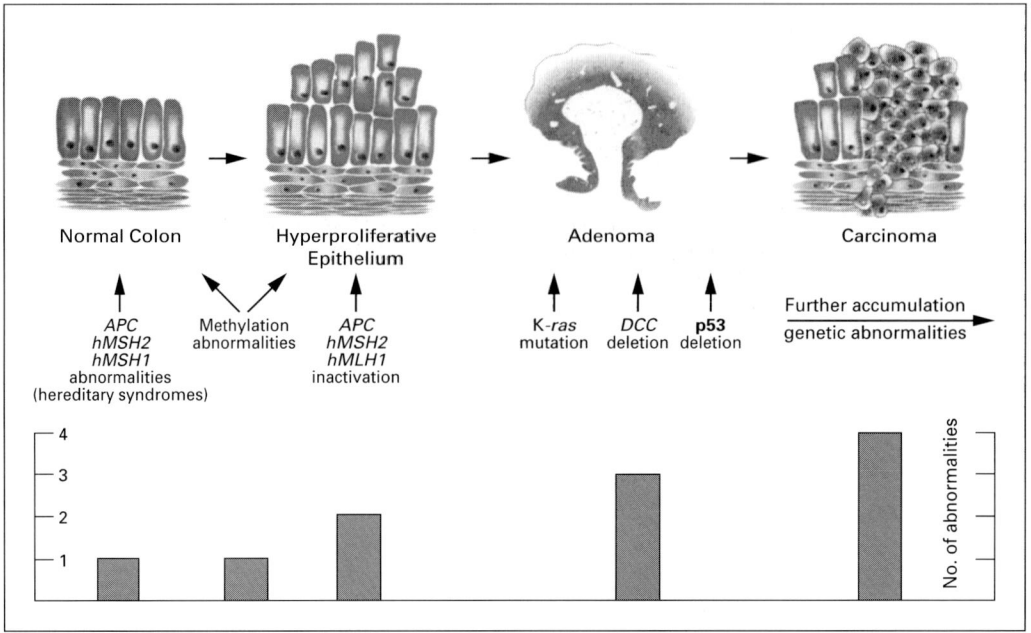

Figure 1. Multistep carcinogenesis of colorectal cancer through accumulation of multiple genetic abnormalities over time.

Genomic instability

In any cancer and most prominently in CRCs numerous genetic alterations occur and are tolerated. Three forms of genomic instability can be distinguished that affect different target genes *(table II)*:

(i) *Chromosomal instability (CIN)* in CRC pathogenesis ("suppressor pathway") is conferred by inactivating mutations of tumour suppressor genes [18], for example by the allelic loss of the adenomatous polyposis coli (APC) gene on chromosome 5 or of the p53 tumour suppressor gene on chromosome 17p or of chromosome 18q genes (SMAD4, SMAD2, DCC). Frequently, tumour DNA has only one copy of these genes. Thus, CRCs develop in the CIN pathway by the clonal expansion of cells that carry a single mutant copy of APC or p53.

(ii) *Microsatellite instability (MSI)* is a form of genomic instability ("mutator pathway") that produces thousands of mutations at repetitive DNA sequences [13, 19-21]. It is found in about 15% of sporadic CRCs, is linked to hereditary nonpolyposis colorectal cancer (HNPCC; 13, 20) and is caused by a loss of the MMR system [22, 23]. These tumours ultimately progress through the accumulation of insertion/deletion mutations in microsatellite sequences of "target genes" that control cell growth, differentiation and proliferation. Once they are inactivated tumour formation follows. Target genes of MSI are encoding proteins with a function central to the biology of the cell, *e.g*, tumour growth factor beta 1 receptor II or insulin-like growth factor 2 receptor *(table II)*.

Table II. Types of Genomic Instability in Colorectal Cancer and Genetic Targets

Chromosomal Instability (CIN)
 APC on chr. 5q: 1 allele mutated, 1 allele lost
 p53 on chr. 17p: 1 allele mutated, 1 allele lost
 SMAD4, SMAD2, DCC on chr. 18q

Microsatellite Instability (MSI)
 Tumour growth factor beta 1 receptor II (TGF-beta 1 RII)
 Insulin-like growth factor 2 receptor (IGF2R)
 HMSH3, hMSH6
 Caspases
 BAX

CpG Island Methylator Phenotype (CIMP)
 hMLH1
 APC
 PTEN
 p16
 p14
 Methylated in tumour (MINT) clones

(iii) *CpG Island methylator phenotype (CIMP)* is also linked to genomic instability ("methylator pathway") and is caused by gene silencing through hypermethylation of CpG islands within promoters [24]. Several genes have been found to be hypermethylated in CRCs, incl. APC *(table II)* as well as hMLH1 which in turn inactivates DNA MMR through hypermethylation, demonstrating the combined action of CIMP and MSI in specific cases.

In summary, CRCs are caused by the accumulation of multiple mutations that modify genes regulating cell division, growth and death. CIN, MSI and CIMP contribute to tumour formation through favouring cell division, growth and survival. Genetic and epigenetic alterations in tumour cells can be specifically identified and used as molecular markers.

CRC – Molecular Markers

Molecular biology and recombinant DNA technology have become an integral part of research related to the diagnosis, therapy and prevention of human diseases. Apart from the better understanding of the molecular basis of inherited and malignant diseases, molecular methods allow the early detection of patients at risk for a given disease. In this context, research during the past few years on the molecular pathogenesis of CRC and its phenotypic precursor lesions (polyps, adenomas) has revealed new insights which allow to identify individuals at risk for the development of the FAP or HNPCC syndrome as well as sporadic CRC.

In the absence of definitive primary prevention programs to identify individuals at risk for CRC development, conventional screening strategies are aimed at the identification of individuals at risk by careful family history, annual screening for fecal occult blood and the clinical detection and removal of CRC precursors (colorectal polyps or adenomas). Molecular markers of cancer, useful for prevention, early diagnosis and staging as well as for the prognosis and optimal therapy are increasingly emerging [25].

Familial adenomatous polyposis (FAP)

FAP is the most common dominantly inherited adenomatous polyposis syndrome. It is characterized by the progressive development of hundreds of adenomatous colorectal polyps and the inevitable development of CRC. The inheritance of FAP was genetically linked to chromosome 5q21 [26, 27]. After the discovery of germ-line mutations of the adenomatous polyposis coli (APC) gene on chromosome 5 in patients with FAP [28, 29], direct genetic testing of presymptomatic individuals became feasible.

In a study of 62 unrelated patients the presence of APC mutations in DNA from peripheral blood mononuclear cells was analyzed in two different ways [30]:

(i) Detection of a truncated APC protein by an *in vitro* synthesized-protein assay demonstrating shorter than normal APC gene products in 51 of the 62 patients with FAP.

(ii) Detection of the reduced expression of one allele of the APC gene by an allele-specific-expression assay, identifying another 3 of the remaining 11 patients with FAP.

The use of these two assays in combination, therefore, identified 54/62 patients with FAP (87%), making the routine molecular diagnosis of FAP in subjects at risk feasible.

Hereditary non-polyposis colorectal cancer (HNPCC)

Similar to the hereditary polyposis syndromes (adenomatous polyposis [FAP, Gardner's syndrome, Turcot's syndrome] and hamartomatous polyposis [Peutz-Jeghers syndrome, neuro-fibromatosis and others]), the HNPCC is an autosomal dominant disease. HNPCC affects predominantly the proximal colon and is characterized by an early age at onset (about 40 years), an accelerated adenoma-carcinoma sequence and the synchronous or metachronous development of mucinous or poorly differentiated colon cancers [13]. HNPCC, therefore, is phenotypically different from FAP with respect to number and location of polyps and CRCs, respectively.

Apart from taking a careful family history to assess conformity with HNPCC criteria as well as performing colonoscopy or follow-up colonoscopy every two years, genetic testing to detect mutations and DNA instability is being done already at some institutions. The discovery and characterization of additional genetic markers of DNA instability will eventually lead to the routine testing of DNA from peripheral blood mononuclear cells to screen individuals at risk for HNPCC.

Sporadic colorectal cancer

Sporadic CRCs account for about 85% of CRCs and parallel the incidence of colorectal polyps or adenomas. The phenotypic changes associated with the development of CRCs are paralleled by genetic changes *(figure 1)* and resulted in the concept that CRC is a multistep genetic disease. Apart from mutations of genes involved in DNA MMR, genetic alterations of three tumour suppressor genes have been identified in more than 70% of CRCs: the APC gene on chromosome 5 [31], the DCC gene on chromosome 18 [32] and the p53 gene on chromosome 17 [33].

Among the oncogenes the most frequent mutations in CRCs are found in the *ras* gene. Among the three *ras* genes H-, K- and N-*ras*, the most frequently altered *ras* gene is K-*ras*. Missense mutations are found predominantly in codons 12, 13 and 61 *(table III)*. The frequency of *ras* gene mutations correlates with the size of the lesions (adenoma < 2 cm 14%, adenoma > 2 cm 33%) and the degree of dysplasia (mild 0%, moderate 33%, severe or malignant 50%). *Ras* gene mutations, therefore, occur early in CRC development and may be a useful genetic marker for the molecular detection of this malignancy in a potentially curable stage. Further, the presence of a codon 12 GGT to GAT mutation *(table III)* in Duke's B or C CRC predicts a low risk of recurrence while other *ras* gene mutations are associated with a poor prognosis.

Table III. Most Frequent *ras* Gene Point Mutations in Colorectal Cancer

Wild-Type		Mutant	
Gly-12	GGT	GAT	Asp-12
	GGT	AGT	Ser-12
	GGT	TGT	Cys-12
	GGT	GCT	Ala-12
	GGT	GTT	Val-12
Gly-13	GGC	GAC	Asp-13
Gln-61	CAA	CAC	His-61

The molecular detection of *ras* gene mutations as a screening test for early CRC in stool is based on the concept that the mutations occur in 30-50% of growing adenomas and that epithelial cells of the gastrointestinal tract, including cells from tumours, are constantly shed into the gut lumen. It is estimated that the colon sheds about 10^{10} epithelial cells daily and that a lesion of 1 cm^3 accounts for about 1% of these cells. Sidransky *et al.* developed a method for the molecular detection of specific *ras* gene mutations in stool [34]: DNA is extracted from stool and a segment of the K-*ras* oncogene is amplified by PCR. The rare K-*ras* mutations are then identified either by cloning of the PCR product and sequencing or by plaque hybridization of the clones with *ras* mutant-specific oligodeoxynucleotide probes or by direct dot blot hybridization of the PCR product with *ras* mutant-specific oligodeoxynucleotide probes. The mutations found in stool were identical to those found in the subsequently surgically removed tumours. The analyses of DNA extracted from stool detected 90% of all tumours that carried K-*ras* mutations. With respect to the study group as a whole, however, the sensitivity of this molecular screening method for the detection of early CRCs was 33% (8/24) only. Compared to the sensitivity of conventional testing for faecal occult blood, the molecular screening for *ras* gene mutations, therefore, is of no routine clinical use at present. More recent developments include the detection of APC mutations in faecal DNA from patients with colorectal tumours [35] as well as of microsatellite mutations in faecal DNA from patients with proximal colorectal cancers [36], suggesting new approaches for the early detection of colorectal neoplasms. While technically impressive, these methods are clearly not ready for clinical application [37].

Staging

In view of the high sensitivity and specificity of molecular markers for a given cancer, genetic mutation analysis may be useful not only for detecting cancer but also in defining the extent of the disease and determining its prognosis. Indeed, p53 gene mutations were used to follow tumour spread into margins and draining lymph nodes of head and neck cancer patients [38]. Patients with mutation positive surgical-tissue margins or lymph nodes were found to have a high risk of recurrence and a poor overall survival. Similar results were obtained for K-ras or p53 gene mutations in patients with colorectal cancer [39].

Another encouraging type of marker is based on the detection of hypermethylated promoter regions of cancer associated genes in serum from patients with colorectal cancer [40]. Obviously, in principle any tumour-specific molecular marker is a potential candidate for the sensitive and specific detection of malignant cells.

Prognosis

A novel application of molecular markers is the prediction of recurrence of early-stage CRC. Using a new, quantitative approach, allelic imbalance was a better predictor of prognosis than the histopathological stage [41].

Prediction of benefit from therapy

In patients with CRC, the analysis of LOH and MSI at four loci (17p13, 18q22.3, 18q21.1, 5q21) revealed that retention of heterozygosity at one or more 17p or 18q sites was associated with a benefit from adjuvant fluorouracil therapy, suggesting that molecular markers may be predictive factors in treatment decisions [42]. Similarly, in another study fluorouracil-based adjuvant chemotherapy benefited patients with stage II or III CRC with microsatellite-stable tumours or tumours exhibiting low-frequency MSI but not those with tumours exhibiting high-frequency MSI [43].

Predictive cancer genomics and proteomics

With the completion of the sequencing of the human genome [1, 2] and the further development of novel analytical tools, *e.g*, DNA and RNA microarray analyses, it is now possible to detect changes in gene expression in normal and cancer cells of tens of thousands of genes in one experiment. High throughput mass spectroscopy further allows to compare protein profiles between normal and cancerous cells and tissues.

Table IV. Molecular Markers of FAP, HNPCC and Sporadic Colorectal Cancer

Disease Entity	Genetic Screening
FAP	Analysis of APC gene and protein in peripheral blood mononuclear cells
HNPCC	Analysis of *hMSH2, hMLH1, hPMS1, hPMS2* genes in peripheral blood mononuclear cells
Sporadic CRC	Microsatellite mutations in DNA from stool APC mutations in DNA from stool

The molecular classification of lymphomas [44], breast cancers [45-47] as well as GI cancers, such as esophageal cancer [48, 49], stomach cancer [50, 51], CRC [52-54], pancreatic cancer [54, 56] and HCC [57-59] by gene expression profiling has yielded remarkable first results that are highly relevant for the assessment of the patients' prognosis as well as the optimal therapeutic strategy. These approaches should eventually lead to a personalized profile relevant for the patient's optimal clinical management [60].

Summary and perspectives

With the better understanding of the genetic events leading to malignant transformation of normal cells, molecular markers will increasingly allow to identify individuals at risk of cancer development as well as improve (early) diagnosis, staging, assessment of prognosis and the selection of the optimal therapeutic strategy. Thus, molecular markers of cancer are becoming increasingly relevant for patient care and will eventually be an integral part of clinical medicine. For the clinician/surgeon, therefore, a basic understanding of molecular oncogenesis and of the principle and clinical relevance of molecular markers are essential to implement strategies to prevent, diagnose and treat different types of cancer. These aspects should translate into better patient care and a reduction of morbidity and mortality from GI cancer.

References

1. Lander ES, Linton LM, Birren B, *et al*. Initial sequencing and analysis of the human genome. *Nature* 2001; 409: 860-921. (Errata, *Nature* 411: 720; 412: 565.)
2. Venter JC, Adams MD, Myers EW, *et al*. The sequence of the human genome. *Science* 2001; 291: 1304-51. (Erratum, *Science* 2001; 292: 1838.)
3. Guttmacher AE, Collins FS. Genomic medicine – a primer. *N Engl J Med* 2002; 347: 1512-20.
4. Morales CP, Souza RF, Spechler SJ. Halmarks of cancer progression in Barrett's esophagus. *Lancet* 2002; 360: 1587-9.
5. Bergsland EK. Molecular mechanisms underlying the development of hepatocellular carcinoma. *Semin Oncol* 2001; 28: 521-31.
6. Rubin BP, Singer S, Tsao C, *et al*. KIT activation is a ubiquitous feature of gastrointestinal stromal tumours. *Cancer Res* 2001; 61: 8118-21.

7. Demetri GD, von Mehren M, Blanke CH, *et al.* Efficacy and safety of imatinib mesylate in advanced gastrointestinal stromal tumours. *N Engl J Med* 2002; 347: 472-80.
8. Hanahan D, Weinberg RA. The hallmarks of cancer. *Cell* 2000; 100: 57-70.
9. Fearon ER, Vogelstein B. A genetic model for colorectal tumorigenesis. *Cell* 1990; 61: 759-67.
10. Rustgi AK, Podolsky DK. The molecular basis of colon cancer. *Annu Rev Med* 1992; 43: 61-8.
11. Rustgi AK. Hereditary gastrointestinal polyposis and nonpolyposis syndromes. *N Engl J Med* 1994; 331: 1694-702.
12. Boland RC. Molecular basis for stool-based DNA tests for colorectal cancer: a primer for clinicians. *Rev Gastroenterol Disord* 2002; 2: S12-9.
13. Lynch HT, de la Chapelle A. Hereditary colorectal cancer. *N Engl J Med* 2003; 348: 919-32.
14. Sieber OM, Lipton L, Crabtree M, *et al.* Multiple colorectal adenoma, classic adenomatous polyposis, and germ-line mutations in MYH. *N Engl J Med* 2003; 348: 791-9.
15. Marra G, Jiricny J. Multiple colorectal adenomas – is their number up? *N Engl J Med* 2003; 348: 845-7.
16. Emery J, Lucassen E, Murphy M. Common hereditary cancers and implications for primary care. *Lancet* 2001; 358: 56-63.
17. Vogelstein B, Fearon ER, Kern SE, *et al.* Allelotype of colorectal carcinomas. *Science* 1989; 244: 207-11.
18. Lengauer C, Kinzler KW, Vogelstein B. Genetic instability in colorectal cancers. *Nature* 1997; 386: 623-7.
19. Ionov Y, Peinado MA, Malkhosyan S, *et al.* Ubiquitous somatic mutations in simple repeated sequences reveal a new mechanism for colonic carcinogenesis. *Nature* 1993; 363: 558-61.
20. Aaltonen LA, Peltomaki P, Leach FS, *et al.* Clues to the pathogenesis of colorectal cancer. *Science* 1993; 260: 812-6.
21. Thibodeau SN, Bren G, Schaid D. Microsatellite instability in cancer of the proximal colon. *Science* 1993; 260: 816-9.
22. Fishel R, Lescoe MK, Rao MRS, *et al.* The human mutator gene homolog MSH2 and its association with hereditary nonpolyposis colon cancer. *Cell* 1993; 75: 1027-38. (Erratum *Cell* 1994; 77: 167.)
23. Leach FS, Nicolaides NC, Papadopoulos N, *et al.* Mutations of a mut S homolog in hereditary non-polyposis colorectal cancer. *Cell* 1993; 75: 1215-25.
24. Toyota M, Ohe-Toyota M, Ahuja N, Issa JP. Distinct genetic profiles in colorectal tumours with or without the CpG island methylator phenotype. *Proc Natl Acad Sci USA* 2000; 97: 710-5.
25. Sidranski D. Emerging molecular markers of cancer. *Nature Reviews Cancer* 2002; 2: 210-9.
26. Joslyn G, Carlson M, Thliveris A, *et al.* Identification of deletion mutants and three new genes at the familial polposis locus. *Cell* 1991; 66: 601-13.
27. Kinzler KW, Nilbert MC, Su L-K, *et al.* Identification of FAP locus genes from chromosome 5q21. *Science* 1991; 253: 661-5.
28. Groden J, Thliveris A, Samowitz W, *et al.* Identification and characterization of the familial adenomatous polyposis coli gene. *Cell* 1991; 66: 589-600.
29. Nishisho I, Nakamura Y, Miyoshi Y, *et al.* Mutations of chromosome 5q21 genes in FAP and colorectal cancer patients. *Science* 1991; 253: 665-9.
30. Powell SM, Petersen GM, Krush AJ, *et al.* Molecular diagnosis of familial adenomatous polyposis. *N Engl J Med* 1993; 329: 1982-7.
31. Cottrell A, Bicknell D, Kaklamanis L, Bodmer WF. Molecular analysis of APC mutations in familial adenomatous polyposis and sporadic colon carcinomas. *Lancet* 1992; 340: 626-30.
32. Fearon ER, Cho KR, Nigro JM, *et al.* Identification of a chromosome 18q gene that is altered in colorectal cancers. *Science* 1990; 247: 49-56.
33. Baker SJ, Preisinger AC, Jessup JM, *et al.* p53 gene mutations occur in combination with 17p allelic deletions as late events in colorectal tumorigenesis. *Cancer Res* 1990; 50: 7717-22.

34. Sidransky D, Tokino T, Hamilton SR, et al. Identification of *ras* oncogene mutations in the stool of patients with curable colorectal tumours. *Science* 1992; 256: 102-5.
35. Traverso G, Shuber A, Levin B, et al. Detection of APC mutations in fecal DNA from patients with colorectal tumours. *N Engl J Med* 2002; 346: 311-20.
36. Traverso G, Shuber A, Olsson L, et al. Detection of proximal colorectal cancers through analysis of faecal DNA. *Lancet* 2002; 359: 403-4.
37. Schwartz RS. A needle in a haystack. *N Engl J Med* 2002; 346: 302-4.
38. Brennan JA, Mao L, Hruban RH, et al. Molecular assessment of histopathological staining in squamous cell carcinoma of the head and neck. *N Engl J Med* 1995; 332: 429-35.
39. Hayashi N, Arakawa H, Nagase H, et al. Genetic diagnosis identifies occult lymph node metastases undetectable by the histopathological method. *Cancer Res* 1994; 54: 3853-6.
40. Grady WM, Rajput A, Lutterbaugh JD, Markowitz SD. Detection of aberrantly methylated hMLH1 promotor DNA in the serum of patients with microsatellite unstable colon cancer. *Cancer Res* 2001; 61: 900-2.
41. Zhou W, Goodman SN, Galizia G, et al. Counting alleles to predict recurrence of early stage colorectal cancers. *Lancet* 2002; 359: 219-25.
42. Barratt PL, Seymour MT, Stenning SP, et al. DNA markers predicting benefit from adjuvant fluorouracil in patients with colon cancer: a molecular study. *Lancet* 2002; 360: 1381-91.
43. Ribic CM, Sargent DJ, Moore MJ, et al. Tumour microsatellite-instability status as a predictor of benefit from fluorouracil-based adjuvant chemotherapy for colon cancer. *N Engl J Med* 2003; 349: 247-57.
44. Alizadeh AA, Eisen MB, Davis RE, et al. Distinct types of diffuse large B-cell lymphoma identified by gene expression profiling. *Nature* 2000; 403: 503-11.
45. Huang E, Cheng SH, Dressmann H, et al. Gene expression predictors of breast cancer outcomes. *Lancet* 2003; 361: 1590-6.
46. Ramaswamy S, Prou CM. DNA microarrays in breast cancer: the promise of personalised medicine. *Lancet* 2003; 361: 1576-7.
47. Chang JC, Wooten EC, Tsimelzon A, et al. Gene expression profiling for the prediction of therapeutic response to docetaxel in patients with breast cancer. *Lancet* 2003; 362: 362-9.
48. Selaru FM, Zou T, Shustova V, et al. Global gene expression profiling in Barrett's esophagus and esophageal cancer: a comparative analysis using cDNA microarrays. *Oncogene* 2002; 21: 475-8.
49. Su H, Hu N, Shih J, et al. Gene expression analysis of esophageal squamous cell carcinoma reveals consistent molecular profiles related to family history of upper gastrointestinal cancer. *Cancer Res* 2003; 63: 3872-6.
50. Hasegawa S, Furukawa Y, Li M, et al. Genome-wide analysis of gene expression in intestinal-type gastric cancers using a complementary DNA microarray representing 23,040 genes. *Cancer Res* 2002; 62: 7012-7.
51. Inoue H, Matsuyama A, Mimory K, et al. Prognostic score of gastric cancer determined by cDNA microarray. *Clin Cancer Res* 2002; 8: 3475-9.
52. Suzuki H, Gabrielson E, Chen W, et al. A genomic screen for genes upregulated by demethylation and histone deacetylase ingibition in human colorectal cancer. *Nat Genet* 2002; 31: 141-9.
53. Williams NS, Gaynor RB, Scoggin S, et al. Identification and validation of genes involved in the pathogenesis of colorectal cancer using cDNA microarrays and RNA interference. *Clin Cancer Res* 2003; 9: 931-46.
54. Maxwell PJ, Longley DB, Latif F, et al. Identification of 5-fluorouracil-inducible target genes using cDNA microarray profiling. *Cancer Res* 2003; 63: 4602-6.
55. Logsdon CD, Simeone DM, Binkey C, et al. Molecular profiling of pancreatic adenocarcinoma and chronic pancreatitis identifies multiple genes differentially regulated in pancreatic cancer. *Cancer Res* 2003; 63: 2649-57.

56. Crnogorac-Jurcevic T, Efthimiou E, Nielsen T, et al. Expression profiling of microdissected pancreatic adenocarcinomas. *Oncogene* 2002; 21: 4587-94.
57. Iizuka N, Oka M, Yamada-Okabe H, et al. Differential gene expression in distinct virologic types of hepatocellular carcinoma: association with liver cirrhosis. *Oncogene* 2003; 22: 3007-14.
58. Iizuka N, Oka M, Yamada-Okabe H, et al. Oligonucleotide microarray for prediction of early intrahepatic recurrence of hepatocellular carcinoma after curative resection. *Lancet* 2003; 361: 923-9.
59. Chen X, Cheung ST, So S, et al. Gene expression patterns in human liver cancer. *Mol Biol Cell* 2002; 13: 1929-39.
60. Brenton JD, Caldas C. Predictive cancer genomics – what do we need? *Lancet* 2003; 362: 340-1.

Colitis-Associated Cancer – Time for New Strategies

Fergus Shanahan

Alimentary Pharmabiotic Centre, Department of Medicine, Cork University Hospital and University College Cork, National University of Ireland

Abstract

Colorectal cancer remains a feared and potentially life-threatening complication of both ulcerative colitis or Crohn's colitis. Currently, the main preventive strategy is a secondary one, i.e surveillance colonoscopy usually after 8 years of disease duration, when the risk for neoplasia begins to increase. Despite its widespread acceptance, dysplasia and cancer surveillance is unproven in terms of reducing mortality or morbidity and there is a remarkable lack of uniformity in the manner in which it is practised. In this overview, the pitfalls of dysplasia surveillance are summarised and the need for novel chemopreventive and perhaps pharmabiotic approaches for prevention are highlighted.

Introduction

Patients with long-standing ulcerative colitis and Crohn's disease are at increased risk of developing colorectal cancer. The major risk factors for this are disease extent and duration. The prevalence of cancer appears to rise after 8 years and then becomes exponential after 20 years [1-4]. There is also evidence that the risk may be increased in the presence of primary sclerosing cholangitis [5], a positive family history of sporadic colorectal cancer [6, 7] and backwash ileitis in patients with ulcerative colitis [8].

Effective strategies for preventing colitis-associated cancer will require some fundamental understanding of the mechanisms underlying both the inflammatory process and its associated cancer. Genetic and environmental factors contribute to the pathogenesis of inflammatory bowel disease and colorectal cancer [9, 10]. Although a common inherited factor influencing glycosylation of mucin has been proposed as a link between both forms of inflammatory bowel disease and risk of cancer [11, 12], the weight of evidence does not favour a common genetic link between inflammation and neoplasia of the colon [13]. The two processes are more likely to have a cause and effect relationship [14]. The underlying molecular basis for the linkage is not fully clear, but includes the impact of reactive oxygen and nitrogen species [15], and cytokines [16, 17] generated during the inflammatory process. These can alter the p53 tumour suppressor pathway, and thereby, increase the frequency of mutant cells resistant to apoptosis and promote the accumulation of additional oncogenic mutations.

Difficulties with current preventive strategies

Prophylactic colectomy is the only certain method of avoiding the risk of colorectal cancer, but it is seldom an attractive option. Surveillance colonoscopy is the mainstay of the management of cancer risk in patients with colitis, although it has not been proven to reduce mortality from colorectal cancer [18]. In addition, there are serious questions and pitfalls surrounding surveillance endoscopy for dysplasia and cancer, as it is currently practised [19]. Firstly, it appears that most gastroenterologists have a poor understanding of the term dysplasia. About 80% of American gastroenterologists did not appreciate that dysplasia means neoplasia confined to the epithelium and is not pre-neoplasia [20]. A survey in the United Kingdom showed a similar level of misunderstanding [21].

Secondly, there is a disturbing lack of uniformity in policy and details of surveillance practice amongst different gastroenterologists [20]. For example, the number of biopsies taken is highly variable and this influences sampling error. Thus, it has been estimated that to have a 95% confidence of finding the highest grade of neoplasm (dysplasia or cancer) 65 biopsies are required, and to find the highest degree of dysplasia, 33 biopsies are required [22]. It is doubtful whether many gastroenterologists are as rigorous as this.

Thirdly, even if sufficient samples are taken, the histologic interpretation of the biopsy may be problematic. In nonspecialist centres, the frequency of colonic dysplasia is low; consequently, so also is the experience of the local pathologist. This is important because even with experienced and specialised histologists, the inter-observer agreement for low-grade dysplasia is only about 60% [23].

Fourthly, if clinicians wait for high-grade dysplasia to develop before recommending colectomy, it may be too late to prevent invasive cancer. By the time high grade dysplasia is found, there will be an invasive cancer already present in up to 30% of cases [24]. In addition, several studies have indicated that a predictable progression from low- to high-grade dysplasia through invasive cancer may not be identifiable consistently [25-27]. Finally, even where best practice is observed with regular and rigorous colonoscopic biopsy techniques, colorectal cancer may escape early detection [25].

One conclusion from the available evidence is that the analysis of colonoscopic biopsy specimens by the light microscope alone is too insensitive; molecular markers that are predictive of progression to cancer at an earlier stage are needed. In the absence of reliable biomarkers of increased cancer risk, one has to question whether subjecting patients to a lifetime of annual or biennial colonoscopies is justifiable in terms of its dubious cost-effective impact on mortality.

Primary chemoprevention as a strategy

Since neither early detection of colorectal cancer nor accurate prediction of which patients are at higher risk can be guaranteed with current dysplasia surveillance techniques, the focus should shift toward primary prevention. Given that cancer appears to be the result of the inflammatory process, one might anticipate that effective maintenance of remission would reduce the risk of cancer.

The value of chemoprevention in colonic polyposis is well established and its role in preventing sporadic colorectal cancer is now being explored [28, 29]. The possibility that maintenance therapy with 5-aminosalicylate (5-ASA) might be protective against progression to neoplasia in patients with colitis has been raised by a retrospective case-control study [6]. There is also supportive experimental evidence that 5-ASA can reduce the spontaneous mutation rate at a (CA) 14 microsatellite [30]. In patients with colitis associated with primary sclerosing cholangitis, it has been reported that the risk of cancer can be reduced by ursodeoxycholic acid [31]. This observation requires confirmation, preferably with a prospective study; it may indicate that the relationship between sclerosing cholangitis and enhanced colorectal cancer risk, reflects cause and effect rather than a shared genetic predisposition.

Rationale for a pharmabiotic preventive strategy

Although colitis and cancer do not appear to share a common genetic aetiology, there is the intriguing possibility that environmental factors which prime the inflammatory process in susceptible individuals may also contribute to the pathogenesis of neoplasia. A sobering lesson on the interaction between genetics, host response and gut bacteria has already been learned in the case of *Helicobacteri pylori*, gastric inflammation and gastric cancer. The indigenous gastrointestinal microflora have also been implicated in the pathogenesis of inflammatory bowel disease and in colorectal tumorigenesis [32, 33]. This raises the possibility that modifying the flora or its metabolic activity by dietary prebiotics or food-grade probiotics might offer a preventive strategy against colon cancer.

The intestinal microflora has been shown to be essential for the development of spontaneous colonic adenocarcinoma in experimental knockout mice [34], and colitis-associated cancer in IL-10 knockout mice has been reduced by feeding with probiotics [35]. In humans, there is increasing evidence that the normal flora may influence carcinogenesis both positively and negatively by producing enzymes that convert pre-carcinogens to active carcinogens or, in some instances, transform carcinogens to inactive metabolites. Enzymes implicated in generating carcinogens include glyosidase, β-glucuronidase, azoreductase and nitroreductase [36]. Mechanisms by which probiotics might reduce the risk of colon carcinogenesis have been reviewed in detail elsewhere [37, 38]. These include metabolic effects, alteration of local microflora, and direct effects on the epithelium and the mucosal immune system. Of particular therapeutic potential is the generation of metabolites such as fatty acids, including conjugated linoleic acid (CLA). CLA may be of dietary origin or can be generated by commensals and probiotics. CLA is a natural ligand for peroxisome proliferator-activated receptors (PPAR-alpha and -gamma) and has been shown to have anti-inflammatory and anti-tumourigenic activities [39-41].

Epidemiologic studies of colon cancer risk reduction and consumption of fermented foods including those containing probiotics are difficult to perform and interpret, and have been inconclusive [42]. While controlled clinical trials in humans are desirable, they are, at present, impractical, mainly because of cost and long duration. Instead of studying cancer as an end-point, several surrogate biomarkers of cancer risk have been identified [43]. These include faecal enzymes, known co-carcinogens, and faecal water genotoxicity. Studies of the impact of prebiotics and probiotics on these intermediate markers are underway. While there is evidence for an impact on colon carcinogenesis [44, 45], it requires additional scientific scrutiny and rigorous prospective study.

Acknowledgement

The author is funded in part by the Health Reseach Board of Ireland, the Higher Education Authority of Ireland, Science Foundation Ireland and by the European Union (PROGID: QLKI-2000-00563). He also acknowledges the many stimulating discussions on the present topic with Dr. Charles Bernstein, University of Manitoba, Winnipeg, Canada.

References

1. Ekbom A, Helmick C, Zack M, Adami HO. Ulcerative colitis and colorectal cancer. A population-based study. *N Engl J Med* 1990; 323: 1228-33.
2. Eaden JA, Abrams KR, Mayberry JF. The risk of colorectal cancer in ulcerative colitis: a meta-analysis. *Gut* 2001; 48: 526-35.
3. Ekbom A, Helmick C, Zack M, Adami HO. Increased risk of large-bowel cancer in Crohn's disease with colonic involvement. *Lancet* 1990; 336: 357-9.
4. Bernstein CN, Kliewer E, Wajda A, Blanchard JF. The incidence of cancer among patients with IBD: A population-based study. *Cancer* 2001; 91: 854-62.
5. Shetty K, Rybicki L, Brzezinski A, Carey WD, Lashner BA. The risk for cancer or dysplasia in ulcerative colitis patients with primary sclerosing cholangitis. *Am J Gastroenterol* 1999; 94: 1643-9.
6. Eaden J, Abrams K, Ekbom A, Jackson E, Mayberry J. Colorectal cancer prevention in ulcerative colitis: a case-control study. *Aliment Pharmacol Ther* 2000; 14: 145-53.
7. Nuako KW, Ahlquist DA, Mahoney DW, Schaid DJ, *et al.* Familial predisposition for colorectal cancer in chronic ulcerative colitis: A case control study. *Gastroenterology* 1998; 115: 1079-83.
8. Heuschen UA, Hinz U, Allemeyer EH, *et al.* Backwash ileitis is strongly associated with colorectal carcinoma in ulcerative colitis. *Gastroenterology* 2001; 120: 841-7.
9. Shanahan F, O'Sullivan GC, O'Leary C. Colorectal cancer: still a major killer despite progress on many fronts. *Q J Med* 2000; 93: 131-4.
10. Shanahan F. Crohn's disease. *Lancet* 2002; 359: 62-9.
11. Rhodes JM. Lectins, colitis and colon cancer. *J R Coll Physicians Lond* 2000; 34: 191-6.
12. Rhodes JM. Unifying hypothesis for inflammatory bowel disease and associated colon cancer: sticking the pieces together with sugar. *Lancet* 1996; 347: 40-4.

13. Askling J, Dickman PW, Karlen P, et al. Colorectal cancer rates amongst first-degree relatives of patients with inflammatory bowel disease: a population-based cohort study. *Lancet* 2001; 357: 262-6.
14. Shanahan F. Relation between colitis and colon cancer. *Lancet* 2001; 357: 246-7.
15. Hussain SP, Amstad P, Raja K, et al. Increased p53 mutation load in noncancerous colon tissue from ulcerative colitis: a cancer-prone chronic inflammatory disease. *Cancer Res* 2000; 60; 3333-7.
16. Cordon-Cardo C, Prives C. At the crossroads of inflammation and tumorigenesis. *J Exp Med* 1999; 190: 1367-70.
17. Hudson JD, Shoaibi MA, Maestro R, Canrnero A, Hannon GJ, Beach DH. A pro-inflammatory cytokine inhibits p53 tumour suppressor activity. *J Exp Med* 1999; 190: 1375-82.
18. Bernstein CN. Cancer surveillance in inflammatory bowel disease. *Current Gastroenterology Reports* 1999; 1: 496-504.
19. Shanahan F. Discontent with dysplasia surveillance in ulcerative colitis. *Inflamm Bowel Dis* 1995; 1: 80-3.
20. Bernstein CN, Weinstein WM, Levine DS, Shanahan F. Physicians' perceptions of dysplasia and approaches to surveillance colonoscopy in ulcerative colitis. *Am J Gastroenterol* 1995: 90; 2106-14.
21. Eaden JA, Ward BA, Mayberry JF. How gastroenterologists screen for colonic cancer in ulcerative colitis: an analysis of performance. *Gastrointest Endosc* 2000; 51: 123-8.
22. Rubin CE, Haggitt RC, Burmer GC, et al. DNA aneuploidy in colonic biopsies predicts future development of dysplasia in ulcerative colitis. *Gastroenterology* 1992; 103: 1611-20.
23. Melville DM, Jass JR, Morson BC, et al. Observer study of the grading of dysplasia in ulcerative colitis. Comparison with clinical outcome. *Hum Pathol* 1989; 20: 1008-14.
24. Bernstein CN, Shanahan F, Weinstein WM. Are we telling patients the truth about surveillance colonoscopy in ulcerative colitis? *Lancet* 1994; 343: 71-4.
25. Connell WR, Lennard-Jones JE, Williams CB, Talbot IC, Price AB, Wilkinson KH. Factors affecting the outcome of endoscopic surveillance for cancer in ulcerative colitis. *Gastroenterology* 1994; 107: 934-44.
26. Ransohoff DF, Riddell RH, Levin B. Ulcerative colitis and colonic cancer: problems in assessing the diagnostic usefulness of mucosal dysplasia. *Dis Colon Rectum* 1985; 28: 383-8.
27. Taylor BA, Pemberton JH, Carpenter HA, et al Dysplasia in chronic ulcerative colitis: implications for colonoscopic surveillance. *Dis Colon Rectum* 1992; 35: 950-6.
28. Dannerberg AJ, Altorki NK, Boyle JO, et al. Cyclo-oxygenase 2: a pharmacologic target for the prevention of cancer. *Lancet Oncol* 2001; 2: 544-51.
29. Sharma RA. Translational medicine: targetting cyclo-oxygenase isoenzymes to prevent cancer. *Q J Med* 2002; 95: 267-73.
30. Gasche C, Goel A, Boland CR. 5-aminosalicylic acid (5-ASA) but not acetylsalicylic acid (Aspirin) reduces the spontaneous mutation rate at a (CA)13 microsatellite (MS). *Gastroenterology* 2001; 120: A651.
31. Tung BY, Emond MJ, Haggitt RC, et al. Ursodiol use is associated with lower prevalence of colonic neoplasia in patients with ulcerative colitis and primary sclerosing cholangitis. *Ann Intern Med* 2001; 134: 89-95.
32. Berg RD. The indigenous gastrointestinal microflora. *Trends Microbiol* 1996; 4: 430-5.
33. Shanahan F. Probiotics and inflammatory bowel disease: is there a scientific rationale? *Inflammatory Bowel Disease* 2000; 6: 107-15.
34. Kado S, Uchida K, Funabashi H, et al. Intestinal microflora are necessary for development of spontaneous adenocarcinoma of the large intestine in T-cell receptor β chain and p53 double-knockout mice. *Cancer Res* 2001; 61: 2395-8.
35. O'Mahony L, Feeney M, O'Halloran S, et al. Pro-biotic impact on microbial flora, inflammation and tumour development in IL-10 knockout mice. *Aliment Pharmacol Ther* 2001; 15: 1219-25.
36. Rolfe RD. The role of pro-biotic cultures in the control of gastrointestinal health. *J Nutr* 2000; 130: 396S-402S.

37. Dugas B, Mercenier A, Lenoir-Wijnkoop I, Arnaud C, Dugas N, Postaire E. Immunity and probiotics. *Immunol Today* 1999; 20: 387-90.
38. Rafter J. Lactic acid bacteria and cancer: mechanistic perspective. *Br J Nut* 2002; 88 (Suppl. 1): S89-94.
39. Hontecillas R, Wannemeulher MJ, Zimmerman DR, *et al*. Nutritional regulation of porcine bacterial-induced colitis by conjugated linoleic acid. *J Nutr* 2002; 132: 2019-27.
40. Yu Y, Correll PH, Vanden Heuvel JP. Conjugated linoleic acid decreases production of pro-inflammatory products in macrophages: evidence for a PPAR-g-dependent mechanism. *Biochem Biophys Acta* 2002; 1581: 89-99.
41. Vanden Heuval JP. Peroxisome proliferator-activated receptors: a critical link among fatty acids, gene expression and carcinogenesis. *J Nutr* 1999; 129: 575S-580S.
42. Rafter JJ. The role of lactic acid bacteria in colon cancer prevention. *Scand J Gastroenterol* 1995; 30: 497-502.
43. Gill CIR, Rowland IR. Diet and cancer: assessing the risk. *Br J Nutr* 2002; 88 (Suppl. 1): S73-87.
44. Wollowski I, Rechkemmer G, Pool-Zobel BL. Protective role of probiotics and prebiotics in colon cancer. *Am J Clin Nutr* 2001; 73 (Suppl. 2): 451S-455S.
45. Pool-Zobel B, van Loo J, Rowland I, Roberfroid MB. Experimental evidence on the potential of pre-biotic fructans to reduce the risk of colon cancer. *Br J Nutr* 2002; 87 (Suppl. 2): S273-81.

New developments in diagnosis and management of early and advanced GI malignancy.
G.N. Tytgat, F. Penninckx, eds. John Libbey Eurotext, Paris © 2003, pp. 113-129.

Stress response after laparoscopic surgery

M. Buunen[1], M. Gholghesaei[1], R. Veldkamp[1],
N.D. Bouvy[1], D.W. Meijer[2], H.J. Bonjer[1]

[1] Department of Surgery, Erasmus Medical Center Rotterdam, Rotterdam, The Netherlands
[2] Laboratory of Experimental Surgery, AMC University Hospital of Amsterdam, Amsterdam, The Netherlands

Summary

Background: Laparoscopic surgery is associated with reduced surgical trauma, and therefore with less induction of acute phase response to injury. Diminished impairment of the immune system may prevent surgical infections, port-site metastases and sepsis. The objective of this study was to assess the immunologic consequences of laparoscopic surgery and to highlight controversial aspects. Methods: Literature search on immunologic changes during laparoscopy and open surgery was conducted using Medline and Cochrane databases. Cross-references from the reference list of major articles on the subject were used. We focused on literature published from 1993 until now. Results: Peritoneal immune function seems to be altered by the application of a carbon dioxide pneumoperitoneum. A diminished production of Tumour Necrosis Factor (TNF) by, and phagocytosis capacity of peritoneal macrophages is apparent. The systemic stress response shows a preservation of immune function following laparoscopy in comparison with conventional surgery. A pronounced difference in Delayed Type Hypersensitivity (DTH) response and a diminished reduction of leukocyte antigen expression on lymphocytes sustain the finding of a better preserved immune function. Conclusion: The peritoneal response to laparoscopic surgery shows suppression of host defence mechanism. However the systemic response and the better maintained immune function postoperatively, compensate this shortcoming of laparoscopic surgery.

Background

Laparoscopic surgery has certain advantages over open surgery among which are faster recovery, shorter hospital stay and quicker return to daily activity. The impact of the surgical stress on the immune response is a possible predictive factor of patients' clinical outcome [1-4]. Laparoscopic surgery induces less trauma and is therefore less aggravating for the immune system [5]. In this review, several different aspects of immunology are considered. To improve insight, a distinction was made between local, *i.e.* peritoneal immunity, and systemic immunity. Preservation of the peritoneal and systemic immune system is important to prevent (postoperative-) infections, sepsis and possibly adherence of tumour cells to the port-site wound. There seems to be a general understanding, that open surgery has more impact on the immune system than the laparoscopic approach [6]. Establishing a carbon dioxide pneumoperitoneum mainly causes peritoneal impairment. Peritoneal macrophages seem to produce less cytokines and its intrinsic function (phagocytosis) diminishes in the presence of carbon dioxide [7, 8]. In recent literature, in which researchers are in search of a new gas for the application of a pneumoperitoneum, helium is the most likely substitute. The objective of this study was to assess the immunologic consequences after laparoscopic surgery and to highlight controversial aspects, by reviewing the literature on this subject.

Peritoneal immunity

Two immunological changes within the peritoneal cavity are apparent. Both are probably caused by the application of a carbon dioxide pneumoperitoneum. The first alteration is a diminished production of tumour necrosis factor (TNF) by peritoneal macrophages. The second change of the local immune system is the reduction in phagocytosis activity of peritoneal macrophages.

Insufflation gases

Carbon dioxide (CO_2) is the insufflation gas of choice in laparoscopy. It is preferred above air insufflation, which affects the systemic and peritoneal response to a larger degree than carbon dioxide does [9]. There are some important advantages to its usage; it is transparent, noninflammable, well dissolvable in blood and it has a rapid pulmonary excretion [10]. There are however some disadvantages associated with its usage. *Table I* shows physical alterations associated with the application of a carbon dioxide pneumoperitoneum. Any pneumoperitoneum whether established with carbon dioxide or any other insufflation gas, reduces cardiac output and stroke volume due to increased abdominal pressure [11, 12]. Respiratory acidosis, port-site recurrence, enhanced formation of tumour growth and adhesions (subject of discussion), immunological alterations and possible bacterial translocation are specific carbon dioxide mediated alterations [7, 8, 13-20]. To avoid problems with local immunity some researchers propose the application of helium as an alternative insufflation gas. Helium is an inert gas, and does not cause acidosis, nor is it associated with enhanced tumour growth. Adhesion formation and immunological changes are less after helium compared with changes following carbon dioxide pneumoperitoneum. Several animal studies on the subject of immunologic alterations during pneumoperitoneum, were conducted comparing helium and carbon dioxide insufflation. In each of these studies the poor solubility of helium must be taken into consideration. The poor solubility is inherent to the use of helium, increasing the risk of embolisms. That is why helium insufflation should not be used for laparoscopic operations involving an increased risk of embolism (*e.s.* hepatic resection).

Table I. Alterations associated with the application of pneumoperitoneum with CO_2 as insufflation gas

Cardiovascular[a]	Reduction in CO[b]	Galizia et al. 2001 [11]
	Reduction in SVI[b]	Zuckerman et al. 2001 [12]
Respiratory	Acidosis	Jacobi et al. 2000 [13]
Oncology	Port-site recurrence	Bouvy et al. 1998 [15]
	Tumour growth	Smidt et al. 2001 [17]
Hematology	Activation of tPA[b], adhesions	Nagelschmidt et al. 2001 [16] Jacobi et al. 2001 [14]
Immunology	Diminished production of TNF[b]	West et al. 1996 [7] Iwanaka et al. 1997 [18] Hajri et al. 2000 [8]
	Reduction in phagocytosis of mononuclear phagocytosis system	Gutt et al. 1997 [19]
Microbiology	Bacterial translocation	Erenoglu et al. 2001 [20]

[a] Not solely dependent on pneumoperitoneum, also of Trendelenberg position.
[b] CO = Cardiac Output, SVI = Stroke Volume Index, tPA = tissue Plasminogen Activator, TNF = Tumour Necroses Factor.

Macrophage TNF production

In 1996 West et al. [7] investigated in a murine model production of TNF by peritoneal macrophages stimulated by lipopolysaccharid as an immune enhancer. Despite sufficient production of messenger RNA (mRNA), reversible inhibition of TNF was noticed after 30 minutes of incubation with carbon dioxide. Interleukin-1 (IL-1) production was reversibly inhibited as well, but also showed a diminished production of mRNA. A comparable significant change in cytokine production by macrophages has not been reported in the helium- and air-group. In a study by Watson et al. [9] the production of TNF and superoxide was rather more in the air-group. After 2 hours carbon dioxide peritoneum in rats, Hajri et al. [8] noticed a decline in TNF-production and also a reduction in TNF mRNA. One year later West [21] hypothesized that a reduction of intracellular pH may cause a decrease in the production of cytokines. They concluded that carbon dioxide reduces the pH affecting the inflammatory response in a negative manner.

Kuntz et al. [22] substantiated this finding. The intra-abdominal pH diminishes with appliance of a carbon dioxide pneumoperitoneum. In a rat model they investigated the effect of various gases, pressures and durations of pneumoperitoneum. Carbon dioxide as insufflation gas appears to lower peritoneal-, blood- and subcutaneous pH, more than helium does, which induces smaller changes, in comparison with the carbon dioxide group. The intraperitoneal pH is inversely related to the intra-abdominal pressure.

Peritoneal cell mediated response

In a rat model, Gutt el al. [19] produced evidence of suppressed phagocytosis activity of the mononuclear phagocytosis system when using carbon dioxide. They found significant changes in carbon clearance by phagocytosis between laparoscopy and laparotomy, with a half-life of 16.1 minutes for laparotomy and a half life of 21.91 minutes for laparoscopy. The fastest elimination of carbon particles was found after gasless laparoscopic surgery (half-life of 12.86 minutes). The activity of peritoneal macrophages partly depends on cytokine stimulation, which production is also reduced.

In a murine model, Chekan et al. [23] examined the immune competence of mice based on their ability to clear intraperitoneal administered Listeria Monocytogenes (LM) following carbon dioxide *versus* helium insufflation, or laparotomy. On day 3, they found significant impairment of the intraperitoneal immunity after carbon dioxide insufflation, more so than after helium pneumoperitoneum or after laparotomy. Significantly more bacteria in spleen and liver were found in the laparoscopic group, than in controls. The intraperitoneal immune suppression lasted for 5 days.

Clearance of peritoneal bacteria was also investigated by Balague et al. [24]. They reported a diminished peritoneal macrophage function after intra-abdominal contamination with *Escherichia Coli* suspension, measured by the number of colony forming units obtained in peritoneal fluid and positive blood culture rates.

Other factors

Other factors contributing to the disruption of immunologic balance within the peritoneal cavity are gas pressure and temperature, tissue trauma and mechanical effects. For example, higher levels of cytokines (TNFα, IL-1 and IL-6) were found at room temperature after performing a laparoscopic operation [25].

Systemic stress response

The systemic immune response of a carbon dioxide pneumoperitoneum has been investigated most thoroughly. Results of several studies demonstrate a greater uniformity than peritoneal immunologic changes. Open surgery has more impact on systemic immunity than laparoscopic surgery does, primarily based on clinical trials following cholecystectomies [6]. Variables used to measure the systemic response to injury are mainly cytokine levels, T cell function, T cell subsets, and expression of Major Histocompatibility Complex (MHC) on antigen presenting cells.

Cytokines

The group of cytokines is varied. Their effect is mainly restricted to the area surrounding the producing cell, paracrine or autocrine. Besides activation, cytokines enhance proliferation and differentiation (*e.g.* IL-6, growth factor for B-cells), chemotaxis and occasionally they exhibit cytotoxic activity (*e.g.* INFα and TNFα). The acute-phase response is a good indicator for tissue injury in patient [26]. Production of acute-phase proteins by liver cells often increases a thousand-fold, as does C-reactive protein (CRP). This reaction of liver cells is induced by corticosteroids and cytokines, of which IL-6 is the main activator. The rise in serum IL-1α is one of the early systemic immune events following surgery. It precedes and directs hepatic release of IL-6. IL-6 in turn directs hepatic release of CRP [8]. During recovery levels of acute-phase proteins normalize.

The above mentioned acute phase-reaction is best measured by establishing the levels of CRP and IL-6 [27]. These are the most frequently investigated cytokines. Differences between laparoscopic and open surgery are most pronounced 24 hours postoperative. Three days after surgery, no difference can be found between open and laparoscopic surgery [28]. Postoperative CRP levels are significantly lower after laparoscopy, suggesting a lower burden on immunity [29-33]. No difference was found between mini-laparotomy and laparoscopy [34].

The outcomes of clinical as well as experimental studies show a reduced immune reaction after laparoscopic surgery. This is made clear by a diminished production of cytokines IL-1, IL-6 and CRP. Changes in TNF, IL-8 and acute phase protein fibrinogen, albumin and transferrin are less clear [6]. These results are mainly derived from clinical trials, comparing open cholecystectomy with laparoscopic cholecystectomy.

In the past years, more research has been conducted on other surgical procedures and their impact on the immune system. In a randomized clinical trial conducted by Malik *et al.* [35], no significant changes ($p = 0.066$) were found in CRP concentration between women undergoing laparoscopically assisted vaginal hysterectomy (LAVH) or abdominal hysterectomy (AH). There was a significant increase in IL-6 in patients undergoing AH peaking 2 hours postoperatively and remaining significantly elevated for 12 hours postoperatively, when compared to the IL-6 levels of patients undergoing vaginal hysterectomy (VH) or LAVH ($p < 0.05$).

In a trial by Kishi *et al.* [30], CRP and leukocyte counts (LC) were measured after laparoscopically assisted ileocolectomy (LAC) compared to conventional bowel surgery by patients suffering from morbus Crohn. CRP and LC were both significantly ($p < 0.05$ and $p = 0.05$ respectively) lower after LAC. A difference in stress response was also found following inguinal hernia repair. Concentrations of CRP, malonyldialdehyde (MDA), creatine phosphokinase (CPK) and LC rose in the open as well in the laparoscopic group, but there were significant differences between these two groups. The levels of these proteins and the amount of cells was less disturbed after laparoscopic surgery [31].

Cellular immunity

Cellular immunity consists of non-specific defence and antigen-specific host defence. The first system entails NK cells, granulocytes and monocytes/macrophages, all part of the initial reaction to pathogens. The antigen-specific host defence is primarily represented by T lymphocytes, and is involved with a durable immune reaction.

T cell function: delayed type hypersensitivity response

The Delayed Type Hypersensitivity (DTH) test is of clinical importance to ascertain cross-reaction on T cell level. The tuberculin skin test reaction is well known. In particular T cell function is tested on the basis of DTH-response. It consists of three phases a cognitive phase, an activation phase and an effector phase *(table II)*.

Table II. Delayed Type Hypersensitivity (DTH) test

Cognitive phase	Antigen expression to $CD4^+$ T cells
Activation phase	Cytokine release by $CD4^+$ T cells
Effector phase	Inflammation, differentiation & activation of mononuclear phagocytes

Measurement of the area or magnitude of induration at the site of application, determines the immune response. The bigger the induration of the skin, the more active the immune response is. Postoperative immune suppression takes place in the effector phase of the DTH-response [36]. Absence of DTH-response is associated with a poorer prognosis [37].

Animal studies have shown a better preservation of post operative-operative cell-mediated immune function after laparoscopic surgery compared to laparotomy [5, 36, 38, 39]. This is partly explained by smaller incisions.

A more pronounced difference was found in a prospective non-randomized clinical trial of Schietroma *et al.* [40]. Two groups of patients, open (n = 31) *versus* closed technique (n = 32), underwent cholecystectomy. Until postoperative day three a significantly smaller DTH-response was found in favour of laparoscopy. In a similar study, some years before Schietromas and Kloosterman *et al.* [41] drew a comparable conclusion. On the first postoperative day, they demonstrate a significant diminished reaction on photohemagglutinin (PHA). After 6 days the immune system seems to have recovered from the operation [41].

T cell response: CD4/CD8 expression

T cell metabolism can be expressed in part by measuring the expression of protein molecules on the cell membrane of T lymphocytes during maturation. They are classified according to their reactivity to the same immunologic markers. These clusters are attached to a code: the CD ("cluster of differentiation") code. The codes for leukocyte antigens of T helper cells and cytotoxic T cells are respectively CD4 and CD8.

After any kind of operation CD4/CD8 ratio changes significantly compared to anaesthesia alone. This is due to an increased amount of $CD4^+$ cells and a decrease in $CD8^+$ lymphocytes [42].

These findings are validated in animal studies, *i.e.* rats. From human studies no clear response can be elucidated. A comparison between total laparoscopically performed colorectal resections and open colorectal resections did not demonstrate any significant changes between these operating procedures concerning T cell response. But after laparoscopically assisted colorectal resection the CD4/CD8 ratio was significantly higher compared to conventional colorectal resection [43]. This was confirmed by a randomized clinical trial by Liang et al. [29]. They evaluated clinical outcomes and operative stress of laparoscopically assisted colectomy versus traditional open management of sigmoid complex polyps. Forty-two patients were equally randomized to either open or laparoscopic resection. CD4/CD8 ratio was significantly less elevated as was the total lymphocyte counts (LC), in the laparoscopic group. The investigators concluded, not only on the basis of CD4/CD8 and LC but also on CRP levels and Erythrocyte Sedimentation Rate (ESR) 24 hours after surgery laparoscopically assisted sigmoidectomy to causes less operative stress. They recommend the use of this technique in the management of sigmoid complex polyps.

In a prospective randomized clinical trial by Perttilä et al. [44], patients were divided into two groups for Nissen fundoplication: laparoscopically or by laparotomy. Attention was focused on subsets of lymphocytes. No significant differences were found between the two groups. In both groups the amount of $CD4^+$ T cells and $CD8^+$ T cells increased. Two days postoperative the number of T cells normalized. Walker et al. [45] also observed less $CD4^+$ cells and an increase in $CD8^+$ lymphocytes, contrary to findings in animals. They investigated modulation of lymphocytes after laparoscopic cholecystectomy. The CD4/CD8 ratio decreased due to an increase of $CD8^+$ cells, up till 7 days after surgery. After cholecystectomy in patients with post-necrotic liver cirrhosis or hepatitis C, CD4 andCD8 levels remained unchanged until 24 hours after surgery [46]. Clinical consequences of changes in CD4/CD8 ratio remain relatively unknown.

Two kinds of $CD4^+$ T cells are known, these are T helper 1 (Th1) cells; producing IL-2, IFN-α and TNF-α which in turn enhances cellular immunity and T helper 2 (Th2) cells enhancing the production of immunoglobulin (Ig) by producing IL-4-6, IL-10 and IL-13, therefore maintaining the homeostasis of the host immune system. Following laparoscopic surgery the ratio between these two cells changes. Although clinical relevance is not clear. However in theory, there is a relative shortage of cellular immunity and it is assumed that preservation or elevation of the Th1/Th2 ratio is of benefit to the patient [47].

Monocyte function: HLA-DR expression

Expression of class II Major Histocompatibility Complex (MHC) molecules on antigen presenting cells is a necessity for effective antigen presentation and subsequent elimination of the antigen. In phagocytosis, antigens are incorporated in the cell. The lysosomal system breaks down the antigen into peptides, those peptides bind with HLA class II within the endosomes. The HLA-II-molecule with peptide is expressed on the cell membrane. T helper cells ($CD4^+$) recognize the paired molecules and adheres to it. This leads to an activation of the T cell. Monocyte HLA-DR expression is a reliable marker for infection. Reduced expression of MHC class II molecules, particular HLA-DR, is associated with an impaired ability to eliminate pathogens effectively. Subsequently, it seems to be related with an increased risk of infection [48]. Expression of HLA-DR is reduced in open surgery [49]. HLA-DR expression after laparoscopic surgery is preserved [41]. In 1993, Kloosterman and colleagues demonstrated HLA-DR expression to be significantly less following laparoscopic cholecystectomy than following conventional cholecystectomy. After laparoscopic surgery an increase was noticed, but did not differ significantly from baseline levels. Six days postoperatively the expression returned to preoperative values. More recent studies [40, 49] confirmed these findings. A randomized clinical trial by Hewitt *et al.* [43] comparing laparoscopic-assisted *versus* open surgery for colorectal cancer, showed other values of HLA-DR expression on monocytes. A significant reduction was found after both surgical procedures, with no difference between open and laparoscopic surgery. Restoration was not noticed 7 days postoperatively. After 21 days a complete recovery to baseline was noted.

Systemic phagocytosis function remains unaltered after laparoscopic surgery. Sietses *et al.* [50] compared phagocytosis by polymorphonuclear lymphocytes after open laparoscopical Nissen fundoplication. In the laparoscopic group the opsonic capacity was not altered and thereby preserving the ability of polymorphonuclear lymphocytes to phagocytose bacteria.

In a murine model Lee *et al.* [51] evaluated cell-mediated immunity by examining lymphocyte proliferation rates after laparotomy *versus* carbon dioxide insufflation. Lymphocyte proliferation rate was significantly lower than in both control and insufflation groups. Between control and insufflation group no differences were observed.

Particles entering the circulatory system are not removed by circulating macrophages. Macrophages residing in liver (Kupffer cells) and spleen take care of the clearance of these particles. Opsonisation enhances this elimination process. The role of fixed tissue macrophages, reticulo-endothelial system (RES), is hardly investigated. From what is known, the RES experiences no suppression when a carbon dioxide pneumoperitoneum is established. TNFα and IL-6 production by Kupffer cells which make up 80 percent of the RES is not altered significantly in a rat model [52].

Oncology and laparoscopy

Most literature on oncologic laparoscopic surgery is based on colorectal resections *(table III)*. Laparoscopy was long time associated with an increased risk of metastasis of the abdominal wall at the site of incisions, the so-called port site metastasis. This was considered to be related to mechanical contamination of the port-site wound.

In 1991, a prospective laparoscopic registry was initiated under the auspices of the American Society of Colon and Rectal Surgeons. For the duration of one year, patients undergoing laparoscopic colon resection were voluntarily entered and followed. Recurrences were evaluated by the primary surgeon and reported to the registry. A total of 480 patients were included and followed for one year. Wound recurrence was identified in 5 patients making for an overall incidence of 1.1 percent [53]. This rate of incidence is comparable with wound recurrence rates after open surgery, which is between 0.6 to 1.5 percent [54, 55], depending on definition of such recurrence. It seems that the incidence of wound recurrences after laparoscopic colon resection seems to be low. Although follow-up was short, 80% of recurrences became manifest within the first year.

Table III. Stress response after colorectal resections

Delgado [58]	2001	RCT	To compare acute phase postoperative response in patients diagnosed with colon neoplasm undergoing either open or laparoscopic resection.
Fukushima [59]	1996	Clinical trial	To compare effects of open and laparoscopic colectomy on cytokine and stress hormone responses.
Hewitt [43]	1998	Clinical trial	To test the hypothesis of an immunologic advantage for laparoscopic assisted resection.
Leung [69]	1999	Clinical trial	Review results of lap-assisted colorectal resection.
Leung [71]	2000	Clinical trial	To compare the systemic cytokine response after laparoscopic ass. resection with those after open resection of rectosigmoid.
Liang [29]	2002	Clinical trial	To evaluate outcomes and operative stress of lap-assisted colectomy *versus* traditional open method.
Mehigan [63]	2001	Clinical trial	To study perioperative immune response in patients undergoing lap-assisted or open colorectal surgery.
Nishiguchi [60]	2001	Clinical trial	To measure stress response to laparoscopic surgery compared with open surgery.
Ordemann [49]	2001	RCT	Investigation of the hypothesis; if short-term benefits of laparoscopy are due to diminished cytokine response and cell mediated immunity.
Schwenk [61]	2000	RCT	To examine the cytokine and acute-phase response after laparoscopic and conventional surgery in a clinical setting.
Sietses [70]	2000	Clinical trial	To study the influence of several laparoscopical procedures on IL-6 and monocyte mediated toxicity.
Tang [64]	2001	RCT	To investigate the metabolic stress response of laparoscopically assisted colorectal resection *versus* open resection.
Vermorken [72]	1999	RCT	To investigate if adjuvant active specific immunotherapy is more benificial than resection alone.
Vukasin [53]	1996	Prospective registry	To evaluate the incidence of cancer recurrence after laparoscopic resection of colon cancers.

RCT = Randomized clinical trial.

A recent randomized clinical trial (n = 219) by Lacy *et al.* [56] compared laparoscopy-assisted resection of the colon with open resections. In a median follow-up of 43 months, no significant differences were found between the two operating procedures concerning tumour recurrence. Tumour recurrence in the laparoscopy-assisted group was noticed in 18 cases (17%), which was not significantly different (P = 0.07) from the open conventional group, in which 28 cases (27%) were identified. A significant difference was also found in cancer-related mortality. In the open group 21% died compared with 9% mortality in the laparoscopy-assisted group (p = 0.03). The mechanism by which LAC is associated with tumour recurrence is not known. Association with immunological changes might explain their findings.

Still the question, if an impaired local immunity will improve tumour growth, *i.e.* improve metastasis, remains unanswered. Neuhaus reversed this question; would enhancing of local immunity with endotoxin reduce the risk of port-site recurrences? By injecting endotoxin intraperitoneal eighteen hours before operation, it seems possible to lessen this risk [57].

Cytokine response

Changes in patients immune function can be demonstrated in cytokine response, antigen expression, production of immune globulin and in the cell mediated immune system. The cytokine response starts with an increase of acute phase proteins, of which IL-6, CRP and IL-1α are the most investigated. In *table IV* and *table V*, literature on cytokine responses, interleukine-6 and C-reactive protein, is listed [43, 49, 58-62]. Most studies suggest a decreased interleukin-6 response. Only one study reported a higher serum level of IL-6. One study did not find any significant difference. Although IL-6 levels were less impaired, other studies found conflicting data on other immunological parameters (like IL-10, IL-1RA). Literature on CRP levels after colorectal resection is not consistent either *(table V)*. Animal studies did not exhibit a marked difference in CRP response [62]. Also no difference in tumour growth and spread was noticed [8]. An indication of a reduced response to injury in humans was demonstrated in three studies. On the contrary one out of four (randomized-) clinical trials however showed no significant differences [58-61].

Cell mediated immune response

As described previously, the cell-mediated immune system is preserved after laparoscopic surgery. But does a preserved systemic cellular immune system diminish tumour growth? In an athymic mice experiment Allendorf *et al.* [38] investigated if T cell deficiency caused an increase of tumour growth. Immunocompetent and athymic mice, with mouse mammary carcinoma cells injected in the dorsal skin, underwent either laparoscopy or midline laparotomy. Tumours grew much larger in the athymic group. In immunocompetent mice, tumour growth in laparotomy was larger than in the laparoscopy group, which was 1.5 times larger than control. T cell function seems to be necessary in suppressing tumour growth. Laparoscopy is likely to comply with this necessity.

Cell mediated immunity can be assessed in different ways. Gitzelmann *et al.* [39] compared the effects of carbon dioxide pneumoperitoneum and laparotomy on the delayed type hypersensitivity (DTH) response, in a mouse model. All mice were sensitised to keyhole limpet hemocyanin (KLH) and to a mouse mammarian carcinoma cell line (MC2) before surgery. Tumour growth and DTH-response were assessed postoperatively. The DTH-response after laparotomy was significantly lower compared with control and pneumoperitoneum. Tumour growth was significantly increased on days 2 and 3 postoperatively compared with pneumoperitoneum and control. Cellular immunity seems to be more debilitated after laparotomy than after a carbon dioxide pneumoperitoneum, losing the ability to reject immunogenic tumour. Both studies suggest functioning T cells are necessary in efficient resistance to tumour growth.

Table IV. Measurements of plasma interleukin-6 levels (IL-6) in pg/ml[a]

	Preoperative	Serum level Lap	Serum level Open	Significance	Remarks[b]
Delgado 2001 [58]	n.a.	239.5 (49.1-645.7)	372.7 (31.4-3,226)	$p < 0.05$	Colectomy Clinical trial
Fukushima 1996 [59]	n.a.	was significantly higher after laparoscopy		$p < 0.05$	Sigmoid colectomy Clinical trial
Hewitt 1998 [43]	n.a.	173 (sd 156)	313 (sd 294)	NS	Colorectal resection Rand. clin. trial
Kuntz 2000	~ 200	287 ± 180	517 ± 208	$p < 0.015$	Ascending colon resection Rat model
Nishiguchi 2001 [60] (abstract)	n.a.	was significantly lower after laparoscopy		$p < 0.05$	Colorectal resection Clinical trial
Ordemann 2001 [49]	n.a.	was significantly lower after laparoscopy		$p < 0.01$	Colorectal resection Rand. clin. trial
Schwenk 2000 [61]	4.25 (3.4-7.7)	34.0 (25.6-48.7)	50.5 (39.8-75.7)	$p < 0.03$	Colorectal resection Rand. clin. trial

[a] n.a. = not available, sd = standard deviation, NS = not significant, pg/ml = picogram per milliliter.
[b] Rand. clin. trial = Randomized clinical trial.

Table V. Measurements of plasma C-reactive protein (CRP) in mg/dl

	Preoperative	Lap	Open	Significance	Remarks
Delgado 2001 [58]	n.a.	6.9 ± 4.5	9.1 ± 4.8	$p < 0.01$	Colectomy Clinical trial
Fukushima 1996 [59]	n.a.	n.a.	n.a.	NS	Sigmoid colectomy Clinical trial
Nishiguchi 2001 [60] (abstract)	n.a.	was significantly lower after laparoscopy		$p < 0.05$	Colorectal resection Clinical trial
Schwenk 2000 [61]	n.a.	40 (33.0-49.4)	61.2 (52.0-77.9)	$p < 0.002$	Colorectal resection Rand. clin. trial

n.a. = not available, NS = not significant, mg/dl = milligram per deciliter.

Changes in T cell (subset) counts after laparoscopy compared with open conventional surgery, have not been clarified. There is not enough research on T cell counts to make a concise statement on the subject. Most studies report no difference between open and laparoscopically performed colorectal resections in lymphocyte counts. Neither did they find any difference in T cell count or subsets [43, 63, 64]. Ordemann et al. [49] did find an increase in white blood cell count, significantly more so in the conventional group from the first day until the fourth day postoperative ($p < 0.05$). No differences between laparoscopy and open surgery were apparent, in lymphocyte subpopulations expressing CD4 or CD8.

Carbon dioxide and metastasis

The gas used to create a pneumoperitoneum possibly affects tumour growth. Carbon dioxide seems to correlate with reduced peritoneal host defence and reduction in systemic immunity although the alteration is less, compared with open conventional surgery. Carbon dioxide appears to have an intrinsic stimulating effect on *in vitro* tumour growth [17, 65]. Question to be answered; does a pneumoperitoneum with carbon dioxide promote cell growth c.q. metastasis *in vivo*?

Bouvy et al. [15] reported significantly less ($p = 0.04$) renal subcapsular tumour growth after gasless laparoscopy in proportion to carbon dioxide pneumoperitoneum. No differences were found between rats undergoing air or carbon dioxide peritoneal insufflation. Southall et al. [66] corroborated these results in an experiment using mice.

In a rat model, helium insufflation was likely to produce less port site metastases compared with air, carbon dioxide and nitric oxide ($p < 0.0001$) [67]. Overall tumour growth of an implanted tumour seemed to be similar after helium and carbon dioxide insufflation [68].

Clinical aspects

As stated in the introduction a prospective registry was conducted on patients undergoing laparoscopic colon resection. There was no evidence of any increase in wound metastasis after the laparoscopic procedure compared with the incidence after open conventional surgery. In a case control study by Leung et al. [69], a prospective trial was conducted, with operating time, time to resuming normal diet, and hospital stay as the short term endpoints. Operating time was significantly longer ($p < 0.001$), whereas time to resuming normal diet and hospital stay was significantly lower ($p < 0.002$). On the long-term, 21.4 months for the laparoscopy group and 23.5 months for the comparative group, they followed patients on disease-free rate, and survival rate. They did not find any significant differences. One out of 28 patients (0.035%) from the laparoscopic group, and 9 out of 56 patients (0.161%) from the open group had tumour recurrences.

In a randomized clinical trial (n = 39) of Liang et al. [29], clinical outcome after laparoscopically assisted sigmoidectomy *versus* open surgery, was measured by duration of hospitalisation, postoperative no-bowel-movement, -pain and -complications. Significant differences were found in favour of laparoscopy. Duration of hospitalisation was less in the laparoscopic group, 7.0 ± 1.5 *versus* 10.5 ± 2.0 in the conventional group. Bowel movement in the laparoscopic assisted group was noticed 48.0 hours (± 12.5 h) postoperative, in the open conventional group 96.0 hours (± 18.4) ($p < 0.05$). Pain scores were assessed on postoperative day 1 with the visual analogue scale. Results are 4.2 ± 1.0 cm for laparoscopy and 8.5 ± 1.2 cm after conventional sigmoidectomy ($p < 0.05$). Postoperative complications are also diminished after laparoscopically assisted surgery. The only complication noticed after this operating procedure was fever (defined as 101°F orally on two consecutive readings 12 hours apart after the first 48 hours). After conventional sigmoidectomy seven complications were described; two cases of postoperative fever, two wound infections, one urinary tract infection, one anastomotic leakage and one myocardial infarction.

The randomized clinical trial from Lacy *et al.*, reported also the clinical aspects of colectomies. The duration of intervention was longer for laparoscopy-assisted colectomy ($p = 0.001$), morbidity was lower ($p = 0.001$), as was the duration of hospital stay ($p = 0.005$) and the time of initiation of oral intake ($p = 0.001$).

As there is still conflicting data no correlation could be found between clinical outcome and immunological changes after laparoscopic surgery.

Conclusion

Conventional open surgery as well as laparoscopic surgery affects the immune status of the patient. The trauma induced by open surgery is substantially increased compared to laparoscopic surgery and is therefore more aggravating for the immune system.

The peritoneal response after laparoscopic surgery seems to be characterized by a brief period of immune suppression due to carbon dioxide insufflation. Peritoneal macrophage functioning is affected, probably because of the effect of carbon dioxide on pH in peritoneal fluid. Not only a diminished production of cytokines has been noticed, a decline in the intrinsic functioning of this monocyte (*i.e* phagocytosis) was apparent. Helium seems to be a favourable substitute except for its property of insolubility and therefore should not be considered an alternative for carbon dioxide in surgery with risk of embolism.

The systemic stress-response is less affected after laparoscopic surgery in comparison with conventional surgery. This difference was found in cytokine and cell mediated immune responses in both animal experiments and clinical trials. Not only does the laparoscopic approach preserve systemic immunity after cholecystectomy. It seems to maintain this immunity after other surgical procedures. Serum C-reactive protein and interleukin 6 levels are appreciably lower after laparoscopy compared to laparotomy. This suggests an immune advantage after laparoscopic surgery.

Furthermore, other cytokine parameters do not show a marked difference between the two operating procedures. There is mixed evidence of less immunosuppression, but no real effect is evident. The DTH response, as a quantity for T cell mediated immune response, also shows a marked difference between different operating procedures. The response is distinct and in favour of laparoscopy. An effective elimination of pathogens from the abdomen requires a reasonable presence of HLA-DR molecules in and on monocytes.

After conventional surgery the expression of these molecules is declined, but after laparoscopic surgery this expression is maintained. Sietses *et al.* [70] showed that there is not a delay in the systemic clearance of pathogens, thus supporting the hypothesis that, although a small reduction was noticeable in laparoscopic surgery, the systemic immunity was not altered.

The immunologic findings after colorectal resections for malignancies seem to be the same as after other surgical indications. Carbon dioxide as insufflation gas may enhance tumour growth, helium (a possible alternative insufflation gas) on the contrary is associated with less port site metastasis. The immune fonction seems to play a role in the brawl against tumour metastasis as stimulation of the immune system with the administration of endotoxin may reduce the risk of port site recurrences [57]. No clinical research to date could prove an increase in tumour metastasis after laparoscopy. Also no proof was found for the opposite. In the future large randomized clinical trials should be able to give more information on tumour metastasis, clinical outcome and the possible correlation with the immune system.

References

1. Christou NV, Meakins JL, MacLean LD. The predictive role of delayed hypersensitivity in preoperative patients. *Surg Gynecol Obstet* 1981; 152 (3): 297-301.
2. Hershman MJ, *et al.* Monocyte HLA-DR antigen expression characterizes clinical outcome in the trauma patient. *Br J Surg* 1990; 77 (2): 204-7.
3. Poenaru D, Christou NV. Clinical outcome of seriously ill surgical patients with intraabdominal infection depends on both physiologic (APACHE II score) and immunologic (DTH score) alterations. *Ann Surg* 1991; 213 (2): 130-6.
4. Sietses C, *et al.* Immunological consequences of laparoscopic surgery, speculations on the cause and clinical implications. *Langenbecks Arch Surg* 1999; 384 (3): 250-8.
5. Allendorf JD, *et al.* Postoperative immune function varies inversely with the degree of surgical trauma in a murine model. *Surg Endosc* 1997; 11 (5): 427-30.
6. Gupta A, Watson DI. Effect of laparoscopy on immune function. *Br J Surg* 2001; 88 (10): 1296-306.
7. West MA, Baker J, Bellingham J. Kinetics of decreased LPS-stimulated cytokine release by macrophages exposed to CO_2. *J Surg Res* 1996; 63 (1): 269-74.
8. Hajri A, *et al.* Dual effect of laparoscopy on cell-mediated immunity. *Eur Surg Res* 2000; 32 (5): 261-6.
9. Watson RW, *et al.* Exposure of the peritoneal cavity to air regulates early inflammatory responses to surgery in a murine model. *Br J Surg* 1995; 82 (8): 1060-5.
10. Menes T, Spivak H. Laparoscopy: searching for the proper insufflation gas. *Surg Endosc* 2000; 14 (11): 1050-6.
11. Galizia G, *et al.* Hemodynamic and pulmonary changes during open, carbon dioxide pneumoperitoneum and abdominal wall-lifting cholecystectomy. A prospective, randomized study. *Surg Endosc* 2001; 15 (5): 477-83.
12. Zuckerman R, *et al.* The effects of pneumoperitoneum and patient position on hemodynamics during laparoscopic cholecystectomy. *Surg Endosc* 2001; 15 (6): 562-5.
13. Jacobi CA, *et al.* Cardiopulmonary changes during laparoscopy and vessel injury: comparison of CO_2 and helium in an animal model. *Langenbecks Arch Surg* 2000; 385 (7): 459-66.

14. Jacoby CA, et al. The impact of conventional and laparoscopic colon resection (CO_2 or helium) on intraperitoneal adhesion formation in a rat peritonitis model. *Surg Endosc* 2001; 15 (4): 380-6.
15. Bouvy ND, et al. Effects of carbon dioxide pneumoperitoneum, air pneumoperitoneum, and gasless laparoscopy on body weight and tumour growth. *Arch Surg* 1998; 133 (6): 652-6.
16. Nagelschmidt M, Gerbecks D, Minor T. The impact of gas laparoscopy on abdominal plasminogen activator activity. *Surg Endosc* 2001; 15 (6): 585-8.
17. Smidt VJ, et al. Effect of carbon dioxide on human ovarian carcinoma cell growth. *Am J Obstet Gynecol* 2001; 185 (6): 1314-7.
18. Iwanaka T, et al. Evaluation of operative stress and peritoneal macrophage function in minimally invasive operations. *J Am Coll Surg* 1997; 184 (4): 357-63.
19. Gutt CN, et al. The phagocytosis activity during conventional and laparoscopic operations in the rat. A preliminary study. *Surg Endosc* 1997; 11 (9): 899-901.
20. Erenoglu C, et al. Is helium insufflation superior to carbon dioxide insufflation in bacteremia and bacterial translocation with peritonitis? *J Laparoendosc Adv Surg Tech A* 2001; 11 (2): 69-72.
21. West MA, et al. Mechanism of decreased *in vitro* murine macrophage cytokine release after exposure to carbon dioxide: relevance to laparoscopic surgery. *Ann Surg* 1997; 226 (2): 179-90.
22. Kuntz C, et al. Effect of pressure and gas type on intraabdominal, subcutaneous, and blood pH in laparoscopy. *Surg Endosc* 2000; 14 (4): 367-71.
23. Chekan EG, et al. Intraperitoneal immunity and pneumoperitoneum. *Surg Endosc* 1999; 13 (11): 1135-8.
24. Balague C, et al. Peritoneal response to a septic challenge. Comparison between open laparotomy, pneumoperitoneum laparoscopy, and wall lift laparoscopy. *Surg Endosc* 1999; 13 (8): 792-6.
25. Puttick MI, et al. Comparison of immunologic and physiologic effects of CO_2 pneumoperitoneum at room and body temperatures. *Surg Endosc* 1999; 13 (6): 572-5.
26. Benner R, et al. *Medische immunologie*. Elsevier/Bunge Maarssen, 1998.
27. Cruickshank AM, et al. Response of serum interleukin-6 in patients undergoing elective surgery of varying severity. *Clin Sci (Lond)* 1990; 79 (2): 161-5.
28. Wu FP, Cuesta MA, Sietses C. Randomized clinical trial of the effect of open *versus* laparoscopically assisted colectomy on systemic immunity in patients with colorectal cancer (*Br J Surg* 2001; 88: 801-7). *Br J Surg* 2001; 88 (11): 1545.
29. Liang JT, et al. Prospective evaluation of laparoscopy-assisted colectomy *versus* laparotomy with resection for management of complex polyps of the sigmoid colon. *World J Surg* 2002; 26 (3): 377-83.
30. Kishi D, et al. Laparoscopic-assisted surgery for Crohn's disease: reduced surgical stress following ileocolectomy. *Surg Today* 2000; 30 (3): 219-22.
31. Uzunkoy A, et al. Systemic stress responses after laparoscopic or open hernia repair. *Eur J Surg* 2000; 166 (6): 467-71.
32. Solomon MJ, et al. Randomized clinical trial of laparoscopic *versus* open abdominal rectopexy for rectal prolapse. *Br J Surg* 2002; 89 (1): 35-9.
33. Grande M, et al. Systemic acute-phase response after laparoscopic and open cholecystectomy. *Surg Endosc* 2002; 16 (2): 313-6.
34. McMahon AJ, et al. Comparison of metabolic responses to laparoscopic and minilaparotomy cholecystectomy. *Br J Surg* 1993; 80 (10): 1255-8.
35. Malik E, et al. Prospective evaluation of the systemic immune response following abdominal, vaginal, and laparoscopically assisted vaginal hysterectomy. *Surg Endosc* 2001; 15 (5): 463-6.
36. Trokel MJ, et al. Preservation of immune response after laparoscopy. *Surg Endosc* 1994; 8 (12): 1385-7; discussion 1387-8.
37. Christou NV, et al. The delayed hypersensitivity response and host resistance in surgical patients. 20 years later. *Ann Surg* 1995; 222 (4): 534-46; discussion 546-8.

38. Allendorf JD, et al. Increased tumour establishment and growth after open *versus* laparoscopic surgery in mice may be related to differences in postoperative T-cell function. *Surg Endosc* 1999; 13 (3): 233-5.
39. Gitzelmann CA, et al. Cell-mediated immune response is better preserved by laparoscopy than laparotomy. *Surgery* 2000; 127 (1): 65-71.
40. Schietroma M, et al. Evaluation of immune response in patients after open or laparoscopic cholecystectomy. *Hepatogastroenterology* 2001; 48 (39): 642-6.
41. Kloosterman T, et al. Unimpaired immune functions after laparoscopic cholecystectomy. *Surgery* 1994; 115 (4): 424-8.
42. Gutt CN, et al. Influence of laparoscopy and laparotomy on systemic and peritoneal T lymphocytes in a rat model. *Int J Colorectal Dis* 2001; 16 (4): 216-20.
43. Hewitt PM, et al. Laparoscopic-assisted *versus* open surgery for colorectal cancer: comparative study of immune effects. *Dis Colon Rectum* 1998; 41 (7): 901-9.
44. Pertilla J, et al. Immune response after laparoscopic and conventional Nissen fundoplication. *Eur J Surg* 1999; 165 (1): 21-8.
45. Walker CB, et al. Minimal modulation of lymphocyte and natural killer cell subsets following minimal access surgery. *Am J Surg* 1999; 177 (1): 48-54.
46. Lausten SB, et al. Systemic and cell-mediated immune response after laparoscopic and open cholecystectomy in patients with chronic liver disease. A randomized, prospective study. *Dig Surg* 1999; 16 (6): 471-7.
47. Carter JJ, Whelan RL. The immunologic consequences of laparoscopy in oncology. *Surg Oncol Clin N Am* 2001; 10 (3): 655-77.
48. Cheadle WG, et al. HLA-DR antigen expression on peripheral blood monocytes correlates with surgical infection. *Am J Surg* 1991; 161 (6): 639-45.
49. Ordemann J, et al. Cellular and humoral inflammatory response after laparoscopic and conventional colorectal resections. *Surg Endosc* 2001; 15 (6): 600-8.
50. Sietses C, et al. The influence of laparoscopic surgery on postoperative polymorphonuclear leukocyte function. *Surg Endosc* 2000; 14 (9): 812-6.
51. Lee SW, et al. Time course of differences in lymphocyte proliferation rates after laparotomy *versus* CO_2 insufflation. *Surg Endosc* 2000; 14 (2): 145-8.
52. Vittimberga FJ, et al. Laparoscopic surgery and Kupffer cell activation. *Surg Endosc* 2000; 14 (12): 1171-6.
53. Vukasin P, et al. Wound recurrence following laparoscopic colon cancer resection. Results of the American Society of Colon and Rectal Surgeons Laparoscopic Registry. *Dis Colon Rectum* 1996; 39 (10 Suppl.): S20-3.
54. Hughes ES, et al. Tumour recurrence in the abdominal wall scar tissue after large-bowel cancer surgery. *Dis Colon Rectum* 1983; 26 (9): 571-2.
55. Reilly WT, et al. Wound recurrence following conventional treatment of colorectal cancer. A rare but perhaps underestimated problem. *Dis Colon Rectum* 1996; 39 (2): 200-7.
56. Lacy AM, et al. Laparoscopy-assisted colectomy *versus* open colectomy for treatment of non-metastatic colon cancer: a randomised trial. *Lancet* 2002; 359 (9325): 2224-9.
57. Neuhaus SJ, et al. The effect of immune enhancement and suppression on the development of laparoscopic port site metastases. *Surg Endosc* 2000; 14 (5): 439-43.
58. Delgado S, et al. Acute phase response in laparoscopic and open colectomy in colon cancer: randomized study. *Dis Colon Rectum* 2001; 44 (5) 638-46.
59. Fukushima R, et al. Interleukin-6 and stress hormone responses after uncomplicated gasless laparoscopic-assisted and open sigmoid colectomy. *Dis Colon Rectum* 1996; 39 (10 Suppl.): S29-34.
60. Nishiguchi K, et al. Comparative evaluation of surgical stress of laparoscopic and open surgeries for colorectal carcinoma. *Dis Colon Rectum* 2001; 44 (2): 223-30.

61. Schwenk W, et al. Inflammatory response after laparoscopic and conventional colorectal resections – results of a prospective randomized trial. *Langenbecks Arch Surg* 2000; 385 (1): 2-9.
62. Kuntz C, et al. Short- and long-term results after laparoscopic *versus* conventional colon resection in a tumour-bearing small animal model. *Surg Endosc* 2000; 14 (6): 561-7.
63. Mehigan BJ, et al. Changes in T cell subsets, interleukin-6 and C-reactive protein after laparoscopic and open colorectal resection for malignacy. *Surg Endosc* 2001; 15 (11): 1289-93.
64. Tang CL, et al. Randomized clinical trial of the effect of open *versus* laparoscopically assisted colectomy on systemic immunity in patients with colorectal cancer. *Br J Surg* 2001; 88 (6): 801-7.
65. Gutt CN, et al. CO_2 environment influences the growth of cultured human cancer cells dependent on insufflation pressure. *Surg Endosc* 2001; 15 (3): 314-8.
66. Southall JC, et al. The effect of peritoneal air exposure on postoperative tumour growth. *Surg Endosc* 1998; 12 (4): 348-50.
67. Neuhaus SJ, et al. Wound metastasis after laparoscopy with different insufflation gases. *Surgery* 1998; 123 (5): 579-83.
68. Neuhaus SJ, et al. Influence of gases on intraperitoneal immunity during laparoscopy in tumour-bearing rats. *World J Surg* 2000; 24 (10): 1227-31.
69. Leung KL, et al. Laparoscopic-assisted resection of right-sided colonic carcinoma: a case-control study. *J Surg Oncol* 1999; 71 (2): 97-100.
70. Sietses C, et al. Laparoscopic surgery preserves monocyte-mediated tumour cell killing in contrast to the conventional approach. *Surg Endosc* 2000; 14 (5): 456-60.
71. Leung KL, et al. Systemic cytokine response laparoscopic-assisted resection of rectosigmoid carcinoma: a prospective randomized trial. *Ann Surg* 2000; 231 (4): 506-11.
72. Vermorken JB, et al. Active specific immunotherapy for stage II and stage III human colon cancer: a randomised trial. *Lancet* 1999; 353 (9150): 345-50.

To what extent will *Helicobacter pylori* eradication reduce gastric cancer?

Anthony Axon

Department of Gastroenterology, The General Infirmary at Leeds, Great George Street, Leeds, LS1 3EX, United Kingdom

Introduction

Globally gastric cancer is responsible for over three quarters of a million deaths each year [1] and the increasing age of the population suggests that this mortality rate is set to rise. Once diagnosed the disease carries a dismal prognosis. In most developed countries only 10% of individuals survive for longer than five years. It seems unlikely that advances in surgery and chemotherapy will significantly improve outcomes in the foreseeable future so interventions to reduce mortality should focus upon preventative measures.

Epidemiological and experimental work have identified a number of factors that are associated with the development of gastric cancer. These include a diet high in salt and low in fruit and vegetables. The disease is more common in certain developing countries and especially affects individuals who live in relatively disadvantaged socioeconomic circumstances. A positive family history carries a higher risk. Certain physio-pathological conditions such as bile reflux, pernicious anaemia, hypochlorhydria and the operated stomach also increase the risk. The disease mainly affects older people but in communities where the disease is more prevalent the age of acquisition may be lower. The most important risk factor for gastric cancer is previous infection with *Helicobacter pylori (H pylori)*.

In developing a strategy for prevention it is necessary first to identify those risk factors that are likely to be causative as opposed to surrogate markers. Socioeconomic status may merely reflect the increased prevalence of *Helicobacter* infection in this group or possibly an unsatisfactory diet. Although there appears to be a strong negative association between cancer and a diet rich in fruit and vegetables [2], interventional studies using vitamin supplementation have not, to date, shown any protective effect. When considering possible interventions no measures are available to reduce bile reflux or to influence the genetic constitution of individuals and it is difficult to influence style of life in populations.

Although every effort should be made to encourage a greater consumption of fruit and vegetables the trend in developing countries is to move towards increased consumption of protein and fat. The remaining risk factor is infection with *H pylori*.

H pylori colonizes roughly 50% of the human population. These individuals are at an increased risk of developing cancer. Effective chemo-therapeutic regimens are available for the treatment of *H pylori* gastritis so a feasible preventive strategy would be widespread screening for infection followed by treatment of infected individuals. This approach would be more practicable than attempting to change life style and less expensive than endoscopic population screening for early cancer. In any case primary prevention by removing a risk factor is more desirable than secondary prevention.

This presentation focuses upon the evidence that suggests *H pylori* infection to be a risk factor for cancer as opposed to a simple association and assesses the benefit that might accrue from a population screen and treat strategy.

Helicobacter pylori gastritis – a cause of cancer or merely an association?

Much of the evidence advanced to support the view that *H pylori* is a causative factor in gastric cancer is epidemiological in nature. However, observational epidemiological studies whilst capable of demonstrating an association do not on their own prove that *Helicobacter* is causative for gastric cancer. Indeed it was initially argued that gastritis might predispose patients to infection with the organism rather than *vice versa*. Prospective studies have since shown that the eradication of the infection leads to resolution of the inflammation and that *H pylori* causes gastritis. The only way to prove beyond doubt that *H pylori* infection is responsible for gastric cancer would be either to randomize an uninfected population to iatrogenic infection or placebo and see which group developed cancer, or alternatively to randomize a group of young naturally infected individuals either to *Helicobacter* eradication therapy or placebo and follow for 40 years. In practice ethical considerations would prevent the first approach, the second is hampered by expense, the length of time that it would take as well as certain ethical difficulties. It will probably be many years therefore before we are able to say with absolute certainty that *H pylori* is responsible for gastric cancer. It is even more difficult to compute the degree of risk the infection holds for individuals or populations. This however is the task assigned for this presentation because without being able to calculate the risk it carries it is impossible to speculate to what extent eradication will reduce gastric cancer.

Epidemiological evidence

A large number of studies have drawn attention to the association between *H pylori* gastritis and non-cardia (distal) gastric cancer. However, a major difficulty in their interpretation is that gastric cancer usually occurs in a stomach that has undergone widespread gastric atrophy with intestinal metaplasia [3]. This destructive pathology is believed to be the result of previous *H pylori* infection. Before the stomach reaches this state however parietal cells are destroyed, acid secretion declines, and colonization with "faecal type" and salivary organisms supervenes. *H pylori* which depends upon gastric acid for protection against competitors often disappears and with this the telltale antibodies to *H pylori* infection in the blood also disappear. Bearing in mind that in many parts of the world over half the population are infected with *H pylori* it is not surprising that it was initially difficult to show a strong association between the infection and gastric cancer.

A major step forward was the identification of serum samples that had been "nested" years before during research in other areas. These sera could be reactivated and assessed for *H pylori* antibodies, the outcome of those patients initially positive or negative could then be compared years later. These data convincingly showed a strong association between previous *H pylori* infection and subsequent gastric cancer. A recent meta-analysis of nested studies has shown an odds ratio of around three [4]. Almost certainly this figure underestimates the association because those in whom the serum had been taken more than 15 years earlier had a higher odds ratio than those taken closer in time to the point at which cancer was identified. In other words the organism may well have previously been present in spite of negative serology. The authors of the meta-analysis concluded that an odds ratio of six was more likely to represent the truth. Even this may be an underestimate because studies in Japan assessing younger individuals with cancer and others with "early gastric cancer" as opposed to "advanced cancer" have odds ratios as high as 13 *(table I)* [5, 6]. Odds ratios are not necessarily the best way to estimate the degree of risk that *Helicobacter* infection has in the population. The reason for this is the greater number of individuals in the population infected with the organism the lower will be the odds ratio. It is going to be more easily understood by taking the example of cigarette smoking. If 100% of a population smoked cigarettes it would be impossible to demonstrate epidemiologically that cigarette smoking was the cause of lung cancer because the odds ratio under these circumstances would be one. It is only when the general incidence of an environmental factor does not affect the whole population that differences can be identified, thus in countries with the highest incidence of gastric cancer or in the higher age groups where the infection is more common the odds ratio will be reduced.

Pathological evidence

It is well recognized that non-cardia gastric cancer usually arises in a stomach showing evidence of long-standing gastritis with gastric atrophy and intestinal metaplasia [7]. In these cases the usual histological phenotype of the cancer is "intestinal" and is believed to originate from unstable type III intestinal metaplasia. Non-cardia gastric cancer with the phenotype of "diffuse" infiltration is found in stomachs less severely affected by atrophy and intestinal metaplasia [8]. Nevertheless there is usually a severe corpus predominant *H pylori* inflammation within the stomach [9]. Patients tend to be younger and the lesion is situated closer to the advancing border of inflammation as it progresses from the antrum proximally [10]. Both "intestinal" and "diffuse" cancers are strongly associated with *Helicobacter* infection. It is interesting to speculate that diffuse cancer may arise as a direct result of active inflammation as opposed to mutation in an area of intestinal metaplasia.

Table I. Relationship between gastric carcinoma and seropositivity of anti-*Helicobacter pylori* IgG antibody

	Data sets			
Subjects*	1:2	1:1**	Odds ratio	(95% CI)***
All patients	94	10	13.3	(5.3-35.6)
Men	41	6	6.8	(2.4-18.8)
Women	53	4	32.8	(6.2-330.4)
Early gastric carcinoma patients	36	3	20.8	(3.8-220.4)
Advanced gastric carcinoma patients	58	7	10.8	(3.7-34.8)
Intestinal type gastric carcinoma	14	1	18.0	(1.9-1744.6)
Diffuse type gastric carcinoma	80	9	12.8	(4.7-36.8)
Proximal carcinoma	31	4	11.3	(2.6-68.8)
Distal carcinoma	63	6	14.8	(4.8-53.9)

CI: confidence interval.
* Subjects were patients shown and matched hospital and screening control subjects.
** 1:2 means number of data sets consisting of case and two controls, and 1:1 means that consisting of a case and a control.
*** 95% confidence intervals were calculated by Sato's method[5a]
Reproduced with the kind permission of the journal *Cancer*.

We now appreciate that *H pylori* is the most important causative agent in the development of atrophy and intestinal metaplasia [11-13]. Both the severity of the inflammation and the eventual damage done to the gastric mucosa is greater in those individuals who are infected by the more virulent CagA positive organisms [14]. What is even more interesting however is that the pattern of gastritis varies substantially from individual to individual [15]. Those with a high natural gastric acid secretion develop an antral predominant gastritis with relative sparing of the corpus. This is the phenotype for the development of duodenal ulcer (where again a CagA positive organism will cause greater inflammation and a higher risk of that disease). A corpus predominant gastritis however is what is typically found in individuals who have a relatively low acid secretion such as those who develop gastric ulcer and gastric cancer. Some have argued that the decrease in acid secretion by the stomach is an effect of the gastritis rather than its cause [16]. Certainly there is good evidence showing that those with a corpus predominant gastritis have a relatively lower acid secretion, however work in the last decade has demonstrated that if a patient with antral predominant *H pylori* gastritis is treated with a proton pump inhibitor and rendered hypochlorhydric, the pattern changes to a corpus predominant gastritis with gastric atrophy [17-21]. So whatever the final cause of achlorhydria, the corpus gastritis occurs in patients who initially have relative hypochlorhydria. More recent work still has shown that individuals respond to *H pylori* infection differently depending upon their genetic make-up [22, 23]. The genes involved are those responsible for the production of inflammatory cytokines and include polymorphisms of the IL-1β, IL-1 receptor antagonist, tumour necrosis factor A and IL-10. One way in which the IL-1β polymorphisms exert their deleterious effect is by causing profound hypochlorhydria following infection with the organism.

In summary, the pathological evidence provides strong circumstantial evidence favouring *H pylori* as the major underlying environmental factor responsible for corpus gastritis, atrophy, intestinal metaplasia, hypochlorhydria and cancer.

Animal experiments

It was known as long ago as 1919 that experimental infection of animals with spiral organisms could cause gastric inflammation and ulceration and that the condition could be cured by antimicrobials [24]. Interest in this area was rekindled by the work by Marshall and Warren in the early 1980's [25] and since then a number of *H pylori* strains have been transmitted to experimental animals. Infection is usually accompanied by an inflammatory reaction in the stomach. The major advance in this area was the discovery that the Mongolian gerbil, when infected, developed a gastritis similar to that of human infection and could induce peptic ulceration. Further work has shown that longer standing infection in these animals leads to the development of gastric cancer [26]. More recent studies still that are particularly germane to this presentation have shown that gerbils pretreated with *H pylori* infection and a carcinogen readily developed cancer, but if the *H pylori* is eradicated those animals are relatively protected compared with the controls in whom infection continued [27, 28].

Mechanisms

A great deal of experimental work has been done to identify potential mechanisms whereby *H pylori* may cause cancer. These show that the infection causes hyperproliferation of the gastric mucosa with increased mitoses perhaps increasing the risk of mutation [29]. Infiltration of the mucosa by inflammatory cells elaborates reactive oxygen metabolites which are known to be able to damage DNA [30]. The *H pylori* infection causes a decline in the level of ascorbic acid within the stomach [31]. Normally ascorbic acid is present in the gastric juice at a higher concentration than in the plasma. This concentration difference is abolished by *Helicobacter* infection and in the hypochlorhydric stomach ascorbic acid levels fall to zero. Ascorbic acid may play a role in preventing the conversation of nitrite to N-nitrosomines [32]. N-nitrosomines are known carcinogens and have been postulated as candidate molecules involved in the pathogenesis of gastric cancer.

Helicobacter pylori and the risk of cancer

The data set out above strongly suggests that *Helicobacter pylori* is an important risk factor for the development of most gastric cancer. Indeed it is hard to escape the conclusion that infection is the single most important etiological cause of the disease. It is apparent however that other factors do play a role in its pathogenesis and the real question is whether infection with the organism is a necessary prerequisite for the disease or whether other risk factors such as diet and bile reflux could cause the disease in its absence. In certain cases *H pylori* infection is not a necessary prerequisite. Non-cardia gastric cancer, for example, is negatively associated with the infection. The aetiology of this particular cancer, which affects a tiny vulnerable area of the gastric mucosa accounts for up to 20% of gastric cancer in some countries [33] probably has a totally different aetiology. Similarly certain hereditary gastric cancers appear to arise irrespective of *Helicobacter pylori* infection. In others the disease results from auto-immune gastritis where infection with *Helicobacter pylori* is uncommon. Nevertheless the major burden of gastric cancer is that associated with widespread atrophy and intestinal metaplasia and it does probably arise as a direct result of *H pylori* infection in association with other risk factors which on their own would not lead to the development of this disease. It is difficult to estimate the proportion of cases in which *H pylori* is a necessary prerequisite of the disease in any given population. The reason for this is that the geographical incidence of cancer varies widely and although there is a trend such that countries with a higher prevalence of *H pylori* also have a higher incidence of gastric cancer [34], this does not apply in all cases (the "African enigma"). In certain countries with similar infection rates the incidence of cancer may differ considerably, and this applies to individual countries as well where there is a large multiracial variation [35].

Variation between communities

Geographical differences may be caused by variation in the degree of atrophy and intestinal metaplasia occurring in different infected communities. There is, for example, a general belief that the Japanese develop a more severe gastritis with a more rapid and severe progression than Western populations. To date however few convincing controlled studies have been published in this area [36]. It is nevertheless reasonable to speculate that the severity of *H pylori* gastritis in the community will vary according to the prevalence of more virulent strains (which vary geographically) [37], diet and perhaps the genetic constitution of the individuals. The pattern of the gastritis may be more important than the severity of the inflammation, this may be influenced by such factors as genetics and gastric acidity which itself is affected by a variety of factors including age [38] and linear height [39].

Variations in the incidence of *H pylori* infection, its severity and pattern will all influence the extent to which eradication will reduce the incidence of gastric cancer in a given community. This is not only because of the factors discussed earlier, but also because in a high incidence country cardia cancer, pure hereditary cancer and that due to pernicious anaemia will comprise a smaller proportion of the cancer load compared with that in a community where the overall incidence of *H pylori* related cancer is less. Furthermore, communities may differ according to the age at which irreversible changes take place in the gastric mucosa. It would seem to be a reasonable presumption that communities harbouring *H pylori* gastritis with greater severity will develop irreversible changes of the gastric mucosa at an earlier age than those where the inflammatory damage is less severe. Thus intervention at an earlier age may be necessary to achieve the same proportionate benefit of that in the other community. It does not follow therefore that intervention in a cancer high risk population would necessarily have the same proportionate effect as one with a lower incidence.

At what point would *H pylori* eradication be effective?

H pylori infection occurs in early childhood [40], however there is little benefit in treating individuals who are at high risk of reinfection. The mode of transmission of *H pylori* is unknown. Could it be faecal/oral, oral/oral, gastro/oral (by vomiting) or by water supply? This being the case it is difficult to predict the most suitable age for intervention. It seems reasonable to assume that if the progression to a corpus predominant gastritis with atrophy and intestinal metaplasia could be prevented this would provide the greatest opportunity of preventing cancer. As indicated earlier, in countries where gastric cancer is commoner, the intervention would probably have to be made at an earlier stage than in those with a lower incidence of the disease.

It is possible that "diffuse" type cancer may respond differently to "intestinal" type cancer. Diffuse cancer may be the product of direct inflammation where intestinal type cancer probably follows mutation in intestinal metaplasia. If that is the case (and this is speculative) it may be that *H pylori* eradication would have a greater, immediate effect upon diffuse cancer because of the rapid elimination of the inflammatory reaction, whilst cancers arising from intestinal metaplasia would be less amenable to *H pylori* eradication because intestinal metaplasia reverses slowly, if at all [41].

In spite of the above one would nevertheless expect *H pylori* eradication to have some benefit even if given at a late stage. The reason for this is that once the infection is eradicated the acute inflammatory response disappears almost immediately. In a proportion of individuals gastric acid secretion recovers to some extent and may reduce colonization by faecal and salivary organisms. This, in turn, may reduce the amount of damage to the mucosa. Intestinal metaplasia does not seem to progress once treatment has been given compared with placebo. In those stomachs that are less severely damaged not only will acid secretion improve, but the level of ascorbic acid in the gastric lumen increases, cell turnover declines and the production of reactive oxygen metabolites by inflammatory cells falls.

Interventional studies

The only way to determine the effect of *H pylori* eradication is to perform a prospective randomized clinical trial. Unfortunately attempts to do this have met with problems. The reason for this is that once a patient has been tested for *H pylori* and the nature of the trial has been explained to the patient, few are prepared to enter the placebo arm. Recruitment therefore has been a major drawback with some studies [42, 43] that have been abandoned or are progressing only slowly. If cancer is taken as the end-point large numbers have to be recruited. Alternatively smaller studies are on-going where patients are randomized to treatment or non-treatment and are then followed up endoscopically. In these a primary end-point may be a surrogate marker for cancer such as atrophy or intestinal metaplasia. Three such studies have been reported from China at five years [44-46] and one from Columbia [47], these do show some evidence that *H pylori* eradication may have benefit.

The most persuasive interventional data is from Uemera et al. [48]. They followed up 132 patients diagnosed with early gastric cancer. They provided *H pylori* eradication for 65 and no therapy for 67. After 84 months the intestinal metaplasia score decreased significantly and only one patient developed metachronous cancer. This compared with nine cancers in the non-treated group. This study has been criticized in that it was not blinded, but it remains the most persuasive human controlled study in the literature to date.

Conclusions

The data available implicates *H pylori* gastritis as the most important causative factor for non-cardia gastric cancer. However, the wide variation and incidence of the disease in different populations makes it difficult to predict the benefit that would accrue from *Helicobacter* eradication generally. A better estimate can be made in individual populations but the effectiveness will still be influenced by a series of unknowns, for example, the age at which the intervention should be made, the type of cancer (diffuse or intestinal), the sensitivity of the screening test employed, the rate of successful eradication, the number of individuals who would be prepared to undergo screening and take medication and the avidity with which subjects are pursued to ensure complete eradication by secondary treatment. It would be a reasonable assumption in a Western society that an intervention in early adulthood would prevent nearly all non-cardia cancers in those in whom eradication was achieved, but the benefit to the community would not be realized until 40-60 years had elapsed. Conversely intervention in a high risk group at the age of 50 might produce beneficial results more quickly (to judge from Uemera's data), but it is unlikely that it would totally eliminate the risk of cancer and might only delay its onset. Clearly the greatest benefit would be gained by eradicating or preventing *Helicobacter* infection in early adulthood in countries with the highest risk of cancer.

References

1. Murray CJL, Lopez AD. Alternative projections of mortality and disability by cause 1990-2020 – global burden of disease study. *Lancet* 1997; 349: 1498-504.
2. Committee on Medical Aspects of Food and Nutrition Policy. COMA 1998 Annual Report. London: Department of Health. HMSO. 1999: iv, 1-46.
3. IARC Monographs on the evaluation of carcinogenic risks to humans. Schistosomes, liver flukes and *Helicobacter pylori*. In: International Agency for Research on Cancer Monograph 61, Lyon, France; 1994: 177-240.
4. Helicobacter and Cancer Collaborative Group. Gastric cancer and *Helicobacter pylori*: a combined analysis of 12 case control studies nested within prospective cohorts. *Gut* 2001; 49: 347-53.
5. Kikuchi S, Wada O, Nakajima T, et al. Serum anti-*Helicobacter pylori* antibody and gastric carcinoma among young adults. *Cancer* 1995; 75: 2789-93.
6. Sato T. Confidence limits for the common odds ratio based on the asymptomatic distribution of the Mantel-Haenzel estimator. *Biometrics* 1990; 46: 71-80.
7. Sipponen P, Seppala K. Gastric carcinoma: failed adaptation of *Helicobacter pylori*. *Scand J Gastroenterol* 1992; 27 (Suppl. 93): 33-8.

8. Craanen ME, Blok P, Dekker W, Tytgat GNJ. *Helicobacter pylori* and early gastric cancer. *Gut* 1994; 35: 1372-4.
9. Uemura N, Okamoto S, Yamamoto S, *et al*. *Helicobacter pylori* infection and the development of gastric cancer. *N Engl J Med* 2001; 345: 784-9.
10. Yoshimura T, Shimoyama T, Fukuda S, Tanaka M, Axon ATR, Munakata A. Most gastric cancer occurs on the distal side of the endoscopic atrophic border. *Scand J Gastroenterol* 1999; 34: 1077-81.
11. Asaka M, Kato M, Kudo M, *et al*. Atrophic changes of gastric mucosa are caused by *Helicobacter pylori* infection rather than aging: studies in asymptomatic Japanese adults. *Helicobacter* 1996; 1: 52-6.
12. DeLuca VA, West AB, Haque S, *et al*. Long-term symptom patterns, endoscopic findings, and gastric histology in *Helicobacter pylori* infected and uninfected patients. *J Clin Gastroenterol* 1998; 26: 106-12.
13. Maaroos HI, Vorobjova T, Sipponen P, *et al*. An 18 year follow-up study of chronic gastritis and *Helicobacter pylori* association of CagA positivity with development of atrophy and activity of gastritis. *Scand J Gastroenterol* 1999; 34: 864-9.
14. Parsonnet J, Friedman GD, Orentreich N, Vogelman H. Risk for gastric cancer in people with CagA positive or CagA negative *Helicobacter pylori* infection. *Gut* 1997; 40: 297-301.
15. Lee A, Dixon MF, Danon SJ, *et al*. Local acid production and *Helicobacter pylori*: a unifying hypothesis of gastroduodenal disease. *Eur J Gastroenterol Hepatol* 1995; 7: 461-5.
16. Richter JE. *H pylori*: the bug is not all bad. *Gut* 2001; 49: 319-21.
17. Solcia E, Villani L, Riocca R, *et al*. Effects of eradication of *Helicobacter pylori* on gastritis in duodenal ulcer patients. *Scand J Gastroenterol* 1994; 201 (Suppl.): 28-34.
18. Kuipers EJ, Lundell L, Klinkenberg-Knol EC, *et al*. Atrophic gastritis and *Helicobacter pylori* infection in patients with reflux esophagitis treated with omeprazole or fundoplication. *N Eng J Med* 1996; 334: 1018-22.
19. Meining A, Boseckert H, Caspary WF, *et al*. H_2-receptor antagonists and antacids have an aggravating effect on *Helicobacter pylori* gastritis in duodenal ulcer patients. *Aliment Pharmacol Ther* 1997; 11: 729-34.
20. Berstad AE, Hatlebakk JG, Maartmann-Moe H, *et al*. *Helicobacter pylori* gastritis and epithelial cell proliferation in patients with reflux esophagitis after treatment with lansoprazole. *Gut* 1997; 41: 740-7.
21. Stolte M, Meining A, Schmitz JM, *et al*. Changes in *Helicobacter pylori*-induced gastritis in the antrum and corpus during 12 months of treatment with omeprazole and lansoprazole in patients with gastro-esophageal reflux disease? *Aliment Pharmacol Ther* 1998; 12: 247-53.
22. El-Omar E, Carrington M, Chow W, *et al*. Interleukin-1 polymorphisms associated with increased risk of gastric cancer. *Nature* 2000; 404: 398-402.
23. El-Omar EM, Rabkin CS, Gammon MD, *et al*. Increased risk of non-cardia gastric cancer associated with pro-inflammatory cytokine gene polymorphisms. *Gastroenterology* 2003; 124: 1193-201.
24. Kasai K, Kobayahsi R. The stomach spirochete occurring in mammals. *J Parasitol* 1919; 6: 1-10.
25. Marshall BJ, Warren JR. Unidentified curved bacilli in the stomach of patients with gastritis and peptic ulceration. *Lancet* 1984; i: 1311-4.
26. Watanabe T, Tada M, Nagia H, Sasaki S, Nakao M. *Helicobacter pylori* infection induces gastric cancer in Mongolian gerbils. *Gastroenterology* 1998: 115: 642-8.
27. Shimizu N, Ikehara Y, Inada K, *et al*. Eradication diminishes enhancing effects of *Helicobacter pylori* infection on glandular stomach carcinogenesis in Mongolian gerbils. *Cancer Res* 2000; 60: 1512-4.
28. Nozaki K, Shimizu N, Ikehara Y, *et al*. Effect of early eradication on *Helicobacter pylori* related gastric carcinogenesis in Mongolian gerbils. *Cancer Sci* 2003; 94: 235-9.
29. Lynch DAF, Mapstone NP, Clarke AMT, *et al*. Cell proliferation in *Helicobacter pylori* associated gastritis and the effect of eradication therapy. *Gut* 1995; 36: 346-50.

30. Drake IM, Mapstone NP, Schorah CJ, *et al.* Reactive oxygen species activity and lipid peroxidation in *Helicobacter pylori* associated gastritis: relation to gastric mucosal ascorbic acid concentrations and effect of *H pylori* eradication. *Gut* 1998; 42: 768-71.
31. Sobala GM, Schorah CJ, Sanderson M, *et al.* Ascorbic acid in the human stomach. *Gastroenterology* 1989; 97: 357-63.
32. Guttenplan JB. Inhibition by L-ascorbate of bacterial mutagenesis induced by the two N-nitroso compounds. *Nature* 1977; 268: 368-70.
33. Hansen S, Melby KK, Aase S, Jellum E, Vollset SE. *Helicobacter pylori* infection and risk of cardia cancer and non-cardia gastric cancer. *Scand J Gastroenterol* 1999; 34: 353-60.
34. The EUROGAST Study Group. Epidemiology of, and risk for, *Helicobacter pylori* infection among 3194 asymptomatic subjects in 17 populations. *Gut* 1993; 34: 1672-6.
35. Goh KL, Parasakthi N. The racial cohort phenomenon: seroepidemiology of *Helicobacter pylori* infection in a multiracial South-East Asian country. *Eur J Gastroenterol Hepatol* 2001; 13: 177-83.
36. Bedoya A, Garay J, Sanzon F, *et al.* Histopathology of gastritis in *Helicobacter pylori* infected children from populations at high and low gastric cancer risk. *Hum Pathol* 2003; 34: 206-13.
37. Bravo LE, van Doorn LJ, Realpe JL, *et al.* Virulence associated genotypes of *Helicobacter pylori*: do they explain the African enigma? *Am J Gastroenterol* 2002; 97: 2839-42.
38. Rodbro P, Krasilnikoof PA, Christiansen PM. Parietal cell secretory function in early childhood. *Scand J Gastroenterol* 1967; 2: 209-13.
39. Baron JH. Lean body mass, gastric acid and peptic ulcer. *Gut* 1969; 10: 637-42.
40. Malaty HM, El-Kasabany A, Graham DY, *et al.* Age at acquisition of *Helicobacter pylori* infection: a follow-up study from infancy to adulthood. *Lancet* 2002; 359: 931-5.
41. Dixon MF. Prospects for intervention in gastric carcinogenesis: reversibility of gastric atrophy and intestinal metaplasia. *Gut* 2001; 49: 2-4.
42. Miehlke S, Kirsch C, Dragosics B, *et al. Helicobacter pylori* and gastric cancer: current status of the Austrain Czech German gastric cancer prevention trial (PRISMA-study). *World J Gastroenterol* 2001; 7: 243-7.
43. Forman D. Lessons from ongoing intervention studies. In: Hunt RH, Tytgat GNJ, eds: *Helicobacter pylori* Basic mechanisms to clinical cure 1998. Kluwer Academic Publishers, Dordrecht, The Netherlands 1998: 354-61.
44. Wong BCY, Lam SK, Wong W-M, *et al.* Eradication of *Helicobacter pylori* infection significantly slows down the progression of precancerous lesions in high risk population: a 5 year prospective randomized study. *Gastroenterology* 2001; 122 (Suppl. 1): A588.
45. Zhou L, Sung JYJ, Lin S, *et al.* A five-year follow-up study on the pathological changes of gastric mucosa after *H pylori* eradication. *Chin Med J* 2003; 116: 11-4.
46. Sung JY, Lin SR, Leung WK, *et al.* Curing *H pylori* infection reduce progression of pre-malignant gastric lesions: a prospective randomized study at 5 year follow-up. *Gut* 2002; 51 (Suppl. 2): A91.
47. Correa P, Fontham ETH, Bravo JC, *et al.* Chemoprevention of gastric dysplasia: randomized trial of antioxidant supplements and anti-*Helicobacter pylori* therapy. *J Natl Cancer Inst* 2000; 92: 1881-8.
48. Uemura N, Okamoto S. Effect of *Helicobacter pylori* eradication on subsequent development of cancer after endoscopic resection of early gastric cancer in Japan. *Gastroenterol Clin North Am* 2000; 29: 819-27.

Is antireflux surgery an effective prevention of malignant transformation in GERD?

Lars Lundell

Department of Surgery, Huddinge University Hospital, Stockholm, Sweden

Introduction

Barrett's esophagus would be much more simple and straight forward to treat if not for its well recognised association with adenocarcinoma. The incidence of adenocarcinoma is rising in the western world where more and more institutions report that the numbers of patients with adenocarcinoma of the esophagus now have past those with squamous cell carcinoma. We have learned from epidemiological studies that a variety of risk factors are operational to determine the risk for the development of adenocarcinoma such as frequent, severe and long-lasting symptoms of reflux. A corresponding risk association between Barrett's and chronic reflux was also suggested by the severity of the endoscopic esophagitis and the presence of a hiatus hernia.

Main aspects relevant to the role of surgery in the management of Barrett's esophagus are on one hand to focus on the impact of controlling reflux and to it associated symptoms apart from the issue of defining the surgical options in case of dysplasia and/or early neoplasia. In between these major topics resides the important question if complete reflux control in Barrett's esophagus protects the mucosa from further progression to dysplasia and neoplasia? Having said this we have the question if the intention to treat reflux disease by antireflux surgery prevents dysplasia and neoplasia from occurring and secondly if a per protocol analytic approach is applied, *i.e* if an effective and durable antireflux barrier has been established. These two analytical approaches to the problem are partly independent but also related to each other in terms of elucidation of potential pathogenetic mechanisms.

Recent comprehensive studies applying multivariate analyses on a large cohort of chronic reflux disease patients, found that independent predictors for the presence of Barrett's esophagus were increased esophageal bile exposure, alterations in the geometry of the gastroesophageal junction by a hiatal hernia, a defective lower esophageal sphincter, male gender, the duration of reflux symptoms and a poor esophageal clearance. Of these increased esophageal reflux of bile was the most important predictive factor. Furthermore we have an expanding area of knowledge to find markers to address the issue of cell proliferation and dedifferentiation within the columnar lined esophageal mucosa to correlate and co-vary with dysplasia and neoplasia development within the mucosa. Furthermore, a reduction in the rate of cell proliferation has been demonstrated to occur as a consequence of normalization of esophageal pH. In this context it is important to realise that even small acid and/or bile salt pulses into the esophagus may induce proliferation and decrease the cell differentiation in tissue cultures from patients with Barrett's esophagus. Therefore an important and reasonable assumption, with immediate clinical relevance, is that all long-term therapies should, if possible, also have the therapeutic goal to eliminate abnormal acid exposure to this susceptible columnar mucosa.

How effective are antireflux operations in Barrett's esophagus?

Although Barrett's esophagus is closely associated with reflux disease, our current state of knowledge suggests that only a minority of patients with reflux disease develop Barrett's esophagus. The aim of antireflux surgery is to restore, as closely as possible, a normally functioning hiatal – lower esophageal sphincter complex, allowing an unimpeded passage of swallowed material, while at the same time preventing liquid and solid gastric contents from refluxing into the esophagus.

It is currently not an issue that patients with Barrett's esophagus who have reflux symptoms should be selected for surgery on the basis their symptoms and their response to medications and not because they have a columnar lined esophagus.

The issue of how effective antireflux surgery is in Barrett's patients is still controversial. Some investigators have reported recurrent or persisting reflux from 20 up to 64% of operated cases, when patients have been followed from three years and onwards after similar procedures. Following these reports a pre-operative diagnosis of long-segment Barrett's esophagus appears to predict higher recurrence rates and sub-optimal postoperative outcomes *(table I)*.

Some clinical researches have therefore advocated a tailored approach to antireflux surgery, whereby patients with complicated GERD, by the development of anatomical-functional abnormalities including Barrett's esophagus, should undergo an open thoracic approach with intra operative assessment of esophageal length to determine the best treatment option. Correspondingly, the transabdominal open or laparoscopic approach is reserved for patients with uncomplicated GERD. Many studies, however, recently challenged this concept by both using the laparoscopic and open antireflux operation technology. Many laparoscopic antireflux surgical reports present excellent results with an average mortality of 0.1% and morbidity of 5% and recurrent reflux in between 1-8% of the patients follow-up for a period of up to 36 months. In addition, recent publications from major institutions present data to suggest that the pre-operative diagnosis of Barrett's

Table I. Results of anti reflux surgery in patients with Barretts esophagus

Reference	n	mean follow up (years)	Success rate (%)
28	10	4	40
29	10	4	90
30	8	2	75
31	35	3	77
32	37	5	81
33	21	1.8	90
34	29	5	–
35	19	3	79
36	56	5.5	75
37	32	5	90
38	113	6.5	82
39	45	2	–
40	14	2	90
41	38	2	92
42	50	5	74
42	20	5	95
43	20	2.5	85
44	161	9	42
45	152	4.8	39
45	75	4.8	70
45	210	4.8	91
46	81	2	80
48	15	12	90

esophagus does not expose those patients to poorer outcomes and higher recurrence rates. In a recent trial, Watson and co-workers from Australia found that nearly all patients, even those with pre-operative diagnosis of Barrett's esophagus, could be successfully treated with a laparoscopic antireflux procedure with a recurrence rate of 3.7% during a medium follow-up of 2 years. These authors also presented a normalisation of acid exposure time during ambulatory 24-hour pH monitoring re-enforcing the functional outcome. In another recent series with five years follow-up in patients with long-segment Barrett's esophagus, no differences were found in clinical outcome compared to non Barrett's cases but in similar studies often objective data on the level of reflux control were not available.

It is uncertain why there is a discrepancy between the surgical results in patients with Barrett's esophagus. It is possible, perhaps even likely, that some institutions present data from patients representing a less severe spectrum who are referred earlier in the disease process with the undoubted success of the operative approach. Another possible difference may be the longer follow-up in some of the studies. Presently it can be concluded that there is no conclusive evidence to suggest that all patients with Barrett's esophagus should be treated differently from patients without columnar metaplastic changes. There is a continuing need for studies focusing on factors that predict poor outcomes following antireflux surgery.

Prevention of neo-plastic transformation by control of reflux?

The long duration between development of Barrett's esophagus and its malignant degeneration is important to bare in mind since it suggests that there is a significant time during which therapeutic and/or preventive interventions may have the potential to be effective. There are, however, a number of very important questions, which have to be specifically addressed when discussing the different options available in cancer prevention. Firstly it has to be considered whether the respective therapies can prevent the occurrence of columnar metaplasia, secondly if the extent of columnar metaplasia can be reduced (regression), thirdly if the occurrence of intestinal metaplasia and dysplasia can be prevented and finally if regression of established dysplastic lesions is possible?

Histological identification of dysplasia within Barrett's mucosa is at present the most reliable way of identifying patients who are already harbouring adenocarcinoma or are at risk of developing one. Although the extent of columnar metaplasia may be prognostically important there are difficulties in studying this specific parameter prospectively in clinical trials. Similarly, the loss of the "at risk" mucosa, *i.e* intestinal metaplasia, in patients with Barrett's esophagus is also rare. However, the majority of patients with intestinal metaplasia of the cardia may be of significance, since it has been reported that the cardia loose its intestinal metaplasia after well functioning fundoplication operations.

All studies designed to address preventive aspects are exposed to specific methodological problems since the length of Barrett's esophagus, as determined by the measurement of landmarks, may be influenced by surgery per se. In particular, the position of the end of the tubular esophagus may be shifted by the fundoplication and approximation of the crura and this may give false impression of regression. It is important to know that careful studies have indicated that regression tended not to be observed at the time of the first and second postoperative endoscopy but rather after that more than two years had elapsed. The median length of Barrett's esophagus in patients, in whom regression occurred, was similar before operation and one year afterwards, but there was a steady decline between the measurements recorded at two and seven years after the operation. Data have been presented to show that a late progression of Barrett's esophagus may be associated with failures of the surgical procedures to control reflux, observations which may have importance for the design of long-term follow-up strategies *(figure 1)*.

Careful review of the literature suggest that regression of columnar lined epithelium is influenced by good symptomatic response and effective and objectively maintained control of reflux.

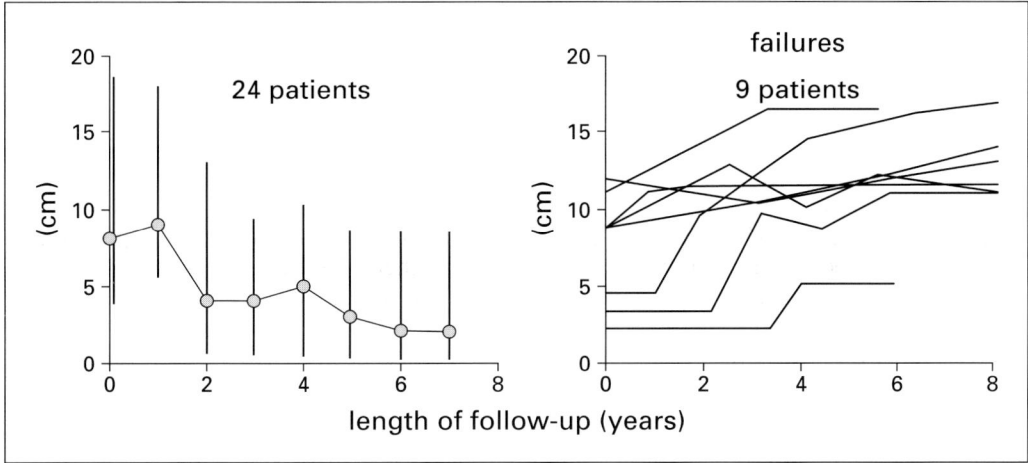

Figure 1. The effect of antireflux surgery on the extent of CLE in patients with a long-term functioning repair compared to those having failure (after Sagar *et al.* 1995).

Does antireflux surgery prevent from dysplasia and cancer?

This question cannot be addressed directly based on the obvious methodological issues and difficulties, which have to be taken into account. The optimal design of a prospective clinical trial to answer a similar question would require: pre-entry characterisation and mapping of both the underlying disease in general and the Barrett's epithelium in particular. Application of a proper definition of anatomical, endoscopic landmarks and rigid protocols for tissue sampling. Furthermore a similar clinical protocol requires a long term follow-up (5-10 years) with repeated endoscopies and biopsy taking to which must be added objective assessment of the level of reflux control both in the short- and long-term perspective. Review in the surgical literature brings into focus two points which require attention and one is the fact that only a comparatively small number of patients have been followed more than five years after an antireflux operation and furthermore that, at any time during the postoperative period a comparatively small proportion has been investigated in order to assess objectively the level of reflux control (endoscopy ± 24 hour pH-monitoring). In the figure are collected the number of cases in whom dysplasia were revealed in biopsies from the columnar lined esophagus during postoperative follow-up. It can be seen that a very small number of cases were found in whom high-grade dysplasia has been documented which is far fewer than the expected rate in a corresponding untreated cohorts of Barrett's patients *(figure 2)*.

Coming to the delicate question of direct cancer prevention, additional methodological problems emerge. Although we need to clarify the eventual reversibility of the step from high-grade dysplasia to neoplasia. A reasonable working hypothesis would currently be that this process is irreversible. Furthermore, it can be concluded that this process is slow. The immediate implications of these assumptions are that when assessing the occurrence

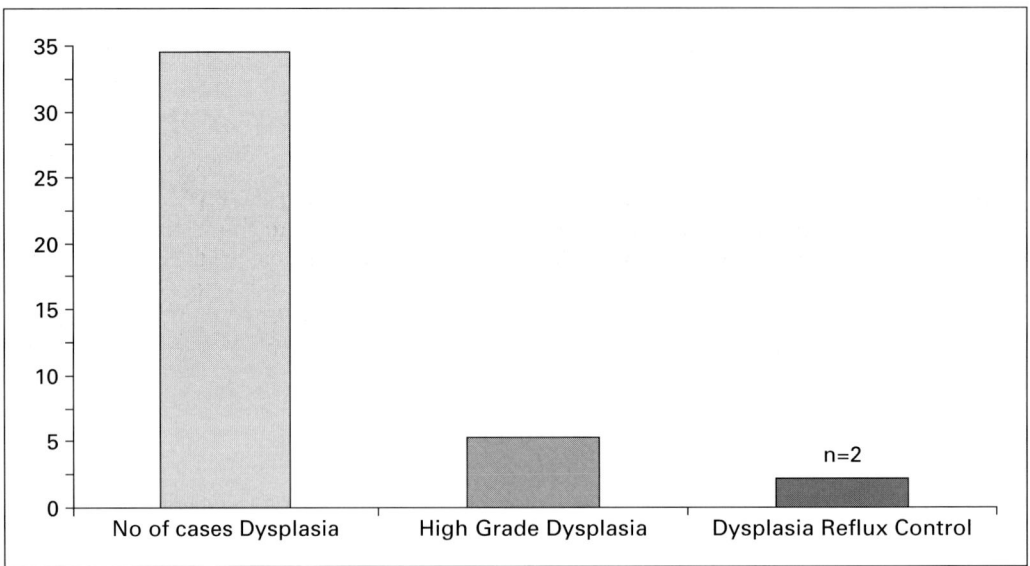

Figure 2. Literature review over the occurrence of dysplasia in CLE after well functioning antireflux operations.

of cancer after induction of effective therapy, a certain time must elapse before *de novo* neoplasia can be accepted as being casually related or affected by the instituted therapy (avoidance of so called prevalent neoplasia).

Addressing the pivotal question of cancer prevention by antireflux surgery, the intention to treat analysis has initially to be applied. By reviewing the relevant surgical literature until 2002, some 20 publications could be scrutinized with a reasonably well-characterized study population and combined with a fair follow-up. Applying a similar analysis the problem of heterogeneity has also to be recognized. An estimated incidence of adenocarcinoma after antireflux surgery undoubtedly converges towards the same level as previously published in untreated or medically treated Barrett cohorts. The outcome of a similar analytical approach is recently supported by the nationwide epidemiological study from Sweden where the incidence of adenocarcinoma in operated patients did not differ from that of the control population.

Review of the literature shows that the majority of cases of adenocarcinoma occurring after previous antireflux surgery have been diagnosed five years or less after the operation. More importantly, however, is that those patients where an objective assessment of reflux control had been carried out, only seven patients developed an invasive carcinoma. All except one of these latter patients had a cancer diagnosed within five years of the operation. In fact only one Barrett's case can be found in the surgical literature where an adenocarcinoma has developed more than five years after a well functioning antireflux operation. In the recent epidemiological study of a large cohort of patients after antireflux operations, where the same incidence of adenocarcinoma was found as in the controls, it should be realized that among those ten patients who, after an alleged antireflux operation developed a new carcinoma, none had any data to document the effectiveness of the antireflux repair.

In this context it should also be emphasised that the trend towards increased risk over time was not existing in those having antireflux surgery as compared to those having an untreated "chronic reflux disease".

Based on the present state of knowledge it cannot be concluded that antireflux surgery, as it is practised in routine surgical care, prevents from adenocarcinoma. On the other hand, since the most important indication for antireflux operations in Barrett's esophagus is to effectively and durably control symptoms, it is important to objectively assess the efficacy of the antireflux repair. Having done so a potential bonus can be that these patients may be exposed to a low risk of subsequent dysplastic or neo-plastic changes in the metaplastic epithelium. The message so far is, however, that follow-up strategies should be the same irrespective whether an antireflux operation has been carried out or not.

References

1. Cameron AJ, Ott BJ, Payne WS. The incidence of adenocarcinoma in columnar lined (Barrett's) esophagus. *N Engl J Med* 1985; 313: 857-9.
2. Spechler SJ, Robbins AH, Rubins HB, *et al*. Adenocarcinoma and Barrett's esophagus. An overrated risk? *Gastroenterology* 1984; 87: 927-33.
3. Hansson LE, Sparen P, Nyren O. Increasing incidence of both major histological types of esophageal carcinomas among men in Sweden. *Int J Cancer* 1993; 54: 402-7.
4. Parkin DM, Whelan SL, Ferby J, *et al. Cancer incidence in five continents.* Vol VII. IARC scientific publ. No 143, International agency on cancer. Lyon, 1997. pp. 66-8.
5. Lagergren J, Bergström R, Lindgren A, Nyren O. Symptomatic gastroesophageal reflux as a risk factor for esophageal adenocarcinoma. *N Engl J Med* 1999; 340: 825-31.
6. Ye W, Chow WH, Lagergren J, Yin L, Nyren O. Risk of adenocarcinomas of the esophagus and gastric cardia in patients with gastroesophageal reflux disease and after anti reflux surgery. *Gastroenterology* 2001; 121: 1286-93.
7. Campos GMR, DeMeester SR, Peters JH, *et al*. Predictive factors of Barrett esophagus. Multivariate analysis of 502 patients with gastroesophageal reflux disease. *Arch Surg* 2001; 136: 1267-73.
8. Menke Pluymers MBE, Hop WCJ, Dees J, *et al*. Risk factors for the development of an adenocarcinoma in columnar lined (Barrett) esophagus. *Cancer* 1993; 72: 1155-8.
9. Weston AP, Badr AS, Hassanein RS. Prospective multivariate analysis of clinical, endoscopic and histological factors predictive of the development of Barrett's multifocal high grade dysplasia or adenocarcinoma. *Am J Gastroenterol* 1999; 94: 3413-9.
10. Tilanus HW, Attwood SEA. *Barrett's esophagus.* Cluevenar Academical Publisher 2001.
11. Watson DI, Jamieson GG. Antireflux surgery in the laparoscopic era. *Br J Surg* 1998; 85: 1173-84.
12. Peters FTM, Ganesh S, Kuipers EJ, *et al*. Endoscopic regression of Barrett's esophagus during omeprazole treatment. A randomised double blind study. *Gut* 1999; 45: 489-94.
13. Neuman CS, Iqbal TH, Cooper BT. Long term continuous omeprazole treatment of patients with Barrett's esophagus. *Aliment Pharmacol Ther* 1995; 9: 451-4.
14. Ortiz A, Martínez de Haro LF, Parrilla P, Molina J, Bermejo J, Munitiz V. 24-h pH monitoring is necessary to assess acid reflux suppression in patients with Barrett's esophagus undergoing treatment with proton pump inhibitors. *Br J Surg* 1999; 86: 1472-4.
15. Katzka DA, Castell DO. Successful elimination of reflux symptoms does not ensure adequate control of acid reflux in Barrett's esophagus. *Am J Gastroenterol* 1994; 89: 989-91.
16. Kuo B, Castell DO. Optimal dosing of omeprazole 40 mg daily: effects on gastric and esophageal pH and serum gastrin in healthy controls. *Am J Gastroenterol* 1996; 91: 1532-8.

17. Ouatu-Lascar R, Triadafilopoulos G. Complete elimination of reflux symptoms does not guarantee normalization of intraesophageal acid reflux in patients with Barrett's esophagus. *Am J Gastroenterol* 1998; 93: 711-6.
18. Johnson D, Winters C, Spurling T, *et al.* Esophageal acid sensitivity in Barrett's esophagus. *J Clin Gastroenterol* 1987; 9: 23-7.
19. Reid BJ, Haggitt RC, Rubin CE, Rabinovitsch PS. Barrett's esophagus. Correlation between flow cytometry and histology in detection of patients at risk for adenocarcinoma. *Gastroenterol* 1987; 93: 1-11.
20. Nowell PC. The clonal evolution of tumour cell populations. *Science* 1976; 194: 23-8.
21. Lane DP, Benchimol S. p53 Oncogene or anti oncogene? *Genes Dev* 1990; 4: 1-8.
22. Reid BJ, Prevo LJ, Sanchez CA, Galipeau PC. p53-mutant clones are prevalent and undergo variable expansion in Barrett's esophagus with high-grade dysplasia and no cancer. *Am J Gastroenterol* 1999; 94: 2598.
23. Reid BJ, Levine DS, Longton G, Blount PL, Rabinovitsch PS. Predictors of progression to cancer in Barrett's esophagus baseline histology and flow cytometry identify low and high risk patients subsets. *Am J Gastroenterol* 1999; 94: 2598.
24. Zhang F, Subbaramaiah K, Altorki N, Dannenberg AJ. Dihydroxy bile acids activate the transcription of cyclooxygenase -2. *J Bio Chem* 1998; 273: 2424-8.
25. Fitzgerald RC, Omary MB, Triadafilopoulos G. Dynamic effects of acid on Barrett's esophagus: an ex vivo proliferation and differentiation model. *J Clin Invest* 1996; 98: 2120-8.
26. Ouatu-Lascar R, Fitzgerald RC, Triadafilopoulos G. Differentiation and proliferation in Barrett's esophagus and the effects of acid suppression. *Gastroenterology* 1999; 117: 327-35.
27. Shirvani VN, Ouatu-Lascar R, Kaur BS, *et al.* Cyclo-oxygenase 2 expression in Barrett's esophagus and adenocarcinoma: ex vivo induction by bile salts and acid exposure. *Gastroenterology* 2000; 118: 487-96.
28. Brand DL, Yenisaker JT, Gelfand M, *et al.* Regression of columnar esophageal (Barrett's) epithelium after antireflux surgery. *N Engl J Med* 1980; 302: 844-8.
29. Skinner DB, Walther BC, Riddell RH, *et al.* Barrett's esophagus: comparison of benign and malignant cases. *Ann Surg* 1983; 198: 554-66.
30. Starnes VA, Adkins RB, Ballinger JF, *et al.* Barrett's esophagus. A surgical entity. *Arch Surg* 1984; 119: 563-7.
31. DeMeester TR, Attwood SEA, Smyrk TC, *et al.* Surgical therapy in Barret's esophagus. *Ann Surg* 1990; 212: 528-42.
32. Williamson WA, Ellis FHE, Gibb SP, Shahian DM, Aretz T. Effect of antireflux operation on Barrett's mucosa. *Ann Thorac Surg* 1990; 49: 537-42.
33. McEntee GP, Stuart RC, Byrne PS, *et al.* An evaluation of surgical and medical treatment of Barrett's esophagus. *Gullet* 1991; 1: 169-72.
34. McCallum RW, Polepalle S, Dawenport K, *et al.* Role of anti reflux surgery against dysplasia in Barrett's esophagus. *Gastroenterology* 1991; 100: A121.
35. Attwood SEA, Barlow AP, Norris TL, Watson A. Barrett's esophagus: effect of antireflux surgery on symptom control and development of complications. *Br J Surg* 1992; 79: 1050-3.
36. Sagar PM, Ackroyd R, Hosie KB, Pattersson JE, Stoddard CJ, Kingsnorth AN. Regression and progression of Barrett's esophagus after antireflux surgery. *Br J Surg* 1995; 82: 806-10.
37. Ortiz A, Martinez de Haro LF, Parrilla P, *et al.* Conservative treatment *versus* antireflux surgery in Barrett's esophagus: long-term results of a prospective study. *Br J Surg* 1996; 83: 274-8.
38. McDonald ML, Trastek VF, Allen M. Deschamps C, Pairolero PC. Barrett's esophagus: Does an antireflux procedure reduce the need of endoscopic surveillance? *J Thorac Cardiovasc Surg* 1996; 111: 1135-40.
39. DeMeester SR, Campos GMR, DeMeester TR, *et al.* The impact of anti reflux surgery on intestinal metaplasia of the cardia. *J Gastrointest Surg* 1998; 228: 547-56.

40. Low DE, Levine DS, Dail DH, Kozarek RA. Histological and anatomic changes in Barrett's esophagus after antireflux surgery. *Am J Gastroenterol* 1999; 94: 80-5.
41. Patti MG, Arcentino M, Feo CV, et al. Barrett's esophagus. A surgical disease. *J Gastrointest Surg* 1999; 3: 397-404.
42. Hofstetter WL, Peters JH, DeMeester TR, et al. Long-term outcome of antireflux surgery in patients with Barrett's esophagus. *Ann Surg* 2001; 234: 532-8.
43. Farrell TM, Smith CD, Metreveli RE, et al. Fundoplication provides effective and durable symptom relief in patients with Barrett's esophagus. *Am J Surg* 1999; 178: 18-21.
44. Csendes A, Burdiles P, Korn O, et al. Late results of a randomised clinical trial comparing total fundoplication *versus* calibration of the cardia with posterior gastropexy. *Br J Surg* 2000; 87: 289-97.
45. Csendes A, Burdiles P, Braghetto I, et al. Early and late results of the acid suppression and duodenal diversion operation in patients with Barrett's esophagus: analysis of 210 cases. *World J Surg* 2002; 26: 556-76.
46. Yau P, Watson DI, Devitte PG, Game PA, Jamieson GG. Laparoscopic antireflux surgery in the treatment of gastroesophageal reflux in patients with Barrett's Esophagus. *Arch Surg* 2000; 135: 801-5.
47. Lundell L, Miettinen P, Myrwold ME, et al. Continued (5 year) follow-up of a randomised clinical study comparing anti reflux surgery and omeprazole in gastro-esophageal reflux disease. *J Am Coll Surg* 2001; 192: 172-9.
48. Hagedorn C, Lonroth H, Rydberg L, Ruth M, Lundell L. Long-term efficacy of total(Nissen-Rossetti) and a posterior partial (Toupet) fundoplication. Results from a randomised clinical trial. *J Gastrointest Surg* 2002; 6: 540-5.
49. Stein HJ, Kauer WKH, Feussner H, Siewert JR. Bile reflux benign and malignant Barrett's esophagus: effect of medical acid suppression and Nissen fundoplication. *J Gastrointest Surg* 1998; 2: 333-41.
50. Jamieson GG, Watson DI. Optimal surgical therapy for reflux disease. In: Tilanus HW, Attwood SEA. *Barrett's esophagus.* Cluevenar Academical Publisher 2001, pp. 137-48.
51. Csendes A, Burdiles P, Korn O. Surgical treatment of duodeno-gastro-esophageal reflux. In: Tilanus HW, Attwood SEA. *Barrett's esophagus.* Cluevenar Academical Publisher 2001, pp. 149-58.
52. Shaheen NJ, Bozymski EM. Does antireflux surgery alter the natural history of Barrett's esophagus? *AJG* 1999; 94: 11-2.
53. Hameeteman W, Tytgat GN, Houthoff HJ, van den Tweel JG. Barrett's esophagus: Development of dysplasia and adenocarcinoma. *Gastroenterology* 1989; 96: 1249-56.
54. Spechler SJ, Goyal RK. Cancer surveillance in Barrett's esophagus: What is the end point? *Gastroenterology* 1994; 106 (1): 275-7.
55. Rabinovitsch PS, Reid BJ, Haggitt RC, Norwood TH, Rubin CE. Progression to cancer in Barrett's esophagus is associated with genomic instability. *Laboratory Investigation* 1988; 60: 65-71.
56. Nigro JJ, Hagen JA, DeMeester TR, et al. Occult esophageal adenocarcinoma. Extent of disease and implications for effective therapy. *Annual of Surgery* 1999; 230 (3), 433-40.
57. Zaninotto H, Pestrny ST, Vodysnini TM, Merigliano S, Ancona E. Esophageal resection for high-grade dysplasia in Barrett's esophagus. *British Journal of Surgery* 2000; 87: 1102-5.
58. van Sandick JW, van Lanschot JJB, Kuiken BW, Tytgat GNJ, Offerhaus GJA, Obertorp H. Impact of endoscopic biopsy surveillance of Barrett's carcinoma. *Gut* 1998: 43: 216-22.
59. McArdle JE, Lewin KJ, Randall G, Weinstein W. Distribution of dysplasias and early invasive carcinoma in Barrett's esophagus. *Hum Pathol* 1992; 23: 479-82.
60. Altorki NK, Sunagawa M, Little AG, Skinner DB. High-grade dysplasia in the columnar-lined esophagus. *Am J Surg* 1991; 161: 97-9, discussion 99-100.
61. Schmidt HG, Riddell RH, Walther B, Skinner DB, Riemann JF. Dysplasia in Barrett's esophagus. *J Cancer Res Clin Oncol* 1985; 110(2): 145-52.
62. DeMeester SR, Campos GMR, DeMeester TR, et al. The impact of an antireflux procedure on intestinal metaplasia of the cardia. *Ann Surg* 1998; 228 (4): 547-56.

63. Öberg S, Johansson J, Wenner J, et al. Endoscopic surveillance of columnar-lined esophagus: frequency of intestinal metaplasia detection and impact of anti reflux surgery. *Ann Surg* 2001; 234: 619-26.
64. Iftikhar SY, James PD, Steele RJC, et al. Length of Barrett's esophagus: an important factor in the development of dysplasia and adenocarcinoma. *Gut* 1992; 33: 1155-8.
65. Avadin B, Sonnenberg A, Schnell TG, et al. Hiatal hernia, Barret's length and severity of acid reflux are all risk factors for esophageal adenocarcinoma. *Am J Gastroenterol* 2002; 97: 1930-6.
66. DeMeester TR. The surgical management of Barrett's esophagus and mucosal ablation. In: *Barrett's esophagus*. An update. Ed. Peracchia A, Bonavina L. EDRA Medical Publishing New Media 1999, pp. 79-92.
67. Isolauri J, Loustarinen M, Viljakka M, Isolauro E, Keyrilainen O, Karvonen AL. Long-term comparison of antireflux surgery *versus* conservative therapy for reflux esophagitis. *Ann Surg* 1997; 225: 295-9.
68. Csendes A, Braghetto I, Burdiles P, et al. Long term results of classic antireflux surgery in 152 patients with Barrett's esophagus: Clinical, radiologic, endoscopic, manometric, and acid reflux test analysis before and late after operation. *Surgery* 1998; 123: 545-57.
69. Katz D, Rothstein R, Schned A, Dunn J, Seaver K, Antonioli D. The development of dysplasia and adenocarcinoma during endoscopic surveillance of Barrett's esophagus. *Am J Gastroenterol* 1998; 93: 536-41.
70. Håkansson HO, Johnsson F, Johansson J, Kjellen G, Walther B. Development of adenocarcinoma in Barrett's esophagus after successful antireflux surgery. *Eur J Surg* 1996; 163: 469-47.
71. Naef AP, Savary M, Ozzello L. Columnar-lined lower esophagus: An acquired lesion with malignant predisposition. Report on 140 cases of Barrett's esophagus with 12 adenocarcinomas. *J Thorac Cardiovasc Surg* 1975; 70: 826-35.
72. Hamilton SR, Hutcheon DF, Ravich WJ, Cameron JL, Paulsson M. Adenocarcinoma in Barrett's esophagus after elimination of gastroesophageal reflux. *Gastroenterol* 1984; 86: 356-9.
73. Pearson FG, Cooper JD, Pattersson GA, Prakash D. Peptic ulcer in acquired columnar lined esophagus. Results of surgical treatment. *Ann Thorac Surg* 1987; 43: 241-4.
74. Pera M, Trastek VF, Carpenter HA, Allen MS, Deschamps C, Pairolero PC. Barrett's esophagus with high-grade dysplasia: An indication for esophagectomy? *Ann Thorac Surg* 1992; 54 (2): 199-204.
75. Parrilla P, Martinez de Haro LF, Ortiz A, et al. Long-term results of a randomised prospective study comparing medical and surgical treatment of Barrett's esophagus. *Ann Surg* 2003; 3: 291-8.
76. Csendes A, Burdiles P, Korn O, et al. Dysplasia and adenocarcinoma after classic antireflux surgery in patients with Barrett's esophagus. *Ann Surg* 2002; 235: 178-85.

Adenocarcinoma of the gastric cardia and gastro-esophageal junction

Kenneth E.L. McColl

University of Glasgow, Scotland, United Kingdom

The cardia is the most proximal region of the stomach, lying immediately below the gastro-esophageal junction. It is lined by columnar epithelium which does not have parietal cells and resembles the epithelium seen in the antral region of the stomach. The epithelium of the cardia region abuts proximally with the squamous mucosa of the distal esophagus and distally with the acid secreting mucosa of the body of the stomach.

There has been considerable debate over the past few years regarding whether the cardia epithelium is a normal anatomical feature or represents a pathological condition. This has been stimulated by the recognition that the cardia epithelium can be very small. Furthermore, it is widely recognized that gastro-esophageal reflux can induce metaplastic columnar mucosa in the distal esophagus resembling that occurring in the cardia. Some groups have therefore proposed that cardia epithelium is always pathological and the consequence of reflux disease [1-4] whereas others believe it to be a normal structure [5-7]. However, an elegant study by De Hertogh *et al.* has recently shown that a small rim of cardia mucosa is present in the foetus prior to the development of gastric acid secretion and this indicates that the cardia mucosa does represent normal anatomy [8]. However, it does appear as though the normal cardia is very small, being less than 1 mm in length [8]. Consequently, more extensive cardia mucosa may represent pathological consequences of reflux disease. From a physiological point of view, it makes sense to interpose a segment of non-acid secreting columnar mucosa between the acid secreting mucosa of the body of the stomach and the squamous mucosa of the esophagus. It will serve as a barrier preventing the esophageal squamous mucosa being damaged by acid being secreted in its immediate vicinity.

The complex epithelial anatomy at the gastro-esophageal junction causes major problems in determining the origin of neo-plastic disease arising at this site. This is due to the fact that several different types of epithelial exist in close proximity. There is the squamous epithelium of the esophagus meeting the columnar cardia mucosa in turn meeting the epithelium of the body region of the stomach. The fact that the cardia mucosa may be less than 1 mm in length means that these three different types of epithelia can all be found within 1 mm of each other. The situation is further complicated by the fact that the squamous mucosa of the distal esophagus is often metaplastic and transformed into either columnar mucosa similar to the cardia mucosa and/or intestinal mucosa which may be similar to small intestine or colonic epithelium. In addition, *H. Pylori* infection may induce intestinal metaplasia of the cardia epithelium and the epithelium of the body of the stomach. When adenocarcinoma occurs at the gastro-esophageal junction, it is therefore impossible to know whether it has arisen from distal esophagus or the cardia mucosa or the mucosa of the proximal body region of the stomach. From a practical point of view, it is therefore convenient to refer to tumours arising in this region as arising from the gastro-esophageal junction. This recognizes that tumours may be arising from the epithelium of the distal esophagus, the original cardia or the most proximal mucosa of the body region of the stomach.

The recent interest in the gastro-esophageal junction has been stimulated by the rising incidence of neo-plastic and pre-neoplastic lesions at this localized site. Over the past 25 years, the incidence of adenocarcinoma at the gastro-esophageal junction has increased more than 4-fold [9-13]. It is also becoming apparent that the anatomical region of the gastro-esophageal junction has a remarkably high propensity to cancer and precancerous lesions. Recent studies indicate that cancer of this site is as common as cancer throughout the whole of the esophagus and the whole of the rest of the stomach which both represent substantially larger areas [14]. In addition, there is a high incidence of metaplasia at this localized site. Gerson et al found intestinal metaplasia at the gastro-esophageal junction in 25% of asymptomatic subjects undergoing screening colonoscopy [15].

It has also become apparent that cancer at the gastro-esophageal junction is aetiologically distinct from the cancer of the rest of the stomach *(figure 1)*. This is demonstrated by the fact that while cancer of the GO junction has been increasing, cancer of the rest of the stomach is decreasing [9-13]. Cancer of the stomach is therefore now reclassified into two types according to its anatomical location. The one type consists of cancer occurring in the cardia region or at the gastro-esophageal junction and the other type occurring more distally and referred to as non-cardia gastric cancer. Another observation indicating different aetiologies for cardia and non-cardia cancer is their association with *Helicobacter pylori* infection. The infection is recognized to be an important risk factor for non-cardia gastric cancer and is thought to be responsible for 75% of non-cardia cancers [16]. In contrast, *H. Pylori* infection is not a risk factor for cancer of the gastro-esophageal junction. Indeed, studies from the west indicate that subjects with *H. Pylori* infection have a reduced risk of cancer at the gastro-esophageal junction [16].

Adenocarcinoma of the gastro-esophageal junction also differs from adenocarcinoma of the rest of the stomach with respect to the underlying gastric phenotype. Cancer of the non-cardia region of the stomach develops in patients with *H. Pylori*-induced atrophic gastritis and hypochlorhydria [17]. This applies to both the intestinal and diffuse type of cancer [17]. In contrast, atrophy and hypochlorhydria are not risk factors for cancer of the gastro-esophageal junction which develops in patients with healthy acid secreting stomachs [18].

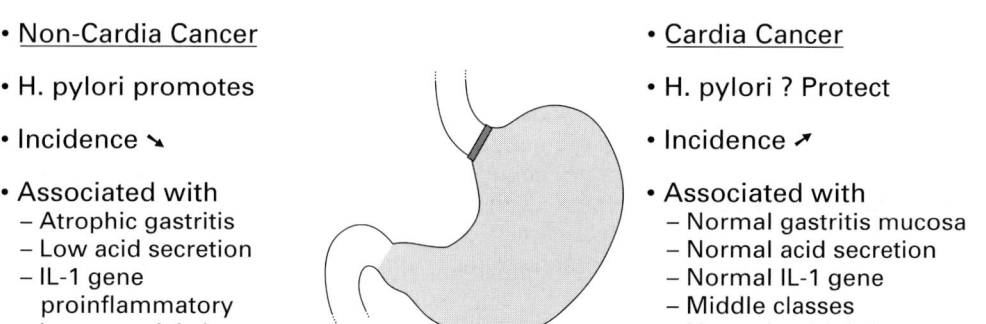

Figure 1. Differences between adenocarcinoma of the gastric carida and cancer of the more distal stomach.

Further differences between the cancers at these two sites is their association with socio-economic status and dietary habits. Adenocarcinoma of the non-cardia stomach is more common in patients of the lower socio-economic status [19]. Whereas, cancer of the gastro-esophageal junction tends to be more common in the middle classes and slightly less common in the socio-economic classes [19]. Cancer of non-cardia region is associated with a diet low in vitamin C and other antioxidants have been recognized to have an increased risk of developing non-cardia gastric cancer [20, 21]. However, there is little evidence of any association between antioxidant intake and cancer of the gastro-esophageal junction [20, 21].

It is therefore clear that cancer of the gastro-esophageal junction is aetiologically distinct from cancer of the rest of the stomach. Substantial advances have been made in our understanding of the aetiology of non-cardia gastric cancer over the past twenty years. This is recognized to be related to *H. Pylori* infection progressing to atrophy and hypochlorhydria and the contribution to this process of excess salt and low intake of antioxidants [22]. Genetic factors have also been identified which increase a propensity to develop atrophy and hypochlorhydria in response to *H. Pylori* infection and thus further explain the aetiology of non-cardia cancer [23]. However, the aetiology of cancer of the gastro-esophageal junction remains unclear. Several possible aetiological factors need to be considered.

Short segment reflux

There is interest in the possible role of gastro-esophageal reflux on the occurrence of cancer at the gastro-esophageal junction. It is recognized that reflux is associated with an increased risk of metaplasia and neoplasia of the distal esophagus. When this metaplasia extends more than 3 cm above the gastro-esophageal junction, it is referred to as Barrett's esophagus. It is thought that the reflux of acid and pepsin, and possibly bile, damage the squamous mucosa of the distal esophagus transforming it to columnar-type mucosa which in areas becomes intestinal in type. Could metaplasia and adenocarcinoma occurring at the cardia and gastro-esophageal junction also be due to gastric reflux? The association with reflux symptoms is much weaker than with cancer of the more proximal esophagus [24]. In addition, there is little if any association between metaplasia at the gastro-esophageal junction and cardia and reflux symptoms [15].

It is possible, however, that the metaplasia and neoplasia occurring at the cardia and gastro-esophageal junction is due to short segment reflux [25]. The latter term is used for gastric juice traversing the squamo-columnar junction but not fully traversing the lower esophageal sphincter. Recent studies in our unit have indicated that the most distal squamous epithelium of the esophagus is exposed to a substantial amount of acid even in subjects without reflux symptoms [25]. In addition, these studies by Fletcher *et al.* indicate that the cardia region of the stomach is not buffered by food and remains highly acidic after meals [25]. This unbuffered acid pocket which exists at the cardia frequently traverses the squamo-columnar junction *(figure 2)*. This asymptomatic short segment reflux could contribute to the high incidence of metaplasia and neoplasia confined to the gastro-esophageal junction.

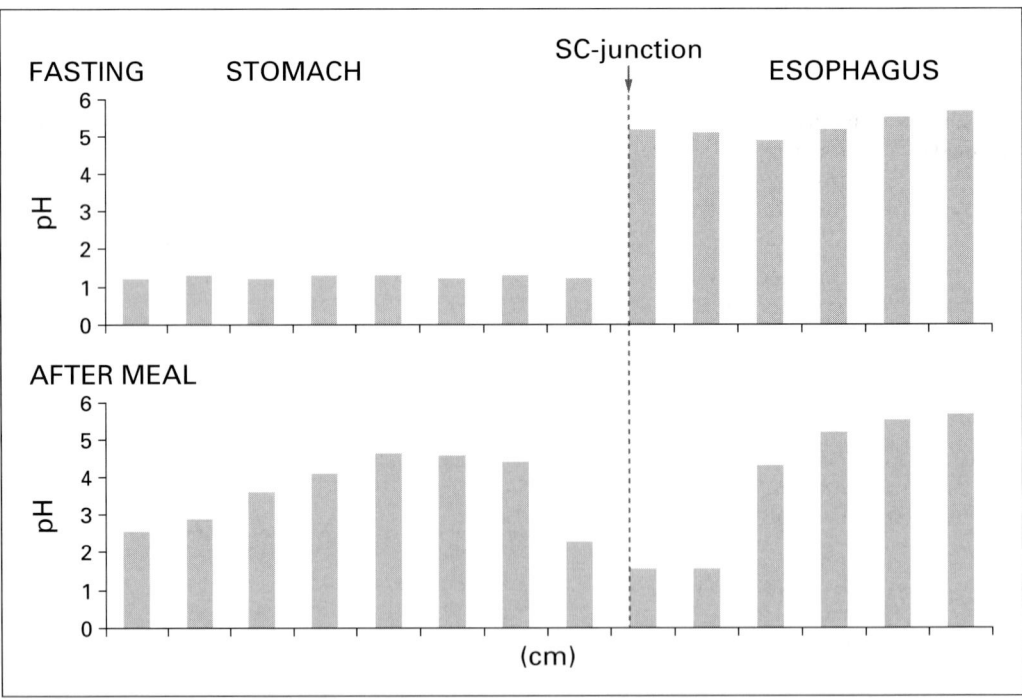

Figure 2. Following a meal, the cardia region of the stomach remains highly acidic and is not protected by the buffering effect of the meal. In addition, the acid pocket at the cardia frequently extends across the squamo-columnar junction even in asymptomatic subjects. From [25].

Though short segment reflux of acid and pepsin and bile would damage the squamous mucosa at the gastro-esophageal junction, it is uncertain whether this process would be sufficient to account for the high incidence of neoplasia at this site. After all, acid, pepsin and bile are not in themselves mutagenic. For example, in duodenal ulcer disease, there is chronic damage of the epithelium of the duodenum by acid, pepsin and bile but no increased incidence of neoplasia. Damage to the epithelium by acid, pepsin and bile will increase epithelial turnover and therefore make the dividing cells more sensitive to DNA damage. In addition, inflammation induced by the epithelial damage may generate radicals which could damage the replicating DNA. However, the inflammatory response to gastro-esophageal reflux is relatively small. One therefore has to consider any source of a mutagenic substance which might act at this particular anatomical site.

Dietary nitrate

For many years there has been interest in the potential role of nitrite in the aetiology of neoplasia of the upper gastrointestinal tract. This is due to the fact that the acidic conditions existing in the stomach can convert nitrite to nitrous acid and *N*-nitroso compounds which are proven carcinogens [26]. The major source of nitrite entering the acid secreting stomach is in swallowed saliva. The nitrite in saliva is derived from dietary nitrate and its enterosalivary recirculation. Thirty per cent of all nitrate absorbed from the diet or generated in the body is taken up from the blood by the salivary glands and secreted into the mouth [27-33]. The main source of dietary nitrate is nitrogenous fertilizers which have been used in increased amounts since the end of the second world war [34-36]. Following its secretion into the mouth about 30% of the nitrate is reduced to nitrite by bacteria on the dorsum of the tongue [37-42]. As a consequence of this chemistry, saliva contains high levels of nitrite for several hours after ingesting nitrate-containing foodstuffs. This nitrite swallowed in the saliva is the main source of nitrite entering the stomach.

On entering the stomach, the acidic pH of gastric juice converts the nitrite to nitrous acid and nitrosating species which can react with 2nd amines and amides to form carcinogenic *N*-nitroso compounds [26]. Thiocyanate, which is present in saliva and gastric juice, catalyses this chemical reaction [43, 44]. The optimum pH for nitrosation in the presence of thiocyanate is 2.5 [43, 44]. The main factor inhibiting the generation of *N*-nitroso compounds from nitrite entering the acidic stomach is ascorbic acid which is actively secreted in gastric juice and ingested in the diet [45-53]. The ascorbic acid rapidly reacts with the nitrosating species reducing them to nitric oxide and in the process is oxidized to dehydroascorbic acid [50-53].

This chemistry indicates that the conditions most favouring *N*-nitroso compound formation within the stomach is an acidic pH of 2.5, the presence of nitrite and thiocyanate and the absence of adequate ascorbic acid.

Previously, it was considered that nitrosation will occur homogeneously throughout the lumen of the stomach. However, the source of the chemicals involved suggest that this may not be the case, but that the conditions favouring nitrosation may be maximal in the site where the nitrite-laden saliva first encounters acidic gastric juice *i.e* the gastro-esophageal junction. If this is the case, then it could provide the source of a mutagen contributing to the high incidence of metaplasia and neoplasia at this site.

We have recently examined the concentrations of the chemicals relevant to nitrosation at different locations in the human upper gastrointestinal tract before and following ingestion of nitrate [54]. This was performed by positioning microdialysis probes in the distal esophagus, cardia region of the stomach as well as mid and distal stomach. At each of these sites, we simultaneously monitored the local pH and concentrations of nitrite, thiocyanate and ascorbic acid. The studies showed that high concentrations of nitrite exist throughout the length of the human esophagus being similar to those in saliva. In addition, we found that the concentration of nitrite was highest in the cardia region of the stomach and the concentration of ascorbic acid lowest in the cardia region. Substantial levels of thiocyanate were present throughout the length of the stomach. These findings indicate that the conditions for luminal generation of *N*-nitroso compounds derived from dietary nitrate is maximal at the gastro-esophageal junction and cardia.

The above studies also indicated a substantial fall in luminal nitrite, concentration between the distal esophagus and proximal stomach. This is most readily explained by the nitrite being reduced to nitric oxide by ascorbic acid. Nitric oxide is itself potentially mutagenic as it can react with oxygen to form nitrosating species at neutral pH. This mechanism is one of the ways in which chronic inflammation is thought to lead to cancer. We therefore proceeded to monitor luminal nitric oxide concentration throughout the length of the esophagus and stomach before and after nitrate ingestion [55]. Again, we found that the highest luminal concentrations occurred at the cardia and gastro-esophageal junction where salivary nitrite first meets acidic gastric juice. Nitric oxide is highly diffusible and will rapidly diffuse into the epithelium and the gastro-esophageal junction and in this way might also contribute to the high incidence of mutagenesis at this anatomical site.

The gastric cardia and gastro-esophageal junction is thus an anatomical region of very active and potentially mutagenic nitrite chemistry *(figure 3)*. The susceptibility of tissues to the mutagenic effects of *N*-nitroso compounds is increased by inflammation [56]. Damage to the most distal esophageal mucosa by short segment reflux of acid, pepsin and bile is likely to increase the epithelium sensitivity to locally generated mutagenic *N*-nitroso compounds.

H. Pylori

The rise in incidence of cancer at the cardia and gastro-esophageal junction has coincided with a fall in incidence of cancer of the more distal stomach. The fall in incidence of the latter has been attributed to the fall in prevalence of *H. Pylori* infection. There has been considerable interest in the possibility that the increase in cancer of the cardia and gastro-esophageal junction might also be related to *H. Pylori* infection and the loss of a protective effect exerted by it. Such a protective effect could be mediated by the ability of *H. Pylori* infection to lower gastric acid secretion as cancer at the gastro-esophageal junction and cardia is associated with normal or high acid secretion [18]. In subjects in whom the infection produces an atrophic pangastritis there is marked suppression of acid secretion

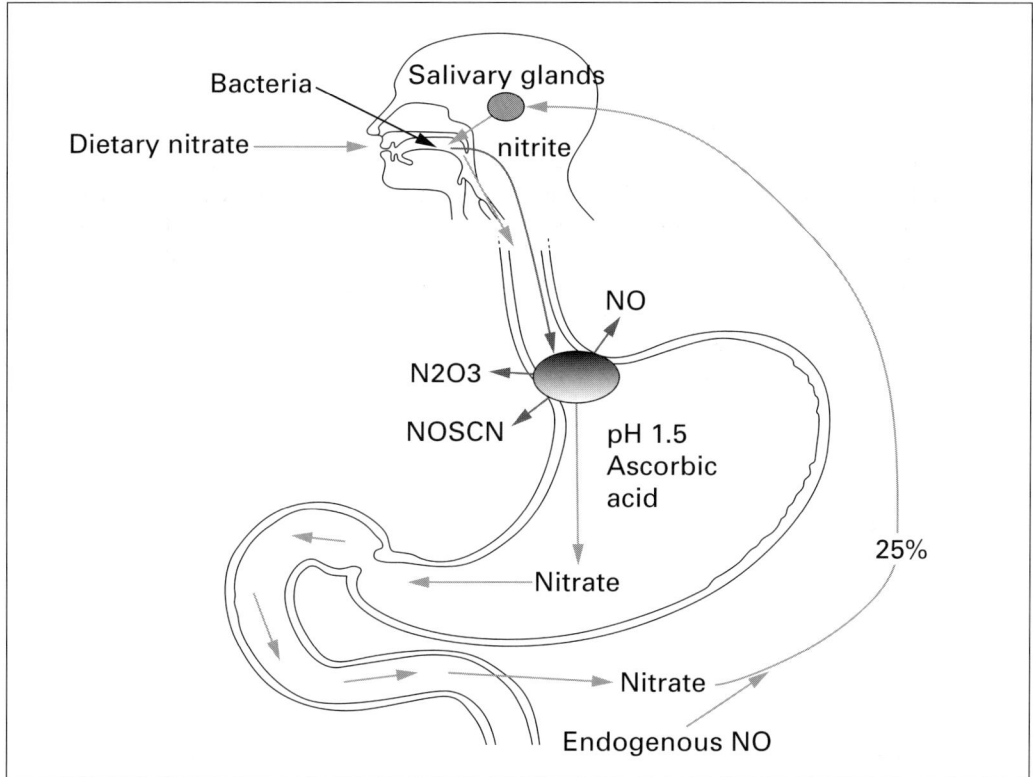

Figure 3. Following its absorption, 30% of dietary nitrate is taken up by the salivary glands and secreted into the mouth. Bacteria on the dorsum of the tongue reduce the nitrate to nitrite. When the nitrate in saliva encounters the acidic gastric juice it is immediately converted to nitrosative species and nitric oxide which may exert mutagenic effects on the adjacent mucosa. This nitrosative chemistry arising from dietary nitrate via salivary nitrite is highly focussed at the gastric cardia and gastro-esophageal junction.

which is only partially reversible by eradicating the infection [57]. Numerous studies have shown that this pattern of gastritis protects against reflux disease [58-62] which may be a factor in the aetiology of gastro-esophageal junction cancer as described above. In the first half of the twentieth century, the prevalence of atrophic pangastritis and hypochlorhydria in *H. Pylori* infected subjects is likely to have been high and thereby explain the low incidence of reflux disease and its complications. It will also have protected from the luminal nitrosative chemistry being focused at the gastro-esophageal junction and cardia as this is also an acid-induced phenomenon. Indirect, but robust evidence that *H. Pylori* predominantly induced atrophic pangastritis and low acid in the early twentieth century is the low prevalence of duodenal ulcer at that time [63]. Duodenal ulceration develops in response to an antral predominant non-atrophic gastritis which stimulates increased acid secretion. As the twentieth century progressed both *H. Pylori* infection and atrophic gastritis in infected subjects has decreased. The consequent rise in acid secretion is likely to have contributed to the rise in cancer of the cardia and gastro-esophageal junction.

References

1. Zhou H, Alba Greco M, Daum F, *et al.* Origin of cardia mucosa: ontogenic consideration. *Pediatr Dev Pathol* 2001; 4: 358-63.
2. Chandrasoma P, Lokuhetty DM, Demeester TR, *et al.* Definition of histopathologic changes in gastroesophageal reflux disease. *Am J Surg Pathol* 2000; 24: 344-51.
3. Chandrasoma P, Der R, Ma Y, *et al.* Histology of the gastroesophageal junction – an autopsy study. *Am J Surg Pathol* 2000; 24: 402-9.
4. Chandrasoma P, Der R, Dalton P, *et al.* Distribution and significance of epithelial types in columnar-lined esophagus. *Am J Surg Pathol* 2001; 25: 1188-93.
5. Zhou H, Alba Greco M, Daum F, *et al.* Origin of cardiac mucosa: ontogenic consideration. *Pediatr Dev Pathol* 2001; 4: 358-63.
6. Glickman JN, Fox V, Antonioli DA, *et al.* Morphology of the cardia and significance of carditis in pediatric patients. *Am J Surg Pathol* 2002; 26: 1032-9.
7. Kilgore SP, Ormsby AH, Gramlich TL, *et al.* The gastric cardia: fact or fiction? *Am J Gastroenterol* 2000; 95: 921-4.
8. Hertogh De G, Eyken Van P, Ectors N, Tack J, Geboes K. On the existence and location of cardia mucosa: an autopsy study in embryos, fetuses and infants. *Gut* 2003; 52: 791-6.
9. Hansson L-E, Sparén P, Nyrén O. Increasing incidence of carcinoma of the gastric cardia in Sweden from 1970 to 1985. *Br J Surg* 1993; 80: 374-7.
10. Blot W, Devesa SS, Kneller RW, Fraumeni Jr JF. Rising incidence of adenocarcinoma of the esophagus and gastric cardia. *JAMA* 1991; 13: 265: No. 10: 1287-9.
11. Powell J, McConkey CC. Increasing incidence of adenocarcinoma of the gastric cardia and adjacent sites. *Br J Cancer* 1990; 62: 440-3.
12. Hansen S, Wiig JN, Giercksky KE, Tretli S. Esophageal and gastric carcinoma in Norway 1958-1992: incidence time trend variability according to morphological subtypes and organ subtypes. *Int J Cancer* 1997; 71: 340-4.
13. Botterweck AAM, Schouten LJ, Volovics A, Dorant E, van den Brandt PA. Trends in incidence of adenocarcinoma of the esophagus and gastric cardia in ten European countries. *Int J Epidemiol* 2000; 29: 645-54.
14. Byrne JP, Mathers JM, Parry JM, Attwood SEA, Bancewicz J, Woodman CBJ. Site distribution of esophagogastric cancer. *J Clin Pathol* 2002; 55: 191-4.
15. Gerson LB, Shetler K, Triadafilopoulos G. Prevalence of Barrett's esophagus in asymptomatic individuals. *Gastroenterology* 2002; 123: 461-7.
16. *Helicobacter* and Cancer Collaborative Group. Gastric cancer and *Helicobacter pylori*: a combined analysis of 12 case control studies nested within prospective cohorts. *Gut* 2001; 49: 347-53.
17. Uemura N, Okamoto S, Yamamoto S, *et al. Helicobacter pylori* infection and the development of gastric cancer. *N Eng J Med* 2001; 345: 11: 784-9.
18. Fischermann K, Bech I, Andersen B. Diagnostic value of the augmented histamine test in cancer of the upper part of the stomach. *Scand J Gastroenterol* 1969; 4: 517-9.
19. Brewster DH, Fraser LA, McKinney PA, Black RJ. Socioeconomic status and risk of adenocarcinoma of the esophagus and cancer of the gastric cardia in Scotland. *Br J Cancer* 2000; 83 (3): 387-90.
20. Terry P, Lagergren J, Ye W, Nyren O, Wolk A. Antioxidants and cancers of the esophagus and gastric cardia. *Int J Cancer* 2000; 87: 750-4.
21. Terry P, Lagergren J, Hansen H, Wolk A, Nyren O. Fruit and vegetable consumption in the prevention of esophageal and cardia cancers. *Eur J Cancer Prev* 2001; 10: 365-9.
22. McColl KEL, El-Omar E. How does *H. Pylori* infection cause gastric cancer? *Keio J Med* 2002; 51: 53-6.

23. El-Omar EM, Carrington M, Wong-Ho C, et al. Interleukin-1 polymorphisms associated with increased risk of gastric cancer. *Nature* 2000; 404: 398-9.
24. Lagergren J, Bergstrom R, Lindgren A, Nyren O. Symptomatic gastroesophageal reflux as a risk factor for esophageal adenocarcinoma. *New Eng J Med* 1999; 340: No. 11: 825-31.
25. Fletcher J, Wriz A, Young J, Vallance R, McColl KEL. Unbuffered highly acidic gastric juice exists at the gastroesophageal junction after a meal. *Gastroenterology* 2001; 121: 775-83.
26. Mirvish SS. Role of N-nitroso compounds (NOC) and N-nitrosation in aetiology of gastric, esophageal, nasopharyngeal and bladder cancer and contribution to cancer of known exposures to NOC. *Cancer Lett* 1995; 93: 17-48.
27. Walker R. Nitrates, nitrites and N-nitroso compounds: a review of the occurrence in food and diet and the toxicological implications. *Food Additives and Contaminants* 1990; 7: 6: 717-68.
28. Bos PMJ, van den Brandt PA, Wedel M, Ockhuizen Th. The reproducibility of the conversion of nitrate to nitrite in human saliva after a nitrate load. *Fd Chem Toxic* 1988; 26: No. 2: 93-7.
29. Wagner DA, Schultz DS, Deen WM, Young VR, Tannenbaum SR. Metabolic fate of an oral dose of ^{15}N-labeled nitrate in humans: Effect of diet supplementation with ascorbic acid. *Cancer Res* 1983; 43: 1921-5.
30. Dougall HT, Smith L, Duncan C, Benjamin N. The effect of amoxicillin on salivary nitrite concentrations: an important mechanism of adverse reactions? *Br J Clin Pharmac* 1995; 39: 460-2.
31. Granli T, Dahl R, Brodin P, Bockman OC. Nitrate and nitrite concentrations in human saliva: variations with salivary flow-rate. *Fd Chem Toxic* 1989; 27: No. 10: 675-80.
32. Bartholomew B, Hill MJ. The pharmacology of dietary nitrate and the origin of urinary nitrate. *Fd Chem Toxic* 1984; 22: No. 10: 789-95.
33. Tannenbaum SR, Weisman M, Fett D. The effect of nitrate intake on nitrite formation in human saliva. *Fd Cosmet Toxicol* 1976; 14: 549-52.
34. Food and Agriculture Organisation of the United Nations (FAO).
35. Wilson WS, Hayes MHB, Vaidyanathan LV. Average fertiliser use and estimates of nitrogen uptake by major arable crops in England and Wales. In: *Managing risks of nitrates to humans and the environment*. Ed: Wilson WS, Ball AS, Hinton RH. Royal Society of Chemistry, Special Publication no. 237, 1999.
36. Hood AEM. Fertiliser trends in relation to biological productivity within the U.K. *Phil Trans R Soc Lond*, 1982; B296: 315-28.
37. Walker R. Nitrates, nitrites and N-nitrosocompounds: a review of the occurrence in food and diet and the toxicological implications. *Food Additives and Contaminants* 1990; 7: 6: 717-68.
38. Bos PMJ, van den Brandt PA, Wedel M, Ockhuizen Th. The reproducibility of the conversion of nitrate to nitrite in human saliva after a nitrate load. *Fd Chem Toxic* 1988; 26: No. 2: 93-7.
39. Wagner DA, Schultz DS, Deen WM, Young VR, Tannenbaum SR. Metabolic fate of an oral dose of ^{15}N-labeled nitrate in humans: Effect of diet supplementation with ascorbic acid. *Cancer Res* 1983; 43: 1921-5.
40. Granli T, Dahl R, Brodin P, Bockman OC. Nitrate and nitrite concentrations in human saliva: variations with salivary flow-rate. *Fd Chem Toxic* 1989; 27: No. 10: 675-80.
41. Bartholomew B, Hill MJ. The pharmacology of dietary nitrate and the origin of urinary nitrate. *Fd Chem Toxic* 1984; 22: No. 10: 789-95.
42. Tannenbaum SR, Weisman M, Fett D. The effect of nitrate intake on nitrite formation in human saliva. *Fd Cosmet Toxicol* 1976; 14: 549-52.
43. Duncan C, Dougall H, Johnston P, et al. Chemical generation of nitric oxide in the mouth from the enterosalivary circulation of dietary nitrate. *Nature Medicine* 1995; 1: 6: 546-51.
44. Lundberg JON, Weitzberg E, Lundberg JM, Alving K. Intragastric nitric oxide production in humans: measurements in expelled air. *Gut* 1994; 35: 1543-6.
45. Fletcher J, Wirz A, Young J, Vallance R, McColl KEL. Unbuffered highly acidic gastric juice occurs at the gastro-esophageal junction following a meal. *Gastroenterology* 2001; 121: 775-83.

46. Pennington JAT. Dietary exposure models for nitrates and nitrites. *Food Control* 1998; 9: No. 6: 385-95.
47. Kim YK, Tannenbaum SR, Wishnok JS. Effects of ascorbic acid on the nitrosation of dialkyl amines. *Advances in Chemistry Series* 1982; 200: 571-85.
48. Chen B, Keshive M, Deen WM. Diffusion and reaction of nitric oxide in suspension cell cultures. *Biophys Journal* 1998; 75: 745-54.
49. Bunton CA. Oxidation of ascorbic acid and similar reductones by nitrous acid. *Nature* 1959; 4655: 163-6.
50. Liu X, Miller MJS, Joshi MS, Thomas DD, Lancaster JR Jr. Accelerated reaction of nitric oxide with O_2 within the hydrophobic interior of biological membranes. *Proc Natl Acad Sci* 1998; 95: 2175-9.
51. Banerjee S, Hawksby C, Miller S, Dahill S, Beattie AD, McColl KEL. Effect of *Helicobacter pylori* and its eradication on gastric juice ascorbic acid. *Gut* 1994; 35: 317-22.
52. Schorah CJ, Sobala GM, Sanderson M, Collis N, Primrose JN. Gastric Juice Ascorbic Acid: Effects of Disease and Implications for Gastric Carcinogenesis. *Am J Clin Nutr* 1991; 53: 287S-93S.
53. Sobala GM, Schorah CJ, Sanderson M, *et al.* Ascorbic acid in the human stomach. *Gastroenterology* 1989; 97: 357-63.
54. Suzuki H, Iijima K, Moriya A, *et al.* Conditions for acid catalysed luminal nitrosation are maximal at the gastric cardia. *Gut* (in press).
55. Iijima K, Henry E, Moriya A, Wirz A, Kelman AW, McColl KEL. Dietary nitrate generates potentially mutagenic concentrations of nitric oxide at the gastroesophageal junction. *Gastroenterology* 2002; 122: 1248-57.
56. Sugiyama A, Maruta F, Ikeno T, *et al. Helicobacter pylori* infection enhances *N*-methyl-*n*-nitrosourea-induced stomach carcinogenesis in the Mongolian gerbil. *Cancer Res* 1998; 58: 2067-9.
57. El-Omar EM, Oien K, El-Nujumi A, *et al. Helicobacter pylori* infection and chronic gastric acid hyposecretion. *Gastroenterology* 1997; 113: 15-24.
58. Koike T, Ohara S, Sekine H, *et al.* Increased gastric acid secretion after *Helicobacter pylori* eradication may be a factor for developing reflux esophagitis. *Aliment Pharmacol Ther* 2001; 15: 813-20.
59. Richter JE, Falk GW, Vaezi MF. *Helicobacter pylori* and gastroesophageal reflux disease: the bug may not be all bad. *Am J Gastroenterol* 1998; 93: 10: 1800-2.
60. Wu JCY, Sung JJY, Ng KWE, *et al.* Prevalence and distribution of *Helicobacter pylori* in gastroesophageal reflux disease: a study from the East. *Am J Gastroenterol* 1999; 94: 7: 1790-4.
61. Koike T, Ohara S, Sekine H, *et al. Helicobacter pylori* infection inhibits reflux esophagitis by inducing atrophic gastritis. *Am J Gastroenterol* 1999; 94: 12: 3468-72.
62. El-Serag HB, Sonnenberg A, Jamal MM, Inadomi JM, Crooks LA, Feddersen RM. Corpus gastritis is protective against reflux esophagitis. *Gut* 1999; 45 (2): 181-5.
63. In: *Peptic ulcer rise and fall.* Edited by Christie DA, Tansey EM. Wellcome Witnesses to Twentieth Century Medicine, vol. 14. Published by Wellcome Trust Centre for the History of Medicine, London, 2002.

Familial cancer syndromes of the gastro-intestinal tract and the role of surgery

G.O. Ceyhan, J. Kleeff, M.W. Büchler, H. Friess

Department of General Surgery, University of Heidelberg, Germany

Abstract

The identification of molecular changes in human malignancies offers the opportunity for early detection, treatment and the ability to estimate the prognosis. Malignant transformation of cells is associated with accumulation of multiple genetic and epigenetic alterations. Molecular analysis has shown that germline tumour suppressor gene inactivation, germline oncogene activation, and disturbance in DNA repair mechanisms are the main parameters which are involved in many hereditary cancer syndromes. During the last few years a number of familial cancer syndromes have been identified, such as familial gastric cancer, familial adenomatous polyposis (FAP), familial juvenile polyposis (FJP), hereditary non-polyposis colon cancer (HNPCC) and hereditary pancreatic cancer. For these hereditary malignancies new surgical treatment strategies have been developed in the last years. This article reviews two major aspects in familial cancer syndromes: surgery dependent on molecular findings and preventive surgery.

Introduction

With the completion of the human genome project, most familial human cancers will be genetically defined. A number of germline or somatic mutations are characterized to affect normal cell growth. In this tumorogenic process two groups of genes are at the centre of interest: proto-oncogenes and tumour suppressor genes (Vogelsang, 2001; Lynch, 2002). Normally the proto-oncogenes promote cell growth. Mutations activate proto-oncogenes to oncogenes, which results in increased cell proliferation and malignant transformation. Tumour suppressor genes act as negative modulators on cell growth and protect cells from malignant transformation. Mutations in tumour suppressors abolish these protective effects. The reason why germline and other somatic mutations influence tumour growth in an organ specific manner, although they are present in all human cells, is still not known.

A number of familial gastrointestinal (GI) cancers are defined as familial gastric cancer, familial adenomatous polyposis (FAP), attenuated familial adenomatous polyposis (aFAP), familial juvenile polyposis (FJP), hereditary non-polyposis colon cancer (HNPCC) and hereditary pancreatic cancer. The early identification of individuals among families with a high risk for cancer development is most important for prevention. For patients at risk, new diagnostic and therapeutic approaches are necessary for early tumour detection and appropriate treatment. The spectrum of surgical options ranges from "wait and see" to extended surgery. Defining the best timing for surgical treatment and the selection of the optimal surgical procedure is still not controversially discussed.

In this article the role of surgery in the treatment of familial gastrointestinal cancer syndromes is summarized.

Familial adenomatous polyposis (FAP)

Detection and surveillance

Familial adenomatous polyposis (FAP) accounts for only < 1% of all colorectal cancers (CRC). The frequency of FAP in the general population is around 1:13500. It results from autosomal dominant germ-line mutations in the gate keeper APC gene on chromosome 5q 21-22 [1]. Approximately 30% of the cases have spontaneous somatic mutations with a newly discovered autosomal recessive disorder caused by mutation of the DNA repair gene MYH [2-4]. Early recognition of the FAP syndrome is of high importance, because of the 100% lifetime risk of developing CRC. The clinical appearance of polyps begins in the second decade, by the average age of 16 and continues with the development of colon cancer at the mean age of 39 years [2]. FAP is clinically characterized by the presence of more than > 100 adenomatous polyps in the colon. The diagnosis is secure, when the patient is a first degree relative of a FAP-positive person and shows typical morphological changes [1]. Then a genetic testing of the APC and of the MYH-mutation should be offered to the patient and his relatives [5, 6]. To optimize the diagnosis of FAP, also thyroid and liver functional tests, and upper gastrointestinal endoscopy should be performed, to exclude extra-colic manifestations like thyroid-, liver-, upper gastrointestinal- and pancreatic cancers which occur at a higher rate in these patients [6].

Once FAP is detected in a patient or in families, a strict organized surveillance program should be initiated [2, 6]. Beginning with the age of 10, yearly sigmoidoscopies with histological verifications should be performed until the age of 35 years, if no polyps are present or when the mutations are genetically excluded [6, 7]. To avoid missing of extra-colic cancers esophago-gastro-duodenoscopies (EGD) should be included starting at infancy or after the age of 30 [6].

Preventive surgery

Repeated removal of large amounts of polyps is not a curing and practical therapy in FAP patients. The standard therapy for FAP patients is the total proctocolectomy with reconstruction of the rectal ampulla with an ileoanal J-Pouch [8]. The ileoanal pouch operation, which was introduced 20 years ago, can be carried out as one stage, or more frequently, as a two stage procedure. It has excellent functional results, a low risk of sexual dysfunction in male patients and a low risk of pouchitis [9-11]. Before the ileoanal pouch procedure was clinically introduced, the standard operation was colectomy with ileorectal anastomosis. This approach led often to adenoma or carcinoma of the remaining rectal stump [12]. Vasen et al. even showed in a collaborative study including 659 FAP patients, that patients with an ileorectal anastomosis have a high risk of dying from rectal cancer [13]. Quality of life measurement did not reveal any differences between the ileorectal and the ileoanal pouch procedure [14]. In both situations the stool-frequency is 3 to 5 defecations per day. It should be emphasized that there might be risk for cancer development in patients with pouch-anal anastomosis if rectal mucosa is left. Therefore patients with total proctocolectomy and ileal pouch-anal anastomosis should be examined yearly by proctoscopies and pouchoscopies [15-17].

Attenuated familial adenomatous polyposis (aFAP)

Detection and surveillance

A subgroup of patients with FAP show fewer colorectal polyps (< 100), which are predominantly located in the right colon, proximal to the splenic flexure. The diagnosis of attenuated FAP is usually established later than of FAP. Detection of polyps is usually at the mean age of 44 and colon cancer is diagnosed at the mean age of 56 [18]. aFAP is associated with mutations of the 5' end of the APC gene between codon 77 and 517 or at the end of the gene distal to codon 1900 [19]. The lifetime colorectal is lower than in FAP patients (80%) [6]. Once polyps or a positive family member is detected the surveillance is equal to conventional FAP.

Preventive surgery

Because there are less polyps in aFAP, the procedure of choice are annual colonoscopies with removal of the polyps. In contrast to FAP patients, when the number of the polyps becomes too numerous or the removed polyps show high grade of atypical cells, surgery should be performed. Colectomy with ileorectal anastomosis is the standard. Since the polyps are localised in the right side of the colon, the rectum can be preserved. However, yearly rectoscopies are necessary to detect early neoplasias in the rectal mucosa [6, 20]. The follow up of the extracolic manifestations follows the same protocol as mentioned for FAP patients.

Familial juvenile polyposis syndrome

Detection and surveillance

Familial juvenile polyposis (JPS) is an autosomal dominant disorder, which is characterized by multiple polyps in the entire gastrointestinal tract, with an increased risk for developing gastrointestinal cancer. The population prevalence is about 1:50000. JPS is in part caused by germ line mutations of the MADH4/SMAD/DPC4 (18q21.1) and BMPR1A (10q22-23) genes [21, 22]. The clinical image of JPS can vary from single polyps (> 3-10) in the colon to multiple polyps throughout all the gastrointestinal tract. The appearance of benign clinical syndromes, like bleeding or obstruction, usually occurs before the age of 30. Malignant transformation is observed after the 4th life decade [23]. The lifetime risk of colon cancer for JPS is approximately 40% and the risk of gastric and duodenal cancer is 15-21% [21]. The surveillance in JPS patients should not solely rely on molecular genetic analysis. The reason for this is that a number of juvenile patients with JPS do not exhibit the above mentioned mutations. The familial history and clinical (pathological) criteria's should lead to the diagnosis and initiate the appropriate surveillance.

Preventive surgery

Because of the rarity of JPS and the limited experience in therapeutic strategies, no precise standard is presently defined. The cancer risk of JPS is high, so that a close surveillance with histological examinations should be carried out. In patients with multiple polyps, repeated polypectomies raises the risk of complications (perforations, bleedings). In these cases early preventive surgery is an option [25]. This can include early gastrectomy and colectomy with ileorectal anastomosis. Like in aFAP the colonic polyps in JPS are localized more on the right side, so a proctocolectomy is not the standard. Follow up postoperative endoscopies must be performed in all patients [6, 24, 25].

Hereditary non-polyposis colon cancer (HNPCC)

Detection and surveillance

The hereditary non-polyposis colon cancer syndrome, also known as "Lynch-Syndrome" is an autosominal dominant genetic disorder resulting from mutations in one of the mismatch repair genes: hMSH2, hMLH1, PMS2, hMSH5 or hMSH6. Mutations in MLH1 and MSH2 account for 70-90% of all mutations in registered HNPCC-families [26]. The incidence of HNPCC is about 1:2000 and is therefore the most common hereditary colon cancer syndrome [6]. In the Lynch I syndrome colorectal cancer is the predominant manifestation. The Lynch II syndrome displays a range of extra-colonic tumours, such as endometrial carcinoma and tumours involving the stomach, small bowel, hepatobiliary tract, pancreas, breast, ovaries, urologic tract, brain, or skin [26-29]. Typical features for HNPCC are:

a) the early onset of colorectal cancer by the median age of 46,
b) a total lifetime colorectal cancer risk of > 80% and 13-20% risk for gastric cancer,
c) right sided localization of colorectal cancer,
d) and common synchronic or metachronic colorectal cancer [6, 25-29].

The clinical diagnostic criteria are defined by the Amsterdam criteria I and II and the enhanced Bethesda criteria [30-32] *(table I)*.

Table I. HNPCC criteria

Amsterdam I (all criteria must be fulfilled)	Amsterdam II (all criteria must be fulfilled)
1. One member diagnosed with CRC < 50 years 2. Two affected generations 3. Three affected relatives, one of thema 1st degree relative of the other two 4. FAP is excluded 5. Tumours are verified by pathologists	1. Three relatives with a HNPCC-associated cancer 2. One should be a first-degree relative of the other two 3. Amsterdam I
Bethesda (one criteria must be fulfilled) 1. Amsterdam criteria 2. Persons with two types of HNPCC-related cancers (including synchronous or metachronous colon cancer) 3. Individuals with CRC and a first-degree relative with CRC and/or HNPCC-associated extracolic cancer and/or adenoma (cancer at < 45 years of age and adenoma at < 40 years of age) 4. Persons with colon or endometrial cancer before age 45 years 5. Persons with right-sided colon cancer with undifferentiated pattern on histology tests before age 45 years 6. Persons with signet-ring – cell type CRC before age 45 years 7. Individuals with diagnosed colonic adenomas before age 40 years	

HNPCC and aFAP might be difficult to distinguish because of their appearance, predominantly in the right colon. Microsatellite instability (MSI) of HNPCC adenomas and cancer tissues can help to exclude FAP or aFAP [33]. Another striking difference is the outward appearance of the adenomas in HNPCC, which appear as "flat" lesions endoscopically and not as polyps as in FAP or aFAP. The cancer surveillance of HNPCC must be performed in a more frequent manner compared to FAP or in aFAP. It should be noted that HNPCC patients contract benign tumours at roughly the same rate as the general population. However, once an adenoma in the colon or rectum develops, it progresses rapidly because of the inherited DNA repair defect. The adenoma-carcinoma-sequence can develop within less than 2 years, so that annual total colonoscopies are recommended [34]. Colonoscopies may be started at the age of 25 years and repeated annually thereafter in first-degree relatives of HNPCC patients with confirmed mutation in one of the mismatch repair genes [35]. The most frequent extra colic manifestation of HNPCC is endometrial cancer, which should be monitored through regular transvaginal sonographies and measuring CA-125. Additionally, esophago-gastro-duodenoscopies and examinations of the urinary tract should be performed when the familiar history is positive [36].

Preventive surgery

Until now there is no standard procedure to treat colorectal cancer in HNPCC. This is due to the fact that approximately 20% of HNPCC patients never develop colorectal cancer. In these cases, a preventive surgical approach without the presence of colorectal adenomas would be overtreatment [37]. For patients with confined colorectal cancer and HNPCC-germ line mutations, or members of a HNPCC family, surgery should be offered. When colorectal cancer is localized in the right colon, an extended subtotal colectomy and ileorectal anastomosis with well standardized onco-surgical principles is the procedure of choice. When colorectal cancer is found in the left colon or in the rectum, the preferred treatment is a subtotal colectomy or a procto-colectomy with an ileoanal J-pouch. All strategies require lifetime surveillance of the remaining colorectum [20]. The risk of local colorectal cancer relapse is not the only fact which the surgeon has to consider, it is also the danger of the 45% chance of metachronous cancer in the remaining gastrointestinal tract [37]. But again, 55% of all operated HNPCC patients do not develop metachronous cancer, so that a primary extended surgical approach is not recommended [38]. The only recommended preventive surgery in HNPCC is the prophylactic hysterectomy with or without oophorectomy in those women who have completed their family planning and are operated for colorectal cancer [36].

Hereditary diffuse gastric cancer (HDGC)

Detection and surveillance

Gastric cancer remains the second most common cause of cancer death world-wide. 10% of all cases of gastric cancer are due to hereditary diffuse gastric cancer (HDGC) [26]. An autosomal dominant germ line mutation of the calcium dependent E-Cadherin gene, CDH1 on chromosome 16q22.1 is responsible for the HDGC-syndrome. The inactivation of the E-Cadherin complex may permit the invasion in adjacent tissues or the detachment of tumour cells [39-41]. HDGC is characterized by an early onset of the disease in both men and women at the average age of 38 years. The lifetime risk of diffuse gastric cancer is 70% in men and 80% in women [42, 43]. Gastric cancer can also appear in other hereditary cancer syndromes like, HNPCC, Li Fraumeni syndrome (LFS), FAP, aFAP and in the Peutz Jeghers syndrome (PJS).

The first diagnosis of HDGC in early stages is difficult, because symptoms first appear when the tumour reaches late stages. When hereditary gastric cancer is obvious, due to the patients history or mutation analysis, first-degree relatives should undergo annual esophago-gastro-duodenoscopies. The surveillance is very difficult, since endoscopy rarely detects non advanced forms of the disease. HDGC starts usually with a submucosal spread of single cells or clustered island of cells and not with grossly visible exophytic tumour like in FAP or in HNPCC [41]. First experiences in the USA and Canada show, that in nearly all prophylactic removed stomachs of patients with E-Cadherin germ line mutations, which had no lesions on endoscopy, histological pre-stages of neoplasia or early gastric cancers were already present [43].

Preventive surgery

Although 20-30% of all CDH1-mutation carriers will never develop a HDGC, the standard therapy is total gastrectomy [40-44]. The surveillance is, as mentioned, not absolutely reliable in this syndrome and until reliable monitoring is guaranteed, total gastrectomy remains the treatment of choice. Data about when gastrectomy should be performed are still sparse. The decision for gastrectomy should be a team decision between clinicians, genetics and the patient. In general total gastrectomy should not be performed before the age of 18 years [45, 46]. Patients who reject the surgical approach must be under very close surveillance of repeated esophago-gastro-duodenoscopies with multiple biopsies (deep) every 6 to 12 months. Radical eradication of *Helicobacter pylori* should additionally be considered if the patient is infected.

Hereditary pancreatic cancer (HPC)

Detection and surveillance

Hereditary pancreatic cancer (HPC) is associated with a number of different inherited diseases and syndromes and has a wide heterogenicity. A single mutation which causes HPC does not exist and the real number of families with HPC still remains unclear. Until now no certain criteria or standardized definitions are established, which allow to distinguish between sporadic pancreatic cancer and HPC. Inherited syndromes that are associated with an increased risk of pancreatic cancer include: HNPCC, hereditary chronic pancreatitis, FAP, familial atypical multiple mole melanoma syndrome (FAMMM), Peutz-Jeghers syndrome, familial breast cancer associated with BRCA2 mutations, ataxia-telangiectasia syndrome, and cystic fibrosis [47]. The centre of interest for the surveillance of HPC is hereditary chronic pancreatitis. Hereditary pancreatitis is an autosomal dominant disorder most commonly caused by mutations in the cationic trypsinogen gene (R122H, N291). The development of pancreatic cancer in hereditary chronic pancreatitis is increased to several thousand fold compared to the general population and the risk begins to increase at about the age of 40 [48, 49].

Once pancreatic cancer is diagnosed it usually presents in an advanced stage in 85-90%, of the patients precluding curative resection [50]. It is difficult to detect pancreatic cancer at an early stage, since the first appearance of focal dysplasia or carcinoma in situ is usually not recognized. To detect HPC at an early stage, a strict surveillance has to be carried out. Persons who have a high lifetime risk to develop pancreatic cancer, like the above mentioned groups must be closely monitored. The currently accepted workup for suspected pancreatic malignancies includes, first, the screening with conventional endoscopic ultrasonography. Endoscopic ultrasonography, which is a sensitive and specific technique for the detection of pancreatic adenocarcinomas [51-53] may be used for detecting suspicious lesions, including 1) heterogeneous parenchyma with 1 to 2 mm echogenic foci scattered throughout, 2) hyperechoic nodules of 2 to 4 mm size, 3) hyperechoic main duct walls, 4) and distinct masses in the pancreatic parenchyma.

However, experience in the detection of dysplasia is still very limited and the difficulty is that similar changes can be seen in patients with chronic pancreatitis [54]. Nevertheless esophago-gastro-duodenoscopies, when performed by experienced investigators, is a safe procedure and together with fine needle aspiration cytology of focal lesions it provides high sensitivity [55, 56] [20, 21]. ERCP – which seems to be the next more useful imaging modality – should be used only when there are changes in the esophago-gastro-duodenoscopies or in the presence of symptoms (persistent epigastric pain, steatorrhoea, jaundice, diabetes mellitus) [54, 57]. Computertomography seems to be ineffective for surveillance of patients with the risk of hereditary pancreatic cancer since findings in CT in the presence of dysplasia could be normal or suggestive of chronic pancreatitis. In

Table II. Incidence and appearance of associated cancers in hereditary disorder

	Colo-rectal	Duodenal/Gastric	Thyroid	Hepatic/Bile duct	Pan-creatic	Ovarian/Endometric	Urinary
FAP	100%	5-10%/0,5%	2%	1,6%	2%		
aFAP	> 90%	5-10%/0,5%	2%	1,6%	2%		
HNPCC	> 80%	13-19%		3,3%		9-12%/43-60%	4-10%
JPS (no incidence)	50%	++ ++			++		
HGC (no incidence)	++					++ (breast-Ca)	++ (prostate)

addition, due to the fact that dysplasia is multifocal and occurs normally in the small and medium-sized pancreatic ducts, without affecting the main pancreatic duct [54, 58] detection is almost impossible. However, CT should be performed when esophago-gastro-duodenoscopies and ERCP findings are positive.

Preventive surgery

The goal of surveillance of patients with a risk of hereditary pancreatic cancer is to diagnose dysplastic lesions before they develop into invasive cancer, and to proceed to total duodenopancreatectomy. False positive findings of dysplastic changes will lead to unnecessary early pancreatic surgery with all the associated risks. Although morbidity and mortality rates of total pancreatectomy in centres of pancreatic surgery are low, the resultant diabetes mellitus that the patient will develop is not at all trivial or insignificant. The multifocal nature of dysplastic lesions precludes any type of operation that would preserve pancreatic tissue. In a recent report, atypical ductal hyperplasia was found incidentally in three patients who underwent partial pancreatic resection, all of whom subsequently developed cancer in the remaining pancreas within 17 months, 9 years and 10 years [59]. Inasmuch as pancreatic cancer is frequently associated with intraductal proliferative lesions, it has been postulated that once dysplasia is present in the pancreatic parenchyma, pancreatic cancer will develop, just as there is progression from adenoma to infiltrating carcinoma of the colon. Taking this concept into consideration, prophylactic whole-organ resection seems to be the preferred treatment. Concerning prophylactic pancreatectomy in high-risk patients, several factors have to be taken into serious consideration:

1) the perioperative morbidity and mortality associated with the operation,
2) the potential for the patient to develop diabetes mellitus,
3) the fact that we do not know the exact risk for the development of cancer and that patients who are at risk may never develop cancer [60, 61].

Table III. Gene mutations, life time risk for cancer development, surveillance and recommended preventive surgery in patients with familial cancer syndrome

	Gene-mutation	Lifetime-cancer-risk	Surveillance	Recommended preventive-surgery
FAP	APC MYH	100%	1. Sigmoidoscopy at age 10-12 years until 30 annual 2. EGD starting at 30 every 2-years	Proctocolectomy + ileoanal-Pouch
aFAP	5' end of the APC gene between codon 77 and 517	> 90%	1. Colonoscopy starting at 10-17 years 2. EGD starting at 30 every 2-years	Total-colectomy + ileo-rectal-anastomosis
HNPCC	hMSH2, hMLH1, PMS2, hMSH5 or hMSH6	> 80%	1. Colonoscopy starting at age of 20-25 until 75 2. EGD starting at 30 every 2-years until 75	Subtotal-or total-colectomy + ileo-rectal-anastomosis
JPS	MADH4/SMAD/DPC4 BMPR1A	50%	1. Colonoscopy starting at 15-18 years every 1-2 years 2. EGD starting at 25 every 3-years	Subtotal-or total-colectomy + ileo-rectal-anastomosis
HGC	CDH1	70%	EGD starting at 30 every 6-12 months	Total gastrectomy
HPC/HP	R122H, N291 (HP)	> 100%	1. EGD starting at age of 35 years annual 2. ERCP if changes in EDG are present	Total pancreatectomy

For the surgical treatment of cancer in the head of the pancreas, the operations which have evolved are the classical-Whipple and the pylorus-preserving-Whipple operation. In a prospective randomized trial performed in our clinic, both techniques proved to be equally radical. No difference in local tumour recurrence and in long-term survival after a median follow-up of 1.5 years were found. In addition, morbidity and mortality and the incidence of delayed gastric emptying were comparable [62].

Summary and conclusion

Optimal timing of surgical intervention in patients with a risk of hereditary cancer diseases is most important for the prevention of the development of malignancies. To achieve this goal an optimal standardized and organized surveillance has to be established, to recognize early pathological changes which ultimately lead to cancer. Best established procedures for surveillance and preventive surgery do exist in FAP. In other hereditary disorders the indication for preventive surgery is often not well defined, as in aFAP, HNPCC, JPS, HGC and HPC. In these cases the lifetime risk to develop cancer is not 100% like in FAP. This fact puts the clinician and surgeon in a difficult situation, because they understand that not all mutation carriers will produce malignancies. They must create an approach so that preventive therapy, in this case radical surgery, would not reduce unnecessarily quality of life. aFAP and HNPCC are often difficult to distinguish and should be controlled regularly by endoscopies, in order to identify severe phenotypes with numerous adenomas. Early preventive surgery is not recommended in these cases [63]. In HGC and in HPC, experiences show that only early radical preventive surgery can exclude or minimize the risk for the development of cancer [43, 59]. Nevertheless, total gastrectomy or total pancreatectomy are procedures which have severe effects on life-quality, even when they are performed in specialized centres.

Continued molecular biology research will help identify patients who are especially at high risk, that could benefit from aggressive surgical intervention. In addition, the gained knowledge from molecular studies, will help to better define the best time point for surgery. An early surgical approach *versus* a late surgical approach has to be evaluated in randomised clinical trials, which will then allow evidence based clinical recommendations for families with hereditary disorders.

References

1. Groden J, Thliveris A, Samowitz W, *et al*. Identification and characterization of the familial adenomatous polyposis coli gene. *Cell* 1991; 66: 589-600.
2. Burt RW. Colon cancer screening. *Gastroenterology* 2000; 119: 837-53.
3. Sieber OM, Lipton L, Crabtree M, *et al*. Multiple colorectal adenomas, classic adenomatous polyposis, and germ-line mutations in MYH. *N Engl J Med* 2003; 348: 791-9.
4. Al-Tassan N, Chmiel NH, Maynard J, *et al*. Inherited variants of MYH associated with somatic G:C-T:A mutations in colorectal tumours. *Nat Genet* 2002; 30: 227-32.
5. NCCN colorectal cancer screening practice guidelines. National comprehensive cancer network. *Oncology* 1999; 13: 152-79.
6. Grady WM. Genetic testing for high-risk colon cancer patients. *Gastroenterology* 2003; 124 (6): 1574-94.
7. Kadmon M, Moslein G, Buhr HJ, Herfarth C. Desmoid tumours in patients with familial adenomatous polyposis (FAP). Clinical and therapeutic observations from the Heidelberg polyposis register. *Chirurg* 1995; 66: 997-1005.
8. King JE, Dzois RR, Lindor NM, Ahlquist DA. Care of patients and their families with familial adanomatous polyposis. *Mayo Clin Proc* 2000; 75: 57-67.
9. Ambroze WL Jr, Dozois RR, Pemberton JH, Beart RW Jr, Ilstrup DM. Familial adenomatous polyposis: results following ileal pouch-anal anastomosis and ileorectostomy. *Dis Colon Rectum* 1992; 35: 12-5.
10. Madden MV, Neale KF, Nicholls RJ, *et al*. Comparison of morbidity and function after colectomy with ileorectal anastomosis or restorative proctocolectomy for familial adenomatous polyposis. *Br J Surg* 1991; 78: 789-92.
11. Nyam DC, Brillant PT, Dozois RR, Kelly KA, Pemberton JH, Wolff BG. Ileal pouch-anal canal anastomosis for familial adenomatous polyposis: early and late results. *Ann Surg* 1997; 226: 514-9; discussion 519-21.
12. Bulow C, Vasen H, Jarvinen H, Bjork J, Bisgaard ML, Bulow S. Ileorectal anastomosis is appropriate for a subset of patients with familial adenomatous polyposis. *Gastroenterology* 2000; 119: 1454-60.
13. Vasen HF, van Duijvendijk P, Buskens E, *et al*. Decision analysis in the surgical treatment of patients with familial adenomatous polyposis: a Dutch-Scandinavian collaborative study including 659 patients. *Gut* 2001; 49: 231-5.

14. Van Duijvendijk P, Slors JF, Taat CW, *et al.* Quality of life after total colectomy with ileorectal anastomosis or proctocolectomy and ileal pouch-anal anastomosis for familial adenomatous polyposis. *Br J Surg* 2000; 87: 590-6.
15. Van Duijvendijk P, Vasen HF, Bertario L, *et al.* Cumulative risk of developing polyps or malignancy at the ileal pouch-anal anastomosis in patients with familial adenomatous polyposis. *J Gastrointest Surg* 1999; 3: 325-30.
16. Church JM, Oakley JR, Wu JS. Pouch polyposis after ileal pouch-anal anastomosis for familial adenomatous polyposis: report of a case. *Dis Colon Rectum* 1996; 39: 584-6.
17. Nugent KP, Spigelman AD, Nicholls RJ, Talbot IC, Neale K, Phillips RK. Pouch adenomas in patients with familial adenomatous polyposis. *Br J Surg* 1993; 80: 1620.
18. Brensinger JD, Laken SJ, Luce MC, *et al.* Variable phenotype of familial adenomatous polyposis in pedigrees with 3' mutation in the APC gene. *Gut* 1998; 43: 548-52.
19. Spirio L, Olschwang S, Groden J, *et al.* Alleles of the APC gene: an attenuated form of familial polyposis. *Cell* 1993; 75: 951-7.
20. Moslein G, Pistorius S, Saeger HD, Schackert HK. Preventive surgery for colon cancer in familial adenomatous polyposis and hereditary nonpolyposis colorectal cancer syndrome. *Langenbecks Arch Surg* 2003; 388: 9-16.
21. Howe JR, Mitros FA, Summers RW. The risk of gastrointestinal carcinoma in familial juvenile polyposis. *Ann Surg Oncol* 1998; 5: 751-6.
22. Howe JR, Bair JL, Sayed MG, *et al.* Germline mutations of the gene encoding bone morphogenetic protein receptor 1A in juvenile polyposis. *Nat Genet* 2001; 28: 184-7.
23. Burt RW. Colon cancer screening. *Gastroenterology* 2000; 119: 837-59.
24. Friedl W, Uhlhaas S, Schulmann K, *et al.* Juvenile polyposis: massive gastric polyposis is more common in MADH4 mutation carriers than in BMPR1A mutation carriers. *Hum Genet* 2002; 111: 108-11.
25. Dunlop MG. British Society for Gastroenterology; Association of Coloproctology for Great Britain and Ireland. Guidance on gastrointestinal surveillance for hereditary non-polyposis colorectal cancer, familial adenomatous polypolis, juvenile polyposis, and Peutz-Jeghers syndrome. *Gut* 2002; 51 (Suppl. 5): V21-7.
26. Lynch HT, Lynch JF. Hereditary cancer: family history, diagnosis, molecular genetics, ecogenetics, and management strategies. *Biochimie* 2002; 84: 3-17.
27. Lynch HT, Smyrk TC, Watson P, *et al.* Genetics, natural history, tumour spectrum, and pathology of hereditary nonpolyposis colorectal cancer: an updated review. *Gastroenterology* 1993; 104: 1535-49.
28. Lynch HT, Lynch PM, Pester J, Fusaro RM. The cancer family syndrome. Rare cutaneous phenotypic linkage of Torre's syndrome. *Arch Intern Med* 1981; 141: 607-11.
29. Watson P, Lynch HT. Extracolonic cancer in hereditary nonpolyposis colorectal cancer. *Cancer* 1993; 71: 677-85.
30. Vasen HF, Mecklin JP, Khan PM, Lynch HAT. The International Collaborative Group on Hereditary Non-Polyposis Colorectal Cancer (ICG-HNPCC). *Dis Colon Rectum* 1991; 34: 424-5.
31. Vasen HF, Watson P, Mecklin JP, Lynch HT. New clinical criteria for hereditary nonpolyposis colorectal cancer (HNPCC, Lynch syndrome) proposed by the International Collaborative group on HNPCC. *Gastroenterology* 1999; 116: 1453-6.
32. Rodriguez-Bigas MA, Boland CR, Hamilton SR, *et al.* A National Cancer Institute Workshop on Hereditary Nonpolyposis Colorectal Cancer Syndrome: meeting highlights and Bethesda guidelines. *J Natl Cancer Inst* 1997; 89: 1758-62.
33. Boland CR, Thibodeau SN, Hamilton SR, *et al.* A National Cancer Institute Workshop on Microsatellite Instability for cancer detection and familial predisposition: development of international criteria for the determination of microsatellite instability in colorectal cancer. *Cancer Res* 1998; 58: 5248-57.

34. Vasen HF, Nagengast FM, Khan PM. Interval cancers in hereditary non-polyposis colorectal cancer (Lynch syndrome). *Lancet* 1995; 345: 1183-4.
35. Lynch HT, Smyrk TC. Hereditary colorectal cancer. *Semin Oncol* 1999; 26: 478-84.
36. Watson P, Vasen HF, Mecklin JP, Jarvinen H, Lynch HT. The risk of endometrial cancer in hereditary nonpolyposis colorectal cancer. *Am J Med* 1994; 96: 516-20.
37. Syngal S, Weeks JC, Schrag D, Garber JE, Kuntz KM. Benefits of colonoscopic surveillance and prophylactic colectomy in patients with hereditary nonpolyposis colorectal cancer mutations. *Ann Intern Med* 1998; 129: 787-96.
38. Schmiegel W, Adler G, Fruhmorgen P, et al. Colorectal carcinoma: prevention and early detection in an asymptomatic population – prevention in patients at risk – endoscopic diagnosis, therapy and after-care of polyps and carcinomas. German Society of Digestive and Metabolic Diseases/Study Group for Gastrointestinal Oncology. *Z Gastroenterol* 2000; 38: 49-75.
39. Guilford P, Hopkins J, Harraway J, et al. E-cadherin germline mutations in familial gastric cancer. *Nature* 1998; 392: 402-5.
40. Dunbier A, Guilford P. Hereditary diffuse gastric cancer. *Adv Cancer Res* 2001; 83: 55-65.
41. Caldas C, Carneiro F, Lynch HT, et al. Familial gastric cancer: overview and guidelines for management. *J Med Genet* 1999; 36: 873-80.
42. Huntsman DG, Carneiro F, Lewis FR, et al. Early gastric cancer in young, asymptomatic carriers of germ-line E-cadherinmutations. *N Engl J Med* 2001; 344: 1904-9.
43. Lewis FR, Mellinger JD, Hayashi A, et al. Prophylactic total gastrectomy for familial gastric cancer. *Surgery* 2001; 130: 612-7.
44. Chun YS, Lindor NM, Smyrk TC, et al. Germline E-cadherin gene mutations: is prophylactic total gastrectomy indicated? *Cancer* 2001; 92: 181-7.
45. Schwarz A. Preventive gastrectomy in patients with gastric cancer risk due to genetic alterations of the E-cadherin gene defect. *Langenbecks Arch Surg* 2003; 388: 27-32.
46. Schwarz A, Beger HG. Gastric substitute after total gastrectomy--clinical relevance for reconstruction techniques. *Langenbecks Arch Surg* 1998; 383 (6): 485-91.
47. Brand RE, Lynch HT. Hereditary pancreatic adenocarcinoma. A clinical perspective. *Med Clin North Am* 2000; 84: 665-75.
48. Lowenfels AB, Maisonneuve P, Whitcomb DC. Risk factors for cancer in hereditary pancreatitis. International Hereditary Pancreatitis Study Group. *Med Clin North Am* 2000; 84 (3): 565-73.
49. Ulrich CD. Consensus Committees of the European Registry of Hereditary Pancreatic Diseases, Midwest Multi-Center Pancreatic Study Group, International Association of Pancreatology: Pancreatic cancer in hereditary pancreatitis: consensus guidelines for prevention, screening and treatment. *Pancreatology* 2001; 1 (5): 416-22.
50. DiMagno EP, Reber HA, Tempero MA. AGA technical review on the epidemiology, diagnosis, and treatment of pancreatic ductal adenocarcinoma. *American Gastroenterological Association. Gastroenterology* 1999; 117 (6): 1464-84.
51. Rosch T, Lorenz R, Braig C, et al. Endoscopic ultrasound in pancreatic tumour diagnosis. *Gastrointest Endosc* 1991; 37: 347-52.
52. Inokuma T, Tamaki N, Torizuka T, et al. Evaluation of pancreatic tumours with positron emission tomography and F-18 fluorodeoxyglucose: comparison with CT and US. *Radiology* 1995; 195: 345-52.
53. Muller MF, Meyenberger C, Bertschinger P, Schaer R, Marincek B. Pancreatic tumours: evaluation with endoscopic US, CT, and MR imaging. *Radiology* 1994; 190: 745-51.
54. Brentnall TA. Cancer surveillance of patients from familial pancreatic cancer kindreds. *Med Clin North Am* 2000; 84: 707-18.
55. Gress F, Gottlieb K, Cummings O, Sherman S, Lehman G. Endoscopic ultrasound characteristics of mucinous cystic neoplasms of the pancreas. *Am J Gastroenterol* 2000; 95: 961-5.

56. Gress F, Gottlieb K, Sherman S, Lehman G. Endoscopic ultrasonography-guided fine-needle aspiration biopsy of suspected pancreatic cancer. *Ann Intern Med* 2001; 134: 459-64.
57. Kekis PB, Friess H, Kleeff J, Buchler MW. Timing and extent of surgical intervention in patients from hereditary pancreatic cancer kindreds. *Pancreatology* 2001; 1: 525-30.
58. Taouli B, Vilgrain V, Vullierme MP, *et al.* Intraductal papillary mucinous tumours of the pancreas: helical CT with histopathologic correlation. *Radiology* 2000; 217: 757-64.
59. Brat DJ, Lillemoe KD, Yeo CJ, Warfield PB, Hruban RH. Progression of pancreatic intraductal neoplasias to infiltrating adenocarcinoma of the pancreas. *Am J Surg Pathol* 1998; 22: 163-9.
60. Hruban RH, Petersen GM, Goggins M, *et al.* Familial pancreatic cancer. *Ann Oncol* 1999; 10 (Suppl. 4): 69-73.
61. Goggins M, Canto M, Hruban R. Can we screen high-risk individuals to detect early pancreatic carcinoma? *J Surg Oncol* 2000; 74: 243-8.
62. Seiler CA, Wagner M, Sadowski C, Kulli C, Büchler MW. Randomized prospective trial of pylorus-preserving *vs.* classic duodenopancreatectomy (Whipple procedure): initial clinical results. *J Gastrointest Surg* 2000; 4: 443-52.
63. Koliopanos A, Wirtz M, Büchler MW, Friess H. The role of surgery in the prevention of familiar cancer syndromes of the gastrointestinal tract. *Dig Dis* 2002; 20: 91-101.

New developments in diagnosis and management of early and advanced GI malignancy.
G.N. Tytgat, F. Penninckx, eds. John Libbey Eurotext, Paris © 2003, pp. 175-182.

Is the novel grading/staging system of neoplasia useful?

K. Geboes

Department of Pathology, K.U. Leuven, Leuven, Belgium

Introduction

Classification of diseases is useful when linked with practical consequences in terms of natural history and management, otherwise it becomes a hollow exercise in semantics [1]. Some 450 years BC, Hippocrates made a distinction between two types of tumours: "carcinos" and "carcinoma" or more usually "benign" and "malignant". The term "malignant" itself in fact was only used for the first time by Fallopio (16th century) in his book *De Tumoribus* for "Cancer Maligno". This distinction between two poles, between good and bad, is a very old distinction which is based upon religious concepts. Manicheism, a religion founded in Persia in the 3th century, proposed a dualistic view and a distinction between two radically opposed poles: spirit and substance. This "two-valued orientation" still largely dominates the thinking about tumours although it is not at all a scientific approach. A scientific classification should be based upon the understanding of a process, adequate measurements using well defined criteria, and aims for practical consequences. Temperature and speed for instance are no longer subdivided into warm and cold or fast and slow, but accurately measured. A good classification requires indeed precision (the degree of variation in assigning a case to a given category) and accuracy (the closeness of the diagnosis to the true clinical state). Precision implies "identification of the **features** or **criteria** for each one of the lesions or categories". Histopathology allows to identify and describe features which can predict the behaviour of a tumour and hence it can help to develop a therapeutic strategy. Precision depends however also on practical **guidelines** indicating how the features should be identified reliably (such as number of samples; number of lymph nodes for a given surgical procedure). The usefulness of pathologic analysis is especially evident in the determination of tumour stage. Staging for colorectal cancer developed gradually since the 1920s. It is essentially based on the determination of the degree of penetration of a cancer into the bowel wall and beyond and infiltration of lymph nodes [2]. The purpose of the present paper is therefore to review the staging of early gastrointestinal epithelial neoplasia (GEN) (including the transition between intraepithelial neoplasia and intramucosal neoplasia; the staging of endoscopic mucosal resections; the importance of lateral (section) margins for endoscopic and surgical resections and the staging and grading of GISTs).

Histopathological features and staging

Several histopathological criteria have been proposed for classification and staging of gastrointestinal tumours *(table I)*. Most of these are still currently routinely used. For some, the use of markers has been considered in order to allow a more reliable identification.

The percentage of the tumour showing formation of gland-like structures is generally used to define the grade and classically a tumour is graded according to the predominant pattern. The prognostic impact of grading is equivocal due to poor standardisation. Furthermore, poorly differentiated areas may be more important for the biologic behaviour of the lesion. For adenocarcinomas of the stomach, the histologic type may well be important for the

Table I. Histopathological features and staging

Feature	Comments
Size of the lesion	Used in staging of endoscopic mucosal resections Used in staging of GISTs
Macroscopy/endoscopy	Used in staging of endoscopic mucosal resections
Degree of penetration	In use in classical staging systems such as Dukes, TNM and for endoscopic resections
Margins (proximal/distal/lateral)	In use in classical staging systems such as Dukes, TNM and for endoscopic resections
Growth pattern	In use in classical staging systems such as Dukes, TNM and for endoscopic resections
Vascular invasion	In use in classical staging systems such as Dukes, TNM and for endoscopic resections
Perineural invasion	
Mitotic activity/proliferation	Used in staging of GISTs (Ki67) Is not shown to be an independent prognostic factor for cancer of the esophagus
Differentiation or histologic grade	In use in classical staging systems such as Dukes, TNM and for endoscopic resections
Histologic type	May be useful for stomach cancer
Lymphocytic infiltration	Has been associated with a better prognosis for cancer of the esophagus and some types of gastric cancer

prognosis. This is illustrated in the classifications according to Lauren, Goseki and Carneiro [3, 4]. The classification according to Goseki, combining tubular differentiation and amount of intracytoplasmatic mucus has prognostic and diagnostic implications. The subdivision in intestinal and diffuse types according to Lauren on the other hand may have diagnostic implications. It has been shown that no detectable fluorodeoxyglucose (FDG) uptake is observed with positron emission tomography (PET) in poorly differentiated tumours (82% out of a series of 96 distal esophageal tumours). An intense hot spot is detected in intestinal type cancer (Lauren) and type I and II (glandular differentiation in Goseki).

Periodical revision of disease classifications is useful and even necessary because of potential shortcomings or new discoveries which can radically alter pre-existing concepts and categorizations of disease. The identification of the ckit protein has indeed radically changed diagnosis, classification and treatment of mesenchymal tumours of the gastrointestinal tract. As a result of new insights several modifications of the Dukes classification for (colo-)rectal cancer have been developed and several adaptations of the TNM system have been proposed.

Historically, staging was performed on surgical specimens. The development of endoscopy has made it possible to identify lesions during other, and perhaps earlier, phases of the disease and made it necessary to deal with such lesions. Furthermore, it became clear that there were major differences in clinical ascertainment and reporting practices between the West and Japan. Such differences need to be clarified and if possible resolved, especially if the results of different studies are to be compared. This implies *a.o.* clear definitions. An example of this is the term "superficial" which is usually used for a cancer limited to the mucosa or the mucosa and submucosa [5]. However, according to some authors, it implies a colorectal lesion which is nonpolypoid, spreads within the mucosal layer, and its mucosal thickness is no greater than twice the thickness of normal mucosa [6]. In the West, such a lesion would be diagnosed as adenoma, because it is common practice to diagnose colorectal cancer only when invasion through the muscularis mucosae has been demonstrated. These differences are the rationale underpinning the development of the Padova and Vienna classifications for gastrointestinal epithelial neoplasia (GEN) while the increased knowledge was the driving force behind an NIH consensus conference for grading and staging of gastrointestinal stromal tumours (GISTs) [7-9].

The new "Vienna classification of epithelial neoplasia"

"Early epithelial neo-plastic lesions" are reported in the West as "dysplasia" and "adenoma". The definition of "dysplasia" has long been very vague (structural changes in the surface epithelium – atypical mucosa). In the 1970s, it was somewhat clarified after the introduction of the World Health Organization (WHO) definition of "unequivocal intraepithelial neoplasia". This approach was followed by an international group studying precursor lesions in chronic idiopathic inflammatory bowel diseases. They defined "dysplasia" as "unequivocal neoplasia confined within the basement membrane". In the recent publication of the WHO classification the term dysplasia has now been replaced by "intraepithelial neoplasia" which is subdivided into low- and high-grade [10].

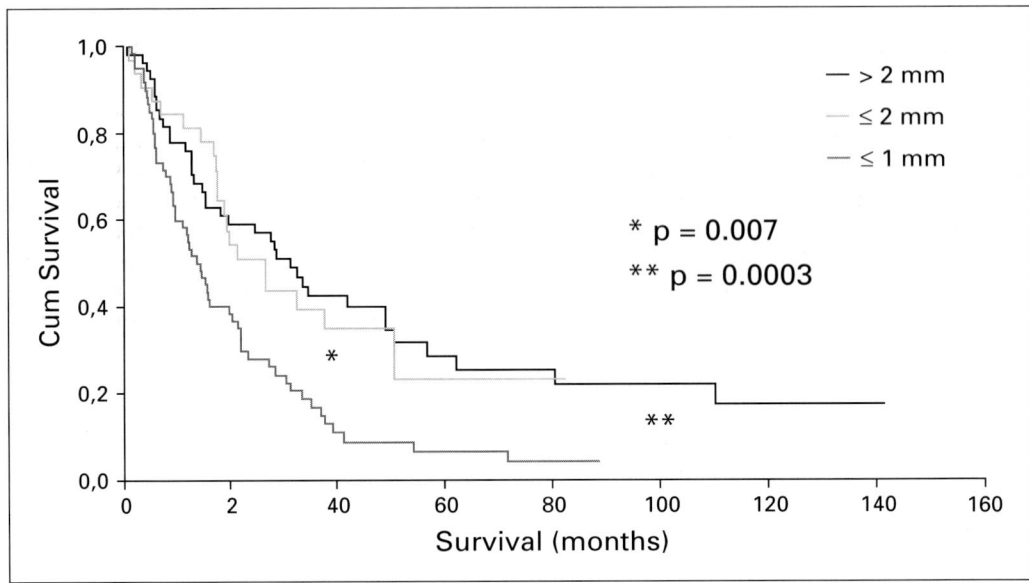

Figure 1. Survival in function of section margin.

Table II. New Vienna classification

Category 1: no neoplasia	Optional surveillance
Category 2: indefinite for neoplasia	Surveillance
Category 3: low-grade non-invasive	Surveilance/local treatment
Category 4: High-grade non-invasive	Local treatment
Category 5: Submucosal invasive	Local/surgical treatment

Western pathologists usually define "malignancy" by "invasion into the lamina propria or submucosa for the esophagus and stomach, and invasion of the submucosa for colorectal carcinoma". Pathologists adopting the Japanese viewpoint make a diagnosis of carcinoma when they see typical changes to the cell nuclei and the architecture of the neoplasia.

The "Vienna classification", developed on the occasion of a pathology workshop held during the World Congress of Gastroenterology in Vienna (1998), represents a preliminary compromise and an attempt to uniform terminology. The advantage of the new classification is that it can be linked to a therapeutic strategy *(table II)* [11].

Yet, the histopathological criteria of the different categories and the guidelines on how to obtain endoscopic biopsies (especially the number) are not clearly verbalised in the original paper. This is however essential, in order to minimize observer variation, to increase acceptance and for (molecular) research and the study of the (histo-)genesis of lesions. The histopathological criteria can be derived from other studies. Carcinoma differs from precursor lesions by the presence of cells with large, vesicular nuclei, irregular conspicuous nucleoli and scalloped nuclear membranes. The nuclear polarity is disrupted and marked cell pleomorphism and aberrant mitosis are present. Structural alterations include budding or branching crypts or tubules and cribriform growth [12]. The number of samples required is however also important. If not enough samples can be studied, it is better to do proper sampling again within a short period. While its practical usefulness is clear, the classification can not yet be considered to be an end-point because the histogenesis of some lesions identified in the Vienna classification as non-invasive and invasive carcinoma is not yet fully understood. A better understanding may come from molecular studies and findings in other tumours.

"Adenoma" is still often used for the identification of a "benign" neo-plastic lesion showing increased proliferation, nuclear atypia and disturbed glandular architecture (changes which represent "malformations" and hence were classified as dysplasia). In the seventies the "polyp – cancer" or "adenoma – carcinoma sequence" has been proposed as an explanation for the pathogenesis of colorectal cancer implying a stepwise process. Later the "colitis – dysplasia – carcinoma sequence" was proposed for a similar process occurring in chronic idiopathic inflammatory bowel diseases. The development of molecular techniques allowed a more refined approach and in the nineties a model for the molecular pathway of colonic carcinogenesis in sporadic cancer was proposed [13].

Vertical tumour growth and staging

It is conceivable that, in the future, the molecular analysis of the processes necessary for tumour progression (and invasion) might change the classification and allow a better diagnosis. At present, it is already clear that "vertical growth" is an important prognostic marker. This is illustrated by the importance of radial (lateral) margins for local recurrence and survival for both (colo-)rectal and esophageal tumours. It is proposed that carcinoma involving the circumferential resection margin and clearance (in mm) should be documented. Presence of carcinoma at less than 1 or 2 mm, depending on the authors, from the circumferential margin is considered to be the criterion for margin involvement. This feature has been included with a margin of 1 mm in the minimum data set of the Royal College [14].

"Vertical growth" is also used as an important prognostic marker for the staging of "endoscopic mucosal resections (EMR)". EMR implies endoscopic resection with curative intent of neo-plastic lesions. Indications for EMR depend on depth of invasion (endosonography), type and size of lesion (endoscopy) and histology. The concept of tumour progression is partially based upon findings in other tumour types. It is long known that malignant melanoma proceeds through successive phases of tumour progression, that each yield increasing growth advantage to the tumour cells. These successive tumour-progression phases comprise 1) the pure (radial) growth phase (RGP) in which cancer spreads in the epidermis resulting clinically in an irregular enlargement; 2) the micro-invasive radial growth phase characterized by invasion of the dermis by single melanoma cell; 3) the vertical growth phase (VGP) characterized by the appearance of expansile nodules in the dermis and 4) the metastasic phase [15]. In the gastrointestinal tract, the "VGP" can be considered to be the invasion in the submucosa.

In the gastrointestinal tract, tumour progression is expressed by the depth of penetration. Penetration in the submucosa is subclassified into 3 grades: namely sm 1, sm 2 and sm 3. Sm 1 is defined as one-third invasion in the superficial submucosal layer, sm 2 as one-third in the medium layer and sm 3 as invasion in the deep layer [16]. Further subclassification into sm 1a, sm 1b and sm 1c is based upon the horizontal expansion of the lesion. These criteria are based on surgical series. In sm 1 lesions, the risk of lymph-node metastases is estimated at 6%. The risk is much higher in sm 2 (45%) and sm 3-type lesions [17]. In addition, sm 2 and sm 3 carcinoma have a high frequency of lymph node metastasis and recurrence [18]. The overall 5-year survival rate does not differ significantly when EMR (77.5%) and surgical resection (84.5%) are compared for sm 1 esophageal cancer. The disease specific survival was equivalent (95.0% for EMR and 93.5% for esophagectomy) [19]. This implies however precise handling and analysis of the specimen after EMR. The histological report must contain type and grade of tumour, depth of invasion and lateral margins. A margin of more than 2 mm is considered safe. Recurrence is observed in 20% if this margin is invaded. Recurrence of 50% is observed if the section edge is invaded.

Gastrointestinal stromal tumours

Gastrointestinal stromal tumours (GISTs) are rare tumours with an annual incidence of 10-20 cases per million, of which 20-30% are malignant. The term GIST was first used to describe these non-epithelial gastric neoplasms, formerly usually known as leiomyoma or leiomyosarcoma, because they lack immunohistochemical features of Schwann cells and ultrastructural characteristics of smooth muscle cells [20]. The discovery of gain-of-function mutations in the KIT proto-oncogene in 1998 was of crucial importance in terms of the classification of these tumours and treatment [21]. These tumours can now be identified using immunohistochemistry and antibodies directed against C-kit (CD-117). As a result, the actual classification of mesenchymal tumours includes:

- Leiomyomas and leiomyosarcoma: rare tumours of the gastrointestinal tract showing specific phenotypical aspects and differentiation of smooth muscle cells;
- Schwannomas and neurofibromas: rare tumours with specific phenotypical aspect and differentiation of Schwann cells or of typical neurofibroma;
- Gastrointestinal stromal tumours (GIST): the vast majority of mesenchymal tumours of the GI that express CD-117, a specific marker of the interstitial cell of Cajal. It is also of note that the previously isolated group of gastrointestinal autonomic nerve tumours (GANT) showing at the ultrastructural level characteristics of the gastrointestinal autonomic plexus is in fact a subgroup of GIST since most of the GANT show same phenotypical and molecular characteristic as the GISTs [22].

Some authors have proposed a more elaborate classification including:

- CD-117 positive tumours (GIST);
- CD117-negative neoplasms showing strong expression (> 50) of several myogenic markers (smooth muscle actin) considered to be gastrointestinal leiomyogenic tumours for which GILT was proposed;
- CD117-negative tumours showing strong expression of S-100 protein and GFAP and PGP9.5 in the absence of myogenic markers regarded as gastrointestinal glial tumours (GIGT) or GINT (when there was concurrent expression of synaptophysin);
- Tumours that were only vimentin positive were classified as gastrointestinal fibrous tumours (GIFT);
- Tumours that strongly expressed CD34 but could not be classified according to other criteria were considered gastrointestinal CD117-negative stromal tumours (GINST).

However, according to other authors, tumours with a null phenotype belong still to the group of GIST [23].

The risk of aggressive behaviour for these tumours is assessed using the size of the lesion and mitotic count. It can be subdivided in very low risk (lesion < 2 cm; mitotic count < 5 per 50 HPF); low (2-5 cm; < 5 per 50 HPF); intermediate (< 5 cm; 6-10 per 50 HPF or 5-1 cm; < 5 per 50 HPF) and high risk (> 5 cm and > 5 per 50 HPF; > 10 cm and any mitotic rate; any size and > 10 per 50 HPF).

Conclusions

Novel grading and staging systems for neoplasia are useful when they have practical consequences. This is exemplified by the Vienna classification for GEN and by the new classification for GISTs. Periodic revision of classifications is needed because of scientific progress. It requires however precision, adequate definition of criteria and guidelines for the application of the systems.

References

1. Dixon MF. Gastrointestinal epithelial neoplasia: Vienna revisited. *Gut* 2002; 51: 130-1.
2. Zinkin LD. A critical review of the classifications and staging of colorectal cancer. *Dis Colon Rectum* 1983; 26: 37-43.
3. Goseki N, Takizawa T, Koike M. Differences in the mode of the extension of gastric cancer classified by histological type: new histological classification of gastric carcinoma. *Gut* 1992; 33: 606-12.
4. Carneiro F, Seixas M, Sobrinho-Simoes M. New elements for an updated classification of the carcinomas of the stomach. *Pathol Res Pract* 1995; 191: 571-84.
5. Ormsby AH, Petras RE, Henrickx WH, Rice TW, Rybicki LA, Richter JE, Goldblum JR. Observer variation in the diagnosis of superficial esophageal adenocarcinoma. *Gut* 2002; 51: 671-6.
6. Jass JR. Histopathology of early colorectal cancer. *World J Surg* 2000; 24: 1016-21.
7. Schlemper RJ, Riddell RH, Kato Y, et al. The Vienna classification of Gastrointestinal Neoplasia. *Gut* 2000; 47: 251-5.

8. Joensuu H, Fletcher C, Dimitrijevic S, Silberman S, Roberts P, Demetri G. Management of malignant stromal tumours. *Lancet Oncology* 2003; 3: 655-9.
9. Fletcher CDM, Berman JJ, Corless C, *et al.* Diagnosis of gastrointestinal stromal tumours: a consensus approach. *Int J Surg Pathol* 2002; 10: 81-9.
10. Hamilton SR, Aaltonen LA (eds). Pathology and genetics of tumours of the digestive system. WHO Classification of Tumours. DARC Press, Lyon.
11. Stolte M. The new Vienna classification of epithelial neoplasia of the gastrointestinal tract: advantages and disadvantages. *Virchows Arch* 2003; 442: 99-106.
12. Rubio C. Gastrointestinal neoplasia. *Gut* 2003; 52: 455-6.
13. Fearon ER, Vogelstein B. A genetic model for colorectal tumourigenesis. *Cell* 1990; 61: 759-67.
14. Mapstone N. Minimum data set for esophageal carcinoma – histopathology reports. Royal College of Pathologists: www.rcpath.org/activities/publications.
15. Clark WH, Elder DE, Guerry D IV, *et al.* The precursor lesions of superficial spreading and nodular melanoma. *Hum Pathol* 1984; 15: 1147-65.
16. Nabeya K, Nakata Y. Topic forum: early esophageal cancer. Extent of resection and lymphadenectomy in early squamous cell esophageal cancer. *Dis Esophagus* 1997; 10: 159-61.
17. Lambert R. Treatment of esophagogastric tumours. *Endoscopy* 2003; 35: 118-26.
18. Araki K, Ohno S, Egashira A, Saeki H, Kawaguchi H, Sugimachi K. Pathologic features of superficial esophageal squamous cell carcinoma with lymph node and distal metastasis. *Cancer* 2002; 15: 570-5.
19. Shimizu Y, Tsukagoshi H, Fujita M, *et al.* Long-term outcome after endoscopic mucosal resection in patients with esophageal squamous cell carcinoma invading the muscularis mucosae or deeper. *Gastrointest Endosc* 2002; 56: 387-90.
20. Mazur MT, Clark HB. Gastric stromal tumours. Reappraisal of histogenesis. *Am J Surg Pathol* 1983; 7: 507-19.
21. Hirota S, Nishida T, Isozaki K, Taniguchi M, Nakamura J, Okazaki T, Kitamura Y. Gain-of-function mutation at the extracellular domain of KIT in gastrointestinal stromal tumours. *J Pathol* 2001; 193: 505-10.
22. Miettinen M, Lasota J. Gastrointestinal stromal tumours: definition, clinical, histological, immunohistochemical, and molecular genetic features and differential diagnosis. *Virchows Arch* 2001; 438: 1-12.
23. Rudolph P, Chiaravalli AM, Pauser U, *et al.* Gastrointestinal mesenchymal tumours – immunophenotypic classification and survival analysis. *Virchows Arch* 2002; 441: 238-48.

Endoscopic mucosal resection for treatment of early gastric cancer. Indication and new technique, IT knife method

Hiroyuki Ono

Endoscopy and GI Oncology Division, Shizuoka Cancer Center Hospital, Japan

Indication

Early gastric cancer (EGC) is defined as that confined to the mucosa or submucosa regardless of the presence or absence of regional lymph node metastasis. It has been increasing in Japan [1], accounting for approximately 60% of all resected cases in our institution. In Japan, the 5-year survival rate of patients with EGC is over 90% after gastrectomy with complete removal of primary and secondary lymph nodes [2, 3]. The incidence of nodal metastasis of intramucosal and submucosal EGC has been reported as 3% and 20% respectively [4], therefore major surgery may be inappropriate in many of these patients. Endoscopic mucosal resection (EMR) has been extended for a treatment of EGC from the beginning of the 1980s. Because EMR is just a local treatment, we should choose appropriate candidates with low possibility of lymph node metastasis. We analyzed about 3,000 patients with solitary, intramucosa, and surgically treated early gastric cancer [5]. An early gastric cancer confined to the mucosa has to meet the following criteria in order to be resected endoscopically:

1. Histologically differentiated adenocarcinoma,
2. Tumour is less than 30 mm in size if it has ulcerative changes. (No limitation of the size if it has no ulcer),
3. Absence of lymphatic vascular involvement.

Table I shows a summary of incidence of lymph node metastasis from intramucosal early gastric cancer. If the cancers satisfy the above criteria, the possibility of lymph node metastasis is less than 1%. In such cases, we can expect curability equal to the surgical treatment.

Table I. Incidence of lymph node metastasis from intramucosal early gastric cancer

Ulcer or ulcer scar	Differentiated type		Undifferentiated type		Lymphatic vascular invasion
	2 cm	2 cm	2 cm	2 cm	
(−)	0/437 0% (0-0.7%)	0/493 0% (0-0.6%)	0/141 0% (0-2.6%)	6/214 2.8% (1.0-6.0%)	ly0, v0
	3 cm	3 cm	52/1041 5.0% (3.8-6.5)		
(+)	0/488 0% (0-0.6%)	7/230 3.0% (1.2-6.2%)			

(): 95% Confidence interval

Evaluation of resected specimens and resectability

The resectability of EMR specimens was carefully evaluated both endoscopically and histopathologically in slices at 2 mm intervals according to the "Japanese Classification of Gastric Carcinoma" [1]. After resection in multiple fragments, resectability was evaluated based on completely reconstructed specimens. The current definition of "Resection EA" [6], which means a high probability of cure, is demonstrated in *table II*. Since submucosal invasion and/or vessel involvement are regarded as a high risk of positive nodes or distant metastasis, surgical intervention was strongly recommended.

Table II. Evaluation of resected specimens by EMR

The following must be confirmed histologically for "complete resection":
1. Intramucosal cancer
2. Well or moderately differentiated type adenocarcinoma
3. No lymphatic or venous invasion
4. No tumour invasion to the lateral margin

Evaluation of invasion to the lateral margin was classified into the following three groups using endoscopic and histopathologic evidence:

1. Complete resection: When the lateral margin was clear endoscopically and pathologically (minimum probability of local recurrence),
2. Incomplete resection: When the tumour definitely invaded to the lateral margin endoscopically and pathologically (high probability of local recurrence),
3. Not evaluable: When the tumour was removed endoscopically, but its lateral margin was not pathologically evaluable due to a burn effect (burned by diathermic treatment), or mechanical damage, or when reconstruction was difficult due to a multi-fragment resection.

Techniques

Most EMRs are performed by the so-called "strip biopsy method" [7] or "Cap method (EMRC)" [8] in Japan. *Figure 1* shows the procedure of "strip biopsy method", however, we had 5 local recurrences in "complete resection", all of which had been resected in multiple fragments by this method. Single-fragment resection is preferable because with multi-fragment specimens it is often difficult to reconstruct the entire lesion. We think it is likely that local recurrence can often be attributed to inappropriate assessment of the multiple fragments of resected specimens.

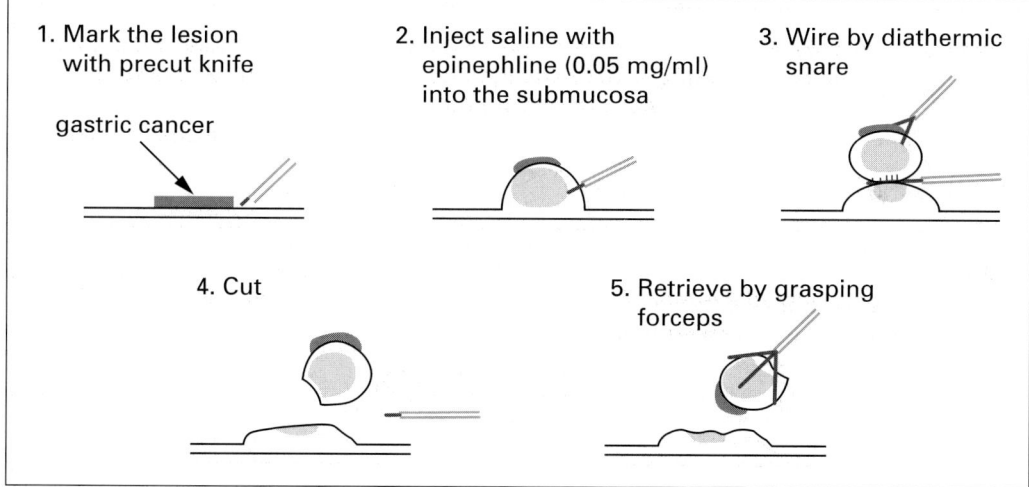

Figure 1. Procedure of EMR

Recently, dramatic developments have occurred in the operational mechanism and design of the accessory apparatus for EMR. To obtain the "complete resection" histologically for large and difficult lesions, we developed a special endoscopic knife in 1996 named Insulation-tipped electrosurgical knife (IT knife, *figure 2*) [9, 10]. This knife can cut submucosa safely and remove a lesion completely. We call this method "Submucosal Dissection; SMD". We also developed an improved technique named "PTA-EMR: Percutaneus Traction-assisted EMR". We raise up a clip attached on the edge of a lesion by a thin retractor through the abdominal wall (like percutaneus endoscopic gastrostomy), and then resect the lesion by IT knife. It can give counter traction to the lesion as well as surgical mucosectomy and can be carried out without systemic anaesthesia.

The rate of complete resection increased extremely in the cases of IT knife method (*table III*).

Table III. Complete Resection Rate – single fragment and cut margin (–) – subjects: lesions in our criteria EMR 1,065 lesions 1987-2002.3

	~ 20 mm	21 ~ 30	31 ~	total
strip biopsy	45% (172/386)	24% (8/34)	0% (0/10)	42% (180/429)
IT knife ('00 ~)	94% (231/245)	90% (57/63)	92% (33/36)	93% (321/344)
(total)	86% (339/395)	76% (86/113)	78% (45/58)	83% (470/566)

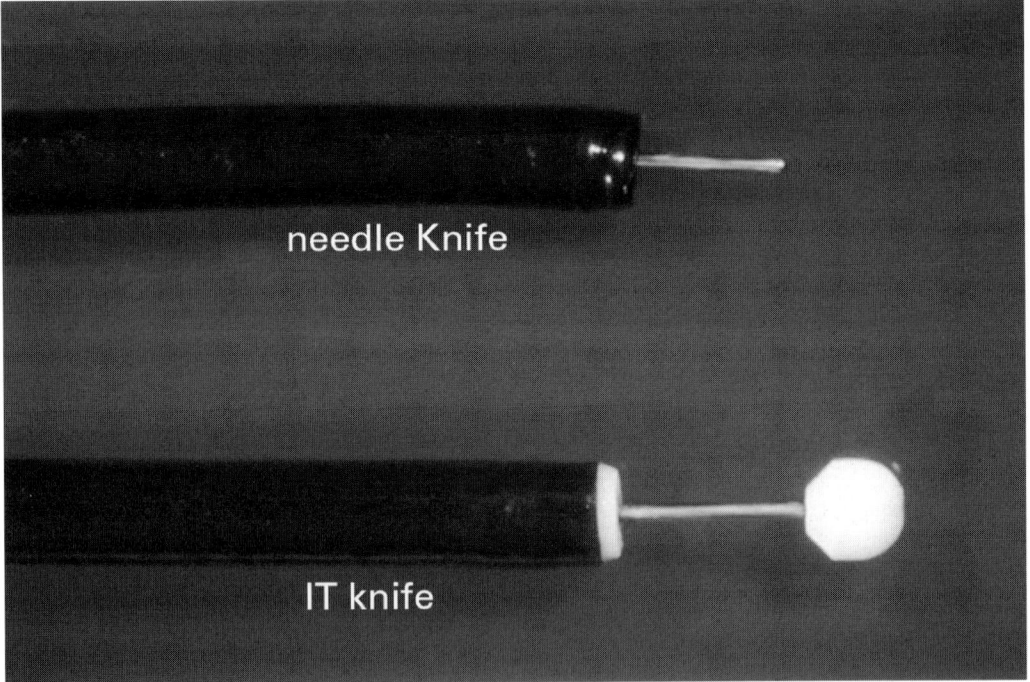

Figure 2. Insulation-tipped electrosurgical knife.

Complications

Bleeding and perforation are two major complications in EMR. Bleeding was almost controllable by endoscopic treatment with ethanol injection, endoscopic clipping (HX5LR-1, Olympus, Japan), and spraying of thrombin solution in the stomach. However, we could not stop the bleeding and referred to our surgeon to stop it surgically. The rate of it was 0.3% (5/1520). There were 82 cases of perforation (5%), the first four were converted to open surgery. Since then, all perforations, except only 1 case, have been successfully treated with endoscopic clipping, intubation of nasogastric tube and administration of antibiotics.

Conclusion

The EMR technique has been developed mainly in Japan, where there is a high incidence of EGC. It is used infrequently in the West. It is important to carefully evaluate the current status of EMR and promote the appropriate use of this technique around the world. The number of patients undergoing EMR is increasing, with about 1,500 procedures performed in our hospital over the past 15 years. Considering that it generally takes one hour for resection and one week for admission, EMR is a minimally invasive procedure (a patient undergoing surgical resection stays about three weeks in our hospital). Our experience suggests that EMR can provide comparable long-term survival rates to traditional therapy, provided that inclusion criteria are strictly adhered to.

Since there are still several unsolved problems in EMR. Patient eligibility for EMR should be considered in relation to the risk of lymph node metastasis. As shown in *table I*, EMR is now applied to EGC with a lower incidence of lymph node metastasis than the mortality rate from surgery for EGC (about less than 1%).

The "Japanese Classification of Gastric Carcinoma" was used for tumour description [1], which is widely used in our country. Western pathologists use the term "high grade dysplasia" for neo-plastic lesions that have not breached the basement membrane to the lamina propria. Japanese pathologists, however, classify them as intramucosal cancer on the grounds that the cells are of malignant type and have the potential to invade [11]. A recent analysis showed that the histological type, macroscopic appearance, degree of invasion and lymph node metastases are the same although more EGCs are detected in Japan than in the West [12]. We usually do EMR for intramucosal cancer in the Japanese criteria, and it is of importance to have the same diagnostic criteria for gastric neo-plastic lesions to propagate EMR around the world.

At all events, a picture is worth a thousand words. I will show a video demonstration of EMR using the IT knife and how to treat complications endoscopically.

References

1. Japanese Research Society for Gastric Cancer. *Japanese Classification of Gastric Carcinoma* (1st edition) Eds: Nishi M, Omori Y, Miwa K, *et al.*, LTD., Tokyo, 1995.
2. Okamura T, Tsujitani S, Korenaga D, *et al.* Lymphadenectomy for cure in patients with early gastric cancer and lymph node metastasis. *Am J Surg* 1998; 155: 476-80.
3. Noguchi Y, Imada T, Matsumoto A, *et al.* Radical surgery for gastric cancer: a review of Japanese experience. *Cancer* 1989; 64: 2053-62.
4. Sano T, Kobori O, Muto T. Lymph node metastasis from early gastric cancer: endoscopic resection of tumour. *Br J Surg* 1992; 79: 241-4.
5. Gotoda T, Sasako M, Yanagisawa A, *et al.* Incidence of lymph node metastasis from early gastric cancer-estimation with a large number of cases at two large centers. *Gastric Cancer* 2000; 3: 219.
6. Japanese Gastric Cancer Association. Japanese classification of gastric carcinoma 2nd English edition. *Gastric Cancer* 1998; 1: 10-24.
7. Tada M, Shimada M, Murakami F. Development of the strip-off biopsy. *Gastroenterol Endosc* 1984; 26: 833-9.
8. Inoue H, Tani M, Nagai K, *et al.* Treatment of esophageal and gastric tumours. *Endoscopy* 1999; 31: 47-55.
9. Gotoda T, Kondo H, Ono H, *et al.* A new endoscopic mucosal resection procedure using an insulation-tipped diathermic knife for rectal flat lesions. *Gastrointestinal Endosc* 1999; 50: 560-3.
10. Ono H, Kondo H, Gotoda T, *et al.* Endoscopic mucosal resection for treatment of early gastric cancer. *Gut* 2001; 48 (2): 225-9.
11. Schlemper RJ, Itabashi M, Kato Y, *et al.* Differences in diagnosis criteria for gastric carcinoma between Japanese and Western pathologists. *Lancet* 1997; 349: 1725-9.
12. Everett SM, Axon ATR. Early gastric cancer in Europe. *Gut* 1997; 41: 142-50.

IV

Secondary liver tumours

Local ablative therapy for liver metastases

Riccardo Lencioni, Chiara Franchini, Laura Crocetti, Dania Cioni

Division of Diagnostic and Interventional Radiology, Department of Oncology, Transplants, and Advanced Technologies in Medicine, University of Pisa; Via Roma 67, I-56125 Pisa, Italy

Introduction

Metastatic disease in the liver usually indicates advanced disease and a poor prognosis. In patients with hepatic metastases from primary malignancies developed in the gastrointestinal tract, particularly colorectal adenocarcinoma, a substantial improvement in long-term survival can be achieved with surgical removal of the metastatic burden. A 5-year survival rate of approximately 20-40% and a 5-year disease-free survival rate of approximately 20-25%, in fact, can be expected in successfully treated patients [1-4]. However, surgery is frequently precluded by the number and location of metastatic nodules or because of other associated medical conditions. Unfortunately, conventional treatment of non-operable or non-resectable patients with systemic or intra-arterial chemotherapy protocols has not been entirely satisfactory in terms of survival outcomes.

Attention has therefore been focused on investigating the effectiveness of minimally invasive techniques for local tumour ablation in treating patients with hepatic metastases who were not surgical candidates. The first technique used for local ablation therapy of liver malignancies has been percutaneous ethanol injection [5]. However, as opposed to hepatocellular carcinoma, alcohol diffusion within metastatic lesions was shown to be uneven, resulting in largely incomplete ablation with necrotic areas and viable tissue irregularly mixed [5]. Therefore, other local ablation methods that seek to achieve more effective tumour necrosis, including laser, microwave, and radio-frequency (RF) thermal ablation, have been developed and tested clinically over the past few years [6]. RF ablation, in particular, has attracted much attention, since recent technological improvements have permitted the creation of thermal necrosis volumes up to 5-7 cm in diameter with a single-probe percutaneous insertion, thus enabling successful ablation of large hepatic tumours in a single treatment session [7]. RF ablation has some merits compared with the other percutaneous techniques: the thermal lesions are larger than those obtained with a microwave electrode, and it is easier to perform than interstitial laser photocoagulation, in which multiple fiber insertions are required. In this article, we review current techniques, indications, and clinical results of RF thermal ablation in the treatment liver metastases.

Technique

The goal of RF ablation is to induce thermal injury to the tissue through electromagnetic energy deposition. In RF ablation, the patient is part of a closed-loop circuit, that includes an RF generator, an electrode needle, and a large dispersive electrode (ground pads). An alternating electric field is created within the tissue of the patient. Because of the relatively high electrical resistance of tissue in comparison with the metal electrodes, there is marked agitation of the ions present in the target tissue that surrounds the electrode, since the tissue ions attempt to follow the changes in direction of alternating electric current. The agitation results in frictional heat around the electrode. The discrepancy between the small surface area of the needle electrode and the large area of the ground pads causes the generated heat to be focused and concentrated around the needle electrode.

The thermal damage caused by RF heating is dependent on both the tissue temperature achieved and the duration of heating. Heating of tissue at 50°-55° C for 4-6 minutes produces irreversible cellular damage. At temperatures between 60° C and 100° C near immediate coagulation of tissue is induced, with irreversible damage to mitochondrial and cytosolic enzymes of the cells. At more than 100°-110° C, tissue vaporizes and carbonizes. For adequate destruction of tumour tissue, the entire target volume must be subjected to cytotoxic temperatures. Thus, an essential objective of ablative therapy is achievement and maintenance of a 50°-100° C temperature throughout the entire target volume for at least 4-6 minutes. However, the relatively slow thermal conduction from the electrode surface through the tissue increases the duration of application to 10-30 minutes. On the other hand, the tissue temperature should not be increased over these values to avoid carbonization around the tip of the electrode due to excessive heating.

In the early experiences with RF ablation, a major limitation of the technique was the small volume of necrosis created by conventional monopolar electrodes. These devices were capable of producing cylindrical lesions not greater than 1.6 cm in diameter. Therefore, multiple electrode insertions were necessary to treat all but the smallest lesions. Subsequently, several strategies for increasing the area of thermal necrosis achieved with RF treatment have been tested, including the use of multi-probe arrays, bipolar arrays, and saline injections during RF application. These devices were shown to increase the volume of coagulation necrosis that can be obtained in a single treatment session. However, such techniques were either technically challenging and time-consuming or produced irregularly-shaped thermal lesions, thereby substantially limiting their clinical usefulness.

A major progress in RF technology was achieved with the introduction of modified electrodes, including cooled-tip electrode needles and expandable electrode needles with multiple retractable lateral-exit prongs on the tip [7]. Cooled-tip electrodes consist of dual-lumen needles with uninsulated active tips, in which internal cooling is obtained by continuous perfusion with chilled saline. Needle cooling is aimed at preventing overheating of tissue nearest to the electrode, which may cause charring, thereby limiting the propagation of RF waves. They are available either as a single needle or as a cluster array with three needles spaced 0.5 cm apart. Expandable needles have an active surface which can be substantially expanded by hooks deployed laterally from the tip. The number of hooks and the length of the hooks deployed may vary according to the desired volume of necrosis. These techniques enabled a substantial and reproducible enlargement of the volume of thermal necrosis produced with a single needle insertion, and prompted the start of clinical application of RF ablation.

At our institution, we currently use 150- or 200-W RF generators and 14-gauge expandable electrode needles (StarBurst XL, RITA Medical Systems). The needle electrode consists of an insulated outer cannula that houses nine curved electrodes of various lengths, that deploy out from the trocar tip. This design decreases the distance between the tissue and the electrodes, thereby ensuring uniform heating that relies less on heat conduction over a large distance. Five of the electrodes are hollow and contain thermocouples in their tips that are used to measure the temperature of the adjacent tissue. Probe-tip temperatures, tissue impedance, and wattage are displayed on the RF generator and graphically recorded by dedicated software, installed on a personal computer.

Maximum power output of the RF generator, amount of electrode array deployed from the trocar, and duration of the effective time of the ablation (time at target temperature) depends on the desired volume of ablation. This is established at the beginning of the procedure with the goal to destroy ideally the visible tumour mass plus a 1-cm safety margin of ablation all around. To perform a typical ablation, two grounding pads are placed on the patient's thighs. The tip of the needle (with retracted electrodes) is advanced under ultrasound guidance to the proximal edge of the lesion, and the electrodes are deployed to 2 cm. The generator is turned on and runs by an automated program. The temperature at the tips of the electrodes are controlled and the peak power is maintained until the temperature exceeds the preselected target temperature (typically between $90°$ and $100°$ C). After the target temperature is achieved, the curved electrodes can be advanced step-by-step to full deployment. When the electrodes are fully deployed, the program maintains the target temperature by regulating the wattage. At the end of the procedure, when the generator runs off, a "cool down cycle" is automatically performed. After retracting the hooks, the coagulation of the needle track can be done (track ablation) by maintaining the temperature above $75°$ C with the aim to prevent any tumour cell dissemination.

In our center, RF ablation is routinely performed percutaneously, although some 15-20% of the procedures are performed with a laparoscopy or laparotomy approach. Typically, the surgical approach is chosen for lesions with a critical size or location, or for combined resection-ablation procedures.

Percutaneous RF ablation is performed by using conscious sedation. The association of an hypnotic drug with an ultrashort half-life analgesic drug allows a mild sedation and the patient, who can co-operate with the operator and bear the pain induced by treatment. Our standard protocol consists in admistering a bolus of ketorolac (0.5-0.8 mg/kg) followed by infusion of propofol (1-2 mg/kg/h) and remifentanil (0.1 mg/kg/min). However, drug posology has to be modulated in relation to the individual patient compliance and to the different phases of the procedure. The infusion of the hypnotic drug can be varied between 0.5 and 2 mg/kg/h to achieve a patient sedation that preserves the ability to do easy actions. The infusion of remifentanil can be varied between 0.05 and 0.15/kg/min to obtain an optimal analgesia. Attention has to be made in order to avoid bolus administration of remifentanil, as this may cause respiratory depression. The procedure is performed under standard cardiac, pressure, and oxygen monitoring with continuous oxygen administration.

A careful post-treatment protocol is to be recommended following RF ablation. The patient is kept under close medical observation and re-scanned with ultrasound 1-2 hours after the procedure. An overnight hospital stay is scheduled. Contrast-enhanced ultrasound performed shortly after the procedure may allow an initial evaluation of tumour response, by showing disappearance of intratumoural signals. Spiral CT obtained 1-3 days after the ablation shows a core of hypoattenuation surrounded by an enhancing rim. The peripheral enhancing rim – which is due to the inflammatory reaction surrounding the area of necrosis – should not be misinterpreted as tumour persistence. Since the enhancing rim tends to disappear over time, spiral CT at 1 month is considered the most reliable method to evaluate the outcome of treatment. If there is imaging evidence of residual tumour, the patient can be considered for repeated RF ablation, provided that requirements for treatment are still met. Follow-up ultrasound and spiral CT studies are usually scheduled at 3- or 6-month intervals.

Indications

Appropriate use of RF ablation can only be done when the therapeutic strategy is decided by a multidisciplinary team and is tailored to the individual patient and to the features of the disease.

The indication for RF ablation is highly dependent on the histology and extension of the primary tumour. The biology and the characteristics of metastatic disease, in fact, limit the applicability of a local therapy like RF. The best indication for RF treatment is represented by metachronous metastases from gastrointestinal malignancies, especially colorectal adenocarcinoma and endocrine tumours. In selected cases, however, patients with liver metastases from other primary neoplasms, such as breast adenocarcinoma, could be considered for RF ablation in the setting of a multidisciplinary approach.

To be considered eligible for treatment by RF thermal ablation, patients must meet some general requirements. First, as RF ablation is a local treatment, disease should be ideally confined to the liver, without evidence of extrahepatic metastases. In addition, the tumour to treat by RF must be a focal, nodular-type lesion. The presence of a clear and easy-to-detect target for needle placement is crucial for the outcome of treatment. The tumour burden must be limited to a maximum of 3-5 lesions smaller than 3-5 cm in the greatest dimension.

Treatment of lesions adjacent to the gallbladder or to the hepatic hilum is at risk of thermal injury of the biliary tract. In contrast, treatment of lesions located in the vicinity of hepatic vessels is possible, since flowing blood usually "refrigerates" the vascular wall, protecting it from thermal injury: in these cases, however, the risk of incomplete ablation of the area of neo-plastic tissue adjacent to the vessel may increase because of the heat loss caused by the vessel itself. Lesions located along the surface of the liver can be considered for RF ablation, although their treatment requires experienced hands and may be associated with a higher risk of complications. Percutaneous treatment of superficial lesions that are adjacent to any part of the gastrointestinal tract must be avoided because of the risk of thermal injury of the gastric or bowel wall. A laparoscopy approach can be considered in such instances.

A careful clinical evaluation of the patient is also necessary to establish the indication for RF ablation, and should include history and full clinical and laboratory assessment. In particular, levels of serum tumour markers, such as carcinoembryonic antigen (CEA) must be measured. Additionally, a staging protocol including at least liver US, abdominal spiral CT or MR imaging, chest spiral CT, and bone scintigraphy must be carried out. PET is also useful, especially to rule out extrahepatic disease. The assessment of coagulation status should be particularly careful. A prothrombin time ratio (normal time/patient's time) greater than 50% as well as a platelet count higher than 50,000/µl are required to keep the risk of bleeding at an acceptable low level.

A careful follow-up protocol is to be recommended following RF ablation. Follow-up studies should be aimed at detecting both the recurrence of the treated lesion (*i.e.*, local recurrence) and possible new lesions developed in other parts of the liver or in other organs. A standard imaging protocol for the follow-up of treated cases should include at least a spiral CT or dynamic MR study of the liver every 3-4 months plus the survey of the possible sites of extrahepatic disease, depending on the primary tumour and the stage of the disease.

Clinical results

In early clinical experiences with RF thermal ablation, patients were treated in the framework of feasibility studies, aimed at analysing safety, tolerability, and local therapeutic effect of the treatment.

Lencioni *et al.* [8] performed a pilot clinical trial, in which 29 patients with 1-4 hepatic metastases 1.1-4.8 cm in diameter (mean, 2.9 cm) from previously resected intra-abdominal primary malignancies were enrolled. All patients were excluded from surgery and had partial or no response to chemotherapy. A total of 127 insertions were performed (mean, 2.4 insertions/lesion) during 84 treatment sessions (mean, 1.6 sessions/lesion) in absence of complications. Complete tumour response – defined as the presence of a unenhancing area of thermal necrosis larger than the treated tumour on posttreatment spiral CT – was seen in 41 (77%) of 53 lesions. After a mean follow-up period of 6.5 months (range 3-9 months), recurrence of the treated lesion was seen in 12% of cases. Solbiati *et al.* [9] assessed feasibility and safety of using dual-lumen, cooled-tip electrodes with a 2-

or 3-cm exposed tip to increase the volume of coagulation necrosis in a series of 29 patients with 44 hepatic metastases ranging from 1.3 to 5.1 cm in diameter. Each tumour was treated in one or two treatment sessions, and technical success – defined as the ablation of all visualized tumours – was achieved in 40 of 44 lesions. However, follow-up imaging studies confirmed complete necrosis of the entire metastasis in only 66% of the cases, while localized progression of disease was observed in the remaining 34%. Only one complication, self-limited haemorrhage, was seen. In the study of De Baere et al. [10], 68 patients with 121 hepatic metastases, mainly of colorectal origin, underwent 76 sessions of RF ablation under sonographic guidance, either percutaneously (47 patients with 88 metastases 10 to 42 mm in diameter) or intraoperatively (21 patients with 33 metastases 5-20 mm in diameter). Procedure efficacy was evaluated with dynamic enhanced CT and MR imaging performed 2, 4, and 6 months after treatment and then every 3 months. Radiofrequency ablation allowed eradication of 91% of the 100 treated metastases that were followed up for 4-23 months (mean, 13.7 months). Tumour control was equivalent for percutaneous radiofrequency ablation (90%) and for intraoperative radiofrequency ablation (94%). Failure to achieve tumour control occurred mostly with the largest tumour nodules. One bilioperitoneum and two abscesses were the major complications encountered after treatment of 121 metastases with a follow-up of more than 2 months.

Recently, data on survival and disease-free survival rates of patients treated by thermal ablation have been reported. In the series of Gilliams and Lees [11], the impact on survival in 69 patients with colorectal metastases – with an average number of 2.9 lesions with a mean diameter of 3.9 cm – was analyzed. All patients had been excluded from surgery. Eighteen (26%) patients had undergone previous hepatic resection and 62 (93%) received chemotherapy at some stage. One-year, 2-year, 3-year, and 4-year survival rates were 90%, 60%, 34%, and 22%. These figures are substantially higher than those achieved with either systemic chemotherapy (48% at 1 year, 21% at 2 years, and 3% at 3 years) or regional chemotherapy (64% at 1 year, 25% at 2 years, and 5% at 3 years), and suggest that thermal ablation therapy improves survival in patients with inoperable but limited liver metastases. Additionally, it has to be considered that recent and ongoing technical refinements are not reflected in these results. In the series of Solbiati et al. [12], 179 metachronous colorectal carcinoma hepatic metastases (0.9-9.6 cm in diameter) were treated with RF ablation in 117 patients. Computed tomographic follow-up was performed every 4-6 months. Recurrent tumours were retreated when feasible. Estimated median survival was 36 months. Estimated 1, 2, and 3-year survival rates were 93%, 69%, and 46%, respectively. Survival was not significantly related to number of metastases treated. In 77 (66%) of 117 patients, new metastases were observed at follow-up. Estimated median time until new metastases was 12 months. Percentages of patients with no new metastases after initial treatment at 1 and 2 years were 49% and 35%, respectively. Time to new metastases was not significantly related to number of metastases. Seventy (39%) of 179 lesions developed local recurrence after treatment. Of these, 54 were observed by 6 months and 67 by 1 year. No local recurrence was observed after 18 months. Frequency and time to local recurrence were related to lesion size.

Recent work was focused on investigating the possible complementary role of RF ablation and surgical resection. Elias et al. [13] performed RF ablation for the treatment of liver tumour recurrence after hepatectomy. Forty-seven patients presenting with local recurrence after hepatectomy for malignant tumours (29 with colorectal secondaries) were treated with percutaneous RF ablation instead of repeat hepatectomy. A retrospective study of the authors' database over two similar consecutive periods showed that RF ablation increased the percentage of curative local treatments for liver recurrence after hepatectomy from 17 to 26 per cent and decreased the proportion of repeat hepatectomies from 100 to 39 per cent. Livraghi *et al.* [14] evaluated the potential role of performing RF ablation during the interval between diagnosis and hepatic metastasectomy as part of this "test-of-time" management approach. Eighty-eight consecutive patients with 134 colorectal carcinoma liver metastases who were potential candidates for hepatic metastasectomy were treated with percutaneous RF ablation. A total of 119 RF ablations were performed. Among all 88 patients, 21 underwent resection after RF ablation (8 were free of disease at the time of last follow-up), 23 remained free of disease after successful RF ablation, and 56 developed untreatable disease progression (44 after RF alone, 12 after RF and surgery). No patient who had been treated with RF ablation became unresectable due to the growth of metastases and there was no evidence of needle track seeding in any patient after RF ablation. Overall, among the 53 patients in whom complete tumour necrosis was achieved after RF ablation therapy, 98% were spared surgical resection: 44% because they have remained free of disease and 56% because they developed disease progression. Overall, among the 35 patients in whom complete tumour necrosis was not achieved after RF ablation therapy, 43% were spared surgical resection.

Other studies investigated the efficacy of combined RF thermal ablation therapy with hepatic arterial infusion chemotherapy (HAI) in the treatment of multiple liver metastases from colorectal cancer. Kainuma *et al.* [15] treated 9 patients with multiple metastases. The number of nodules ranged from 2 to 13 and the size was 0.5-4.8 cm in diameter. RF ablation was performed using a 15-gauge, 4-prong custom RF needle. Treatment temperature was kept at 90-110 degrees C for 5 min. 5-Fluorouracil (5-FU) was administered by weekly 750-1,250 mg/body/5 h as the regimen of HAI. During a 15.2-month follow-up period, 6 of 9 patients survived more than 1 year. Three of the 6 survived more than 2 years. Local recurrence was observed in 5 patients and new lesions in 4. Extrahepatic recurrence was observed in 5 patients. There were no serious complications but one HAI-related cerebral thrombosis. The authors concluded that combined RF ablation with HAI would be effective and safe. This modality provides a new option for the treatment of multiple liver metastases from colorectal cancer. Scaife *et al.* [16] also conducted a study to determine the feasibility of using HAI after RF ablation for colorectal cancer liver metastases. Fifty patients were treated with RF ablation and HAI with or without resection. A median of two lesions per patient, with a median greatest diameter of 2.0 cm, were treated with RF ablation. Postoperative complications, including 1 death, occurred in 11 of 50 patients. Toxicity from HAI was relatively mild. At 20 months' median follow-up, 32% of patients remained disease free. Ten percent of patients had recurrences at the site of RF ablation, 30% developed new liver metastases, and 48% developed extrahepatic disease. RF ablation of colorectal cancer liver metastases followed by HAI is feasible and is associated with acceptable complication and toxicity rates. The high rate of disease recurrence in our patients indicates that novel combinations of regional and systemic therapies are needed to improve patient outcomes.

Several studies have proved the influence of perfusion-mediated tissue cooling on the area of thermal necrosis achievable with RF treatment [17, 18]. Goldberg *et al.* [17] applied RF *in vivo* to normal porcine liver without and with balloon occlusion of the portal vein, coeliac artery, or hepatic artery, and to *ex vivo* calf liver: RF application during vascular occlusion produced larger areas of coagulation necrosis than RF with unaltered blood flow. The same authors demonstrated that intraoperative RF application produced greater coagulation diameter for human hepatic metastases treated during portal inflow occlusion than for tumours treated with normal blood flow. De Baere *et al.* [19] found that RF ablation of liver malignancies performed during balloon occlusion of a hepatic vein or a segmental portal branch created thermal lesions statistically larger than in a matched control group of patients who underwent radiofrequency ablation without vascular occlusion.

Complications following RF ablation of liver malignancies have been recently analyzed in large series. A recent multicenter survey included 2,320 patients with 3,554 lesions [20]. Six deaths (0.3%) were noted, including two caused by multi-organ failure following intestinal perforation; one case each of septic shock following staphylococcus aureus-caused peritonitis, massive haemorrhage following tumour rupture, liver failure following stenosis of right bile duct; and one case of sudden death of unknown cause 3 days after the procedure. Fifty (2.2%) patients had additional major complications. Lencioni *et al.* [21] determined the rate of major and minor complications associated with the use of expandable, multi-probe RF needles in a series of 872 patients with either hepatocellular carcinoma (n = 548) or hepatic metastases (n = 324). Overall, 1,263 lesions were treated. One case of death (mortality rate, 0.1%) caused by multi-organ failure following peritonitis due to colonic perforation occurred in a cirrhotic patient with a superficially-located HCC. Major complications were observed in 27 (3.1%) of 872 patients. Eighteen major complications occurred during the periprocedural time (*i.e.*, within 30 days of the RFA) and included intraperitoneal bleeding requiring treatment (n = 8); hepatic decompensation (n = 3); hepatic abscess (n = 1) and biloma requiring drainage (n = 1); bile duct stenosis requiring stent placement (n = 1); thrombosis of the portal vein (n = 1), the right hepatic vein (n = 1), and the superior mesenteric vein (n = 1); and septicemia (n = 1). Delayed complications were seen in nine patients and included bile duct stricture requiring stent placement (n = 2) and tumour seeding along the needle track (n = 7). Minor complications were observed in 55 (6.3%) of 872 patients.

In summary, RF ablation is a minimally invasive procedure that can achieve effective and reproducible tumour destruction with acceptable morbidity. RF ablation has become a viable alternative or complementary treatment method for patients with hepatic metastases of favourable histotypes who are not candidates for surgical resection. With continued improvement in technology and large-scale clinical experience, this technique has the potential to play an increasingly important role in the clinical management of hepatic metastases.

References

1. Scheele J, Stang R, Altendorf-Hofmann A, Paul M. Resection of colorectal liver metastases. *World J Surg* 1995; 19: 59-71.
2. Brand MI, Saclarides TJ, Dobson HD, Millikan KW. Liver resection for colorectal cancer: liver metastases in the aged. *Am Surg* 2000; 66: 412-5.
3. Bolton JS, Fuhrman GM. Survival after resection of multiple bilobar hepatic metastases from colorectal carcinoma. *Ann Surg* 2000; 231: 743-51.
4. Benevento A, Boni L, Frediani L, Ferrari A, Dionigi R. Result of liver resection as treatment for metastases from noncolorectal cancer. *J Surg Oncol* 2000; 74: 24-9.
5. Bartolozzi C, Lencioni R. Ethanol injection for the treatment of hepatic tumours. *Eur Radiol* 1996; 6: 682-96.
6. Vogl TJ, Muller PK, Mack MG, *et al.* Liver metastases: interventional therapeutic techniques and results, state of the art. *Eur Radiol* 1999; 9: 675-84.
7. Lencioni R, Cioni D, Bartolozzi C. Percutaneous radiofrequency thermal ablation of liver malignancies: techniques, indications, imaging findings, and clinical results. *Abdom Imaging* 2001; 26: 345-60.
8. Lencioni R, Goletti O, Armillotta N, *et al.* Radio-frequency thermal ablation of liver metastases with a cooled-tip electrode needle: results of a pilot clinical trial. *Eur Radiol* 1998; 8: 1205-11.
9. Solbiati L, Goldberg SN, Ierace T, *et al.* Hepatic metastases: percutaneous radio-frequency ablation with cooled-tip electrodes. *Radiology* 1997; 205: 367-73.
10. De Baere T, Elias D, Dromain C, *et al.* Radiofrequency ablation of 100 hepatic metastases with a mean follow-up of more than 1 year. *AJR Am J Roentgenol* 2000; 175: 1619-25.
11. Gillams AR, Lees WR. Survival after percutaneous, image-guided, thermal ablation of hepatic metastases from colorectal cancer. *Dis Colon Rectum* 2000; 43: 656-66.
12. Solbiati L, Livraghi T, Goldberg SN, *et al.* Percutaneous radio-frequency ablation of hepatic metastases from colorectal cancer: long-term results in 117 patients. *Radiology* 2001; 221: 159-66.
13. Elias D, De Baere T, Smayra T, Ouellet JF, Roche A, Lasser P. Percutaneous radiofrequency thermoablation as an alternative to surgery for treatment of liver tumour recurrence after hepatectomy. *Br J Surg* 2002; 89: 752-6.
14. Livraghi T, Solbiati L, Meloni F, Ierace T, Goldberg SN, Gazelle GS. Percutaneous radiofrequency ablation of liver metastases in potential candidates for resection: the "test-of-time approach". *Cancer* 2003; 97: 3027-35.
15. Kainuma O, Asano T, Aoyama H, *et al.* Combined therapy with radiofrequency thermal ablation and intra-arterial infusion chemotherapy for hepatic metastases from colorectal cancer. *Hepatogastroenterology* 1999; 46: 1071-7.
16. Scaife CL, Curley SA, Izzo F, *et al.* Feasibility of adjuvant hepatic arterial infusion of chemotherapy after radiofrequency ablation with or without resection in patients with hepatic metastases from colorectal cancer. *Ann Surg Oncol* 2003; 10: 348-54.
17. Goldberg SN, Hahn PF, Tanabe KK, *et al.* Percutaneous radiofrequency tissue ablation: does perfusion-mediated tissue cooling limit coagulation necrosis? *J Vasc Interv Radiol* 1998; 9: 101-15.
18. Rossi S, Garbagnati F, Lencioni R, *et al.* Percutaneous radio-frequency thermal ablation of nonresectable hepatocellular carcinoma after occlusion of tumour blood supply. *Radiology* 2000; 217: 119-26.
19. De Baere T, Bessoud B, Dromain C, *et al.* Percutaneous radiofrequency ablation of hepatic tumours during temporary venous occlusion. *AJR Am J Roentgenol* 2002; 178: 53-9.
20. Livraghi T, Solbiati L, Meloni MF, Gazelle GS, Halpern EF, Goldberg SN. Treatment of focal liver tumours with percutaneous radio-frequency ablation: complications encountered in a multicenter study. *Radiology* 2003; 226: 441-51.
21. Lencioni R, Veltri A, Guglielmi A, *et al.* Complications of percutaneous radiofrequency ablation of liver malignancies with expandable multi-probe needles: results of a multicenter study. *Radiology* 2003 (in press).

Interstitial laser coagulation: liver metastases

Thomas J. Vogl, Ralf Straub, Kathrin Eichler, Martin Mack

Department of Diagnostic and Interventional Radiology, University Hospital Frankfurt, Johann Wolfgang Goethe-University, Theodor-Stern-Kai 7, D-60590 Frankfurt/Main, Germany

Introduction

The liver plays a central role in the human metabolism and so represents one of the organ systems most often affected, especially by tumourous diseases. The group of colorectal carcinomas metastatically almost exclusively attacks this organ, which, according to studies by Weiss *et al.*, can be attributed to the venous drainage of the intestines through the portal vein [1, 2]. A large number of primary tumours often cause liver metastases as well as bone, lung and brain metastases. After curative treatment of the primary tumour, the liver infestation has a decisive influence on the survival time of affected patients in many cases. The therapeutic strategy for malignant liver lesions is based on a number of factors such as the underlying primary tumour, localization, the stage the tumour has reached, and general factors, such as age or any existing concomitant diseases. In the case of hepatocellular carcinoma [3], when the tumour is at an appropriate stage, liver resection or hemihepatic resection or liver transplant is the essential curative treatment [4]. If there are contra-indications, transarterial chemoembolization [5-8] combined with a local alcohol injection is used as a palliative therapeutic strategy [9-15]. Interstitial procedures such as laser-induced thermotherapy (LITT) or radiofrequency ablation show a high rate of controlling the site of the tumour and are currently clinically evaluated.

Strategies for liver metastases are considerably more complex. Up to now the liver resection of solitary lesions has been the only potential curative treatment [16-26]. Surgical resection is well established in the treatment of liver metastases of colorectal carcinoma, typically yielding 5-year survival rates between 25% and 38%. Two thirds of patients will experience recurrent metastases, and many patients do not benefit from surgery. Data published from studies investigating the efficacy of surgical resection of liver metastases show 1-year survival rates between 71% and 88%; 3-year survival rates between 21% and 46%; and mean survival times between 25 and 35 months. Perioperative mortality ranges from 4.4% to 10% [1-8].

However, the high incidence of new liver metastases following successful resection of metastases – between 60% and 80% – is the challenge for therapeutic alternatives, the goal of which should be to achieve survival statistics similar to those attained with surgery. Ideally such therapeutic alternatives should be less invasive than liver resection; should have a low complication rate; should be possible under local anesthesia (for patients with general contra-indications for surgery); and should be less expensive. All these criteria are met by MR-guided laser-induced thermotherapy (LITT), which has been the subject of growing interest in recent years. For this reason, over the last years there has been great interest in further developments in interstitial procedures such as laser induced interstitial thermotherapy (LITT) and RF ablation.

The present study is based on the analysis of a large prospective series of a percutaneous thermal ablation procedure like LITT for treating hepatic metastases of different primary tumours metastases to the liver.

Technique of laser coagulation

Between June 1993 and May 2003, LITT was performed in 1,291 patients (mean age 59.5 years, range 24 to 89 years) with a total of 2,438 liver metastases and 61 hepatocellular carcinoma. We included patients with different primary tumours like colorectal liver metastases (512 patients, 1,556 metastases), liver metastases from breast cancer (161 patients, 416 metastases), hepatocellular carcinoma (42 patients, 65 lesions), liver metastases from pancreatic cancer (21 patients, 60 metastases) and a variety of other tumours. A total of 9,963 laser applications was performed with a total of 5,892 laser applicators.

A laser application was defined as a laser treatment at one certain position. If the laser applicator was pulled back and another laser treatment was performed to enlarge the coagulative necrosis a second laser application was performed.

We included patients with recurrent liver metastases after partial liver resection, patients with metastases in both liver lobes, patients with locally non-resectable lesions, and patients who had general contra-indications for surgery or who refused surgical resection. The distribution for the different indications varied for different primary tumours *(Figure 1)*.

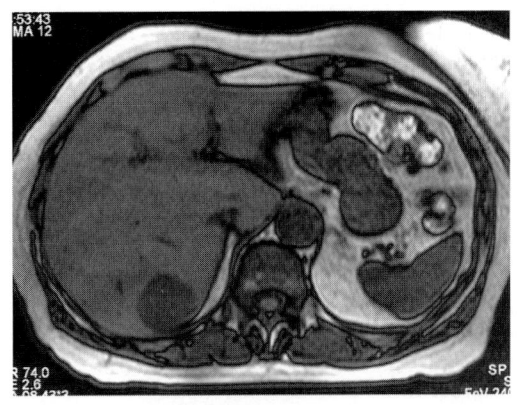

Figure 1. 62-year-old patient with liver metastases from breast cancer.

Figure 1a. Transverse unenhanced T1-weighted GE image (TR/TE = 74/2.6) obtained 2 weeks before laser treatment shows a liver metastasis (arrows) in segment 7 with a maximum diameter of 3.8 cm.

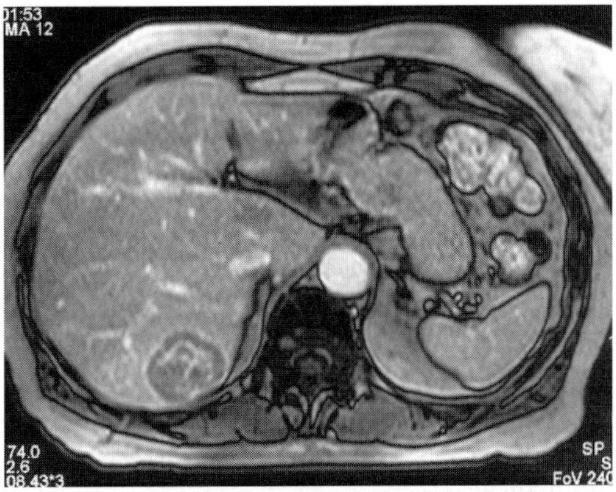

Figure 1b. Transverse contrast-enhanced T1-weighted GE image (TR/TE = 74/2.6) 2 weeks before LITT treatment shows contrast enhancement in the periphery of the metastasis (arrows).

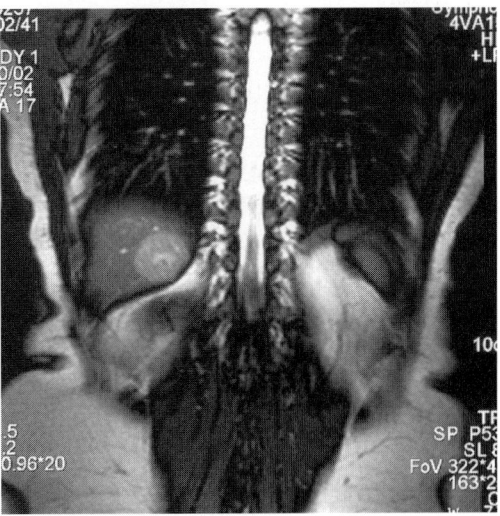

Figure 1c. Coronal unenhanced T2-weighted GE image (TR/TE = 4.5/2.2) obtained 2 weeks before laser treatment shows a liver metastases (arrows) in segment 7 with a maximum diameter of 3.8 cm.

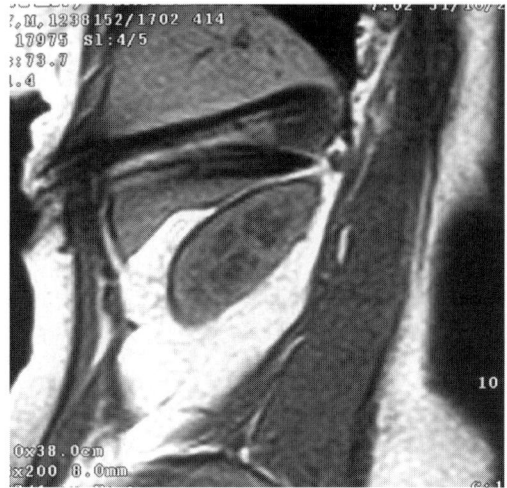

Figure 1d. Sagittal unenhanced T1-weighted FLASH-2D image immediately before starting the LITT treatment shows the metastasis (arrows) and the positioned laser fibers (arrow heads). For better visualization of the application systems a magnetite marker was placed in the protective catheter.

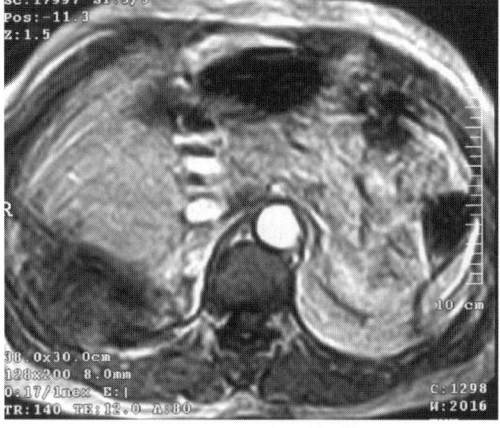

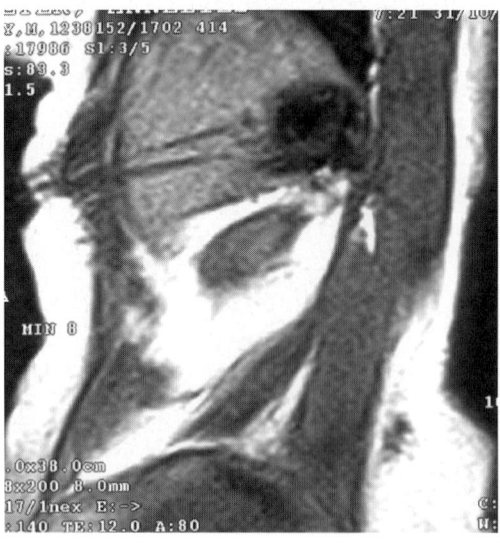

Figures 1e. Transverse and sagittal unenhanced T1-weighted images obtained 20 minutes after starting the laser treatment demonstrates an obvious signal decrease of the lesion and the surrounding tissue (arrows) due to the increase of tissue temperature. The temperature in the center of the lesion is around 110° C; in the peripheral zone the temperature is around 60-70° C.

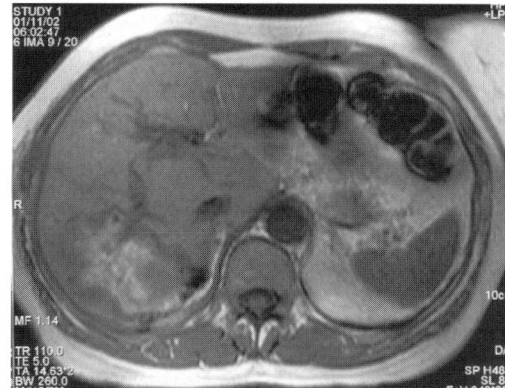

Figure 1f. Transverse unenhanced T1-weighted image obtained 24 hours after laser treatment shows the induced coagulation area (arrows) with some inflammatory changes.

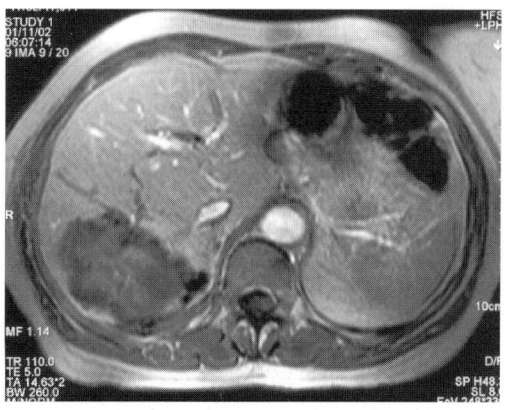

Figure 1g. Transverse contrast-enhanced T1-weighted image 24 hours after laser treatment shows the induced coagulation area (arrows).

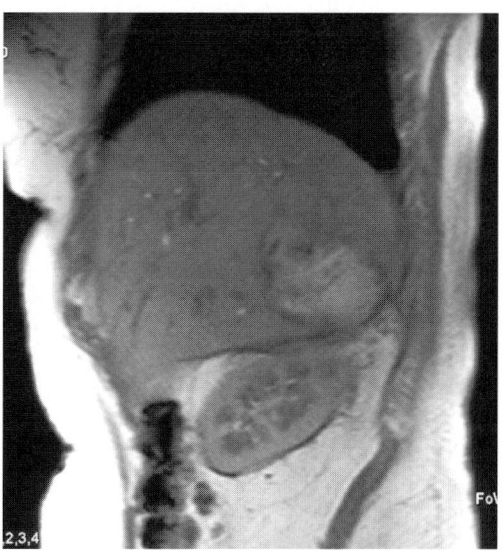

Figure 1h. Sagittal contrast-enhanced T1-weighted GE obtained 24 hours after LITT demonstrates the extension of the necrosis (arrows).

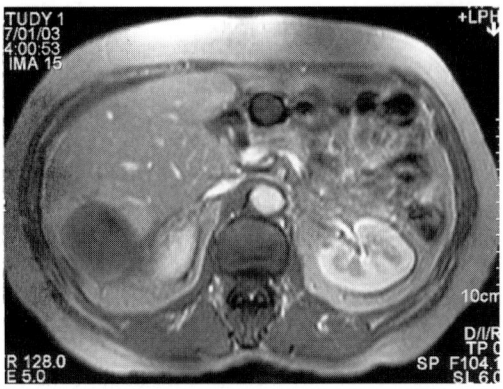

Figure 1i. Transverse contrast-enhanced T1-weighted image 3 months after laser treatment shows the induced coagulation area (arrows).

Laser equipment and application set

Laser coagulation was accomplished using a Neodymium-YAG laser light with a wavelength of 1,064 nm (MediLas 5060, MediLas 5100, Dornier Germering, Germany), delivered through optic fibers terminated by a specially developed diffusor. In the beginning a diffusor tip with a glass dome of 0.9 mm diameter, which was mounted at the end of a 10-m long silica fiber (diameter 400 µm) was used. Since the year 2000 a flexible diffuser tip has been used with a diameter of 1.0 mm, which makes the laser applications much easier due to the fact that the risk of damage to the diffuser tip has dropped to almost zero. The active length of the diffusor tip ranged between 20 and 40 mm in length. The laser power was adjusted to 12 Watts per cm active length of the laser applicator.

The laser application kit (SOMATEX Company, Berlin, Germany) consists of a cannulation needle, a sheath system, and a protective catheter which prevents direct contact of the laser applicator with the treated tissues and allows cooling of the tip of the laser applicator. The closed end of the protective catheter enables complete removal of the applicator even in the unlikely event of damage to the fiber during treatment. This simplifies the procedure and makes it safer for the patient.

The laser itself was installed outside of the MR examination room, and the light was transmitted through a 10-m long optical fiber. All patients were examined using an MR imaging protocol including gradient-echo (GE) T1-weighted plain and contrast-enhanced GD-DTPA 0.1 mmol/kg body weight (b.w). T2-and T1-weighted images were obtained for localizing the target lesion and planning the interventional procedure. The scanners were a conventional 1.5-T system (Siemens, Erlangen, Germany) and a 0.5-T system (Escint).

Imaging during therapy

After informing the patients about potential complications, benefits, and disadvantages of LITT, consent was obtained. The metastasis was localized on computed tomographic scans and the injection site was infiltrated with 20 ml of 1% lidocaine. Under CT guidance the laser application system was inserted using the Seldinger technique. After the patient was positioned on the MRI table, the laser catheter was inserted into the protective catheter. MR sequences were performed in three perpendicular orientations before and during LITT.

MR sequences are performed every 30 seconds to assess the progress in heating the lesion and the surrounding tissue. Heating was revealed as signal loss in the T1-weighted gradient-echo images as a result of the heat-induced increase of the T1 relaxation time. Depending on the geometry and intensity of the signal loss and the speed of heat distribution, the position of the laser fibers, the laser power and the cooling rate were readjusted. Treatment was stopped after total coagulation of the lesion, and a safety margin from 5 to 15 mm surrounding the lesion could be visualized in MR images.

After switching off the laser, T1-weighted contrast-enhanced FLASH-2D images were obtained for verifying the induced necrosis. After the procedure the puncture channel was sealed with fibrin glue. Follow-up examinations using plain and contrast-enhanced sequences were performed after 24 to 48 hours, and every 3 months following the LITT procedure. Quantitative and qualitative parameters, including size, morphology, signal behavior, and contrast enhancement were evaluated for deciding whether treatment could be considered successful, or whether subsequent treatment sessions were required.

Qualitative and quantitative evaluation

Laser-induced effects were evaluated by comparing images of lesions and surrounding liver parenchyma obtained before and after laser treatment with each other, and with those obtained at follow-up examinations. Tumour volume and volume of coagulative necrosis were calculated using three-dimensional MR images and measurements of the maximum diameter in three planes (A, B and C). The volume is calculated using the formula (A × B × C) × 0.5.

The results were tested for significance using the ANOVA test.

Results

All treatments could be performed under local anesthesia and were well tolerated by the patients. All patients treated between June 1993 and September 1998 (n = 278) were hospitalized for 24 to 48 hours after the intervention. All patients treated between October 1998 and May 2003 were treated strictly on an outpatient basis.

Evaluation of the MR thermometry data during MR-guided laser-induced thermotherapy demonstrated that metastatic tissue is very sensitive to heat, showing earlier and more widespread temperature distribution of the delivered thermal energy than does surrounding liver parenchyma *(Figure 1)*. In 90.9% of all cases, the area of obviously decreased signal intensity during LITT treatment was identical with the area, classified as coagulative necrosis on MR images 24 hours after laser treatment. In 8.6% of the cases the size of the coagulative necrosis obtained 24 hours after LITT treatment was larger compared to

MR thermometry images. The difference was 17% in maximum. In 0.6% of the cases the necrosis was smaller on 24 hours control images compared to MR thermometry images. The difference was 15% in maximum.

The mean number of treated metastases per patient was 2.8 (median 2) *(Table 1)*. In 57% of the patients only one or two metastases were treated. In 7% more than 6 metastases were treated in total. The localization of the metastases with respect to the different liver segments showed a quite homogenous distribution of the metastases in the different liver segments taking in account the different volumes of the liver segments.

The evaluation of the distribution of the metastases within the liver is demonstrated in *Figure 4*. 49% of the lesions had a relationship to the liver capsule, 7% had a relationship to the central portal vein structures and only 29% of the metastases were at a location which was classified as easy.

The mean number of inserted laser applicators for the treatment of one metastasis with a reliable safety margin with regard to the size of the metastases showed the following data: In 26.1% of all metastases only one laser applicator was inserted. In 29.8% two laser applicators, in 18.8% three laser applicators, in 18.4% 4 laser applicators, in 5.3% 5 laser applicators and in 1.7% more than 5 laser applicators were necessary for the treatment of a single metastasis with a reliable safety margin.

The approach to the lesion depended on the localization of the lesion. Transpleural approaches were avoided in all cases. The most common approach to lesions located in liver segments 7 and 8 was the angulated lateral approach (65.5% and 82.4%, respectively). The most common approach for lesions located in liver segments 2 and 3 was an approach from ventral (50% and 79%, respectively). An approach was classified as dorsal, lateral or ventral if the angulation of the puncture direction was more than 15° from the scan plane. A transpleural approach was avoided in all cases, therefore the approach to most of the lesions in liver segments 7 or 8 was a lateral angulated approach.

The applied energy per treated metastasis was documented. The mean values of the applied energy were statistically significantly higher in liver metastases from colorectal carcinoma *versus* liver metastases from breast carcinoma and hepatocellular carcinoma (ANOVA test $p < 0.01$).

The volume of the induced coagulative necrosis 24 hours after LITT treatment exceeded the volume of the initial tumour significantly ($p < 0.001$). During follow-up examinations the volume of the induced necrosis was getting smaller again due to resorption and shrinking of the lesion. In the 3-month control the volume of the coagulative necrosis was already roughly half of the initial volume of the necrosis, but still larger than the initial tumour volume. The volume of coagulative necrosis 24 hours after LITT treatment exceeded the initial tumour volume on average by the factor of 13 (range 12-17) for lesions with a diameter of 2 cm or less, by the factor of 8 (range 7.5-8.2) for lesions between 2 and 3 cm in diameter, by the factor of 6 (range 5.3-6.1) for lesions between 3 and 4 cm in diameter, and by the factor of 2.5 (range 1.8-2.7) for lesions larger than 4 cm in diameter. The survival data on our patient material is presented in *Figure 2*.

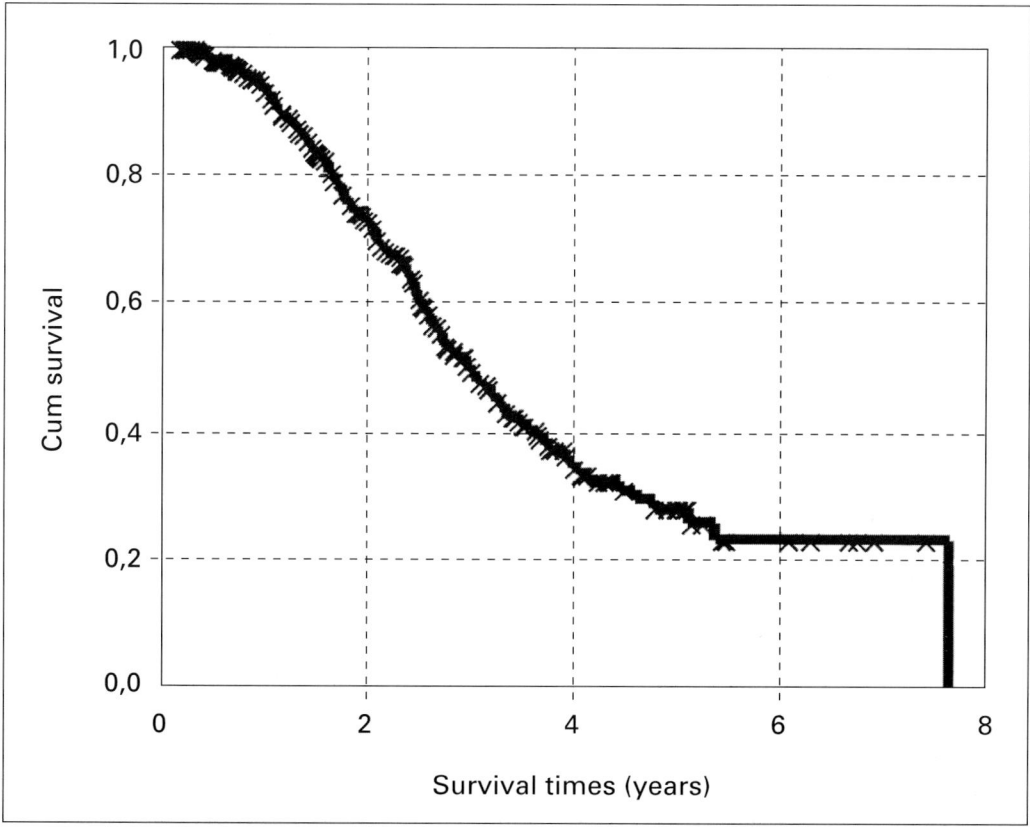

Figure 2a. Survival data of all patients (n = 512) treated with LITT for colorectal liver metastases (n = 1556).

Discussion

Liver metastases are the most common tumours in Europe and the United States and are twenty times more common in Africa, Japan and Eastern countries. The liver is the most common site of metastases. Colorectal cancer is the third leading cause of death in Western communities, outnumbered only by lung and breast cancer. At the time of death, approximately two-thirds of patients with colorectal cancer have liver metastases. Survival in metastatic liver disease depends on the extent of liver involvement and the presence of metastatic tumours. In several studies, liver metastases from colon carcinoma which were confined to one lobe and involved an area of less than 25% of the liver caused death in 6 months when untreated [28]. When 25% to 75% of the liver was involved, survival was 5.5 months; and when more than 75% of the liver was involved, death occurred in 3.4 months.

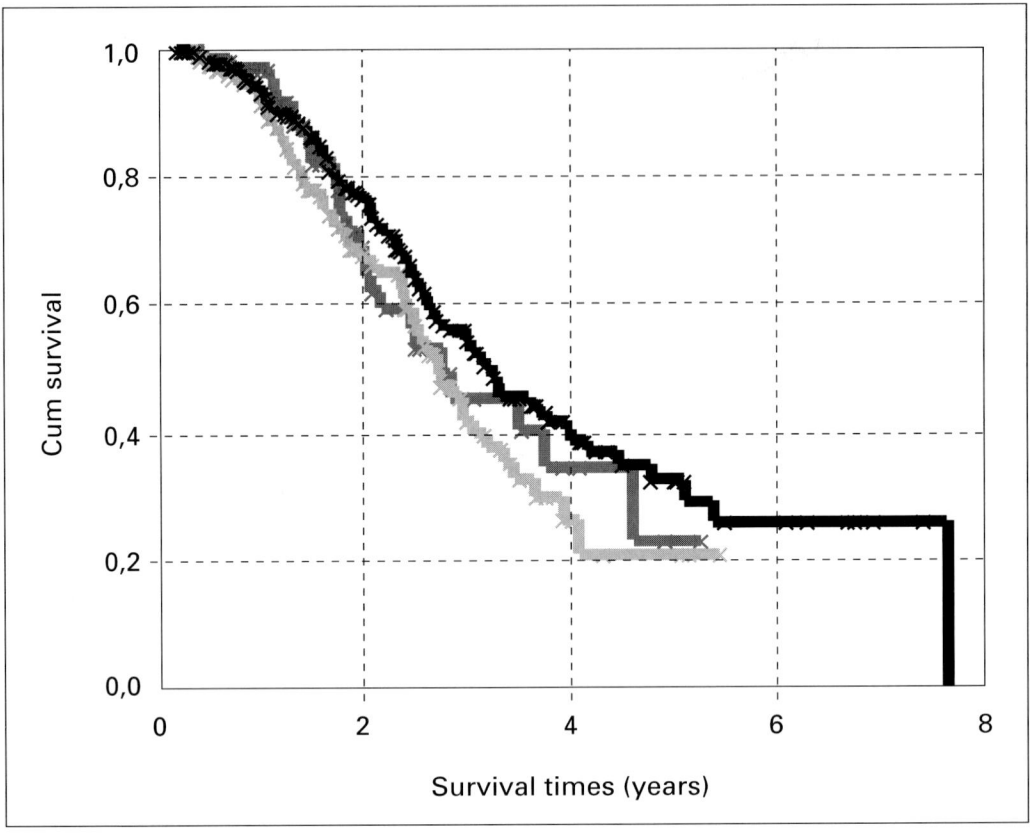

Figure 2b. Comparison of survival of patients with respect to the number of initial metastases (black line = group 1 = 1 or 2 metastases, light grey line = 3 or 4 metastases, dark grey line = group 2 = more than 4 metastases).

Therapeutic alternatives in the treatment of liver metastases include surgery, local ablation as LITT, RF ablation, cryotherapy [29-33], microwave ablation [34] and ethanol injection [10, 12, 13, 35] or oncologic strategies such as systemic or locoregional chemotherapy [36-42]. As a high number of tumours grow in damaged liver parenchyma with reduced hepatic functions, it is important for all methods which damage tumour cells to preserve functional reserve capacity, delaying terminal organ failure for as long as possible.

Therefore many local ablation techniques were developed in order to improve the survival of the patients [6]. Nowadays, the most common technique is RF ablation. Radiofrequency waves (RF waves) have been used since the 1960's for treating intracerebral tumours, controlled stereotaxically. For some years RF treatment has also been used for treating soft tissue, focusing on the treatment of malignant liver tumours. As with LITT a coagulation necrosis is caused through a local temperature increase. Wavelengths between 300 to 500 kHz are introduced into the tissue through mono- or bipolar antennae systems resulting in the target area heating up to temperatures of 90° C, caused by high tissue resistance. In previous studies monopolar systems were used almost exclusively. The

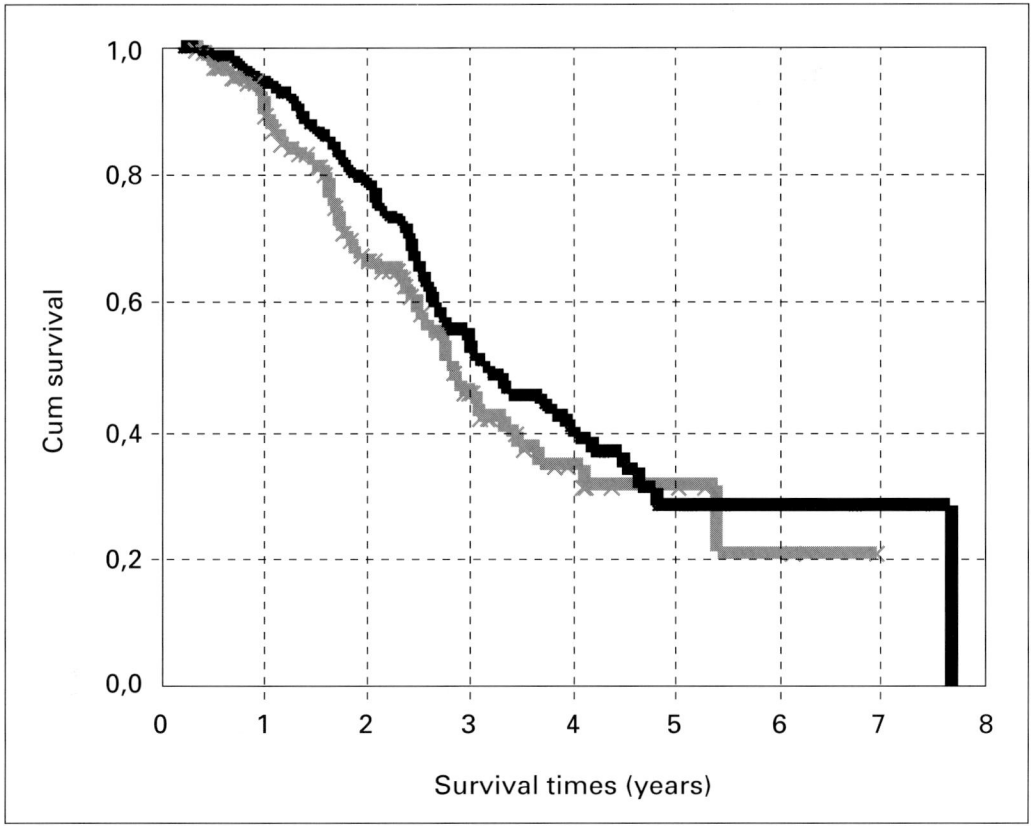

Figure 2c. Comparison of survival of patients with respect to the initial staging of lymph nodes (black line = group 1 = N0 and N1 stage, grey line = group 2 = N2 or N3 stage).

necessity for an external second electrode on patients makes an uncontrolled energy flow outside the required target zone possible in theory, as burns cannot be safely ruled out. Bipolar application systems integrate both poles in one applicator. Cooling the tip of the applicator in RF treatment was introduced to increase the size of the induced necrosis up to 5 cm in diameter.

In 1996 Rossi *et al.* treated 11 patients with 13 metastases using mono- and bipolar systems and the multi-applicator technique. Despite the fact that the tumours were under 3.5 cm in size, one year after the operation only one patient was tumour-free and the relapse rate was around 55%. The findings for the 39 patients with HCC were better, as a relapse rate of only 10% and mean survival times of 44 months have been calculated [43].

In 1997 Solbiati *et al.* published a study of 29 patients with 44 liver metastases (size 1.3-5 cm) of colorectal, stomach, breast, and pancreatic carcinomas. Among them were 20 patients with solitary lesions. The operation took place using cooled systems, and a complete tumour ablation was achieved in 91% of cases. At the 3- and 6-month check-up

66% of the treated lesions were still inactive. A survival rate of 100%, 94% and 86% after 6, 12, and 18 months was documented [44]. Livraghi tried an approach using conventional systems and simultaneous irrigation with NaCl solution with 14 patients with 24 liver metastases (1.2 to 4.5 cm in size) but only 52% of the lesions were inactive after six months [45].

In 1999 Livraghi *et al.* presented a direct comparison of RF therapy (42 patients, 52 lesions) with percutaneous alcohol injection – PAI – (44 patients with 60 tumours) in treating hepatocellular carcinomas. This was the first direct comparison of these two different treatments in similarly structured patient populations. 80% of tumours were removed completely using PAI and 90% using RF (no statistical significance). The main advantage of RF therapy proved to be the smaller number of treatment sessions (1.2 *versus* 4.8). On the other hand a higher complication rate (2% serious, 8% less serious complications *versus* 0% for PAI) was documented [15]. Side effects with regard to punctures are relevant here, *e.g.* pneumothorax or hemothorax (2%), injury of the bile ducts and the gall bladder, intraperitoneal bleeding (8%) and also pleural effusions. Depending on the procedure some cases had to be upgraded from local to general anaesthesia due to severe pain during the energy application.

Our data in a large population of 891 patients with liver metastases from different primary tumours, mainly colorectal carcinomas show a very high local control rate (over 97% in 3- and 6-month control studies) and a very low local recurrence rate. LITT treatment can be performed easily under local anesthesia on an outpatient basis in metastases up to 5 cm in diameter with a 1-cm safety margin, which is very important for a low recurrence rate. Multiple applications can be performed simultaneously.

The wide range of the values of the energy which was applied to the metastases indicates that there is a high variance in heat distribution. Sometimes a couple of minutes are enough to treat a metastasis with a reliable safety margin and sometimes application times of 30 minutes and more are necessary to get the same necrosis in another metastasis of the same size. Therefore reliable nearly online monitoring of treatment is absolutely necessary in order to avoid over- or undertreatment of the metastases. Due to the fact that laser ablation is fully compatible with MRI, which is the most reliable method for thermometry, MRI is very well suited for monitoring thermal ablation like LITT.

The survival rates achieved, which represent the most relevant success criterion for a treatment, are slightly superior in patients with metastases from a colorectal carcinoma or a carcinoma of the breast to those in surgically resected patients. It must be considered, however, that a surgical resection was not or was no longer an option among most of the patients being treated due to metastatic relapse after surgical resection or a bilobibular pattern of infestation. In spite of this it was possible to achieve survival rates comparable to surgical resection among these patients, who are actually in a group with a worse prognosis. Compared with the extensively published historic survival data after surgical metastatic resection, LITT offers a very good further treatment option. Due to the survival data and local tumour control rates achieved so far, in our opinion randomized studies comparing LITT with chemotherapy solely in the case of patients who fulfil the inclusion criteria for LITT are no longer ethically tenable.

In the modern oncological concept of treatment the internationally defined terms of "clinical benefit", "performance status" and "quality of life" are of the utmost importance. That applies predominantly to patients suffering from local and generally advanced tumours that are no longer curative. Above all, however, intensive chemotherapy, systemic or regional, with marked toxic side effects severely affects the quality of life in the majority of cases. Looking at it from this background all the more attention must be paid to the treatment concepts described here, because minimally invasive techniques are applied which adversely affect patients less and shorter-term.

Consequently the prerequisites are given to integrate these new procedures into oncological treatment programs which have been carried out up to now. LITT, which has been used for the past eight years in the clinical routine, can play a great part in modern oncological treatment concepts.

References

1. Weiss L, Grundmann E, Torhorst J, *et al*. Haematogenous metastatic patterns in colonic carcinoma: an analysis of 1,541 necropsies. *J Pathol* 1986; 150: 195-203.
2. Weiss L. *Inefficiency of metastasis from colorectal carcinomas*. Boston, Kluwer Academic Publishers, 1994.
3. Ramsey WH, Wu GY. Hepatocellular carcinoma: update on diagnosis and treatment. *Dig-Dis* 1995; 13: 81-91.
4. Bismuth H, Chiche L, Adam R, Castaing D, Diamond T, Dennison A. Liver resection *versus* transplantation for hepatocellular carcinoma in cirrhotic patients. *Ann Surg* 1993; 218: 145-51.
5. De Cobelli F, Castrucci M, Sironi S, *et al*. Role of magnetic resonance in the follow-up of hepatocarcinoma treated with percutaneous ethanol injection (PEI) or transarterial chemoembolization (TACE). *Radiol-Med-Torino* 1994; 88: 806-17.
6. Dodd GD 3rd, Soulen MC, Kane RA, *et al*. Minimally invasive treatment of malignant hepatic tumours: at the threshold of a major breakthrough. *Radiographics* 2000; 20: 9-27.
7. Kawai S, Tani M, Okumura J, Ogawa M, *et al*. Prospective and randomized clinical trial of lipiodol-transcatheter arterial chemoembolization for treatment of hepatocellular carcinoma: A comparison of epirubicin and doxorubicin (second cooperative study). *Seminars in Oncology* 1997; 24: 38-45.
8. Lorenz M, Waldeyer M, Muller HH. Comparison of lipiodol-assisted chemoembolization *versus* only conservative therapy in patients with nonresectable hepatocellular carcinomas. *Z Gastroenterol* 1996; 34: 205-6.
9. Amin Z, Lees WR, Bown SG. Hepatocellular carcinoma: CT appearance after percutaneous ethanol ablation therapy. *Radiology* 1993; 188: 882-3.
10. Bartolozzi C, Lencioni R. Ethanol injection for the treatment of hepatic tumours. *Eur Radiol* 1996; 6: 682-96.
11. Livraghi T, Lazzaroni S, Vettori C. Percutaneous ethanol injection of small hepatocellular carcinoma. *Rays* 1990; 15: 405-10.
12. Sato M, Watanabe Y, Tokui K, Kawachi K, Sugata S, Ikezoe J. CT-guided treatment of ultrasonically invisible hepatocellular carcinoma. *Am J Gastroenterol* 2000; 95: 2102-6.
13. Shiina S, Tagawa K, Unama T, *et al*. Percutaneous ethanol injection therapy of hepatocellular carcinoma: Analysis of 77 patients. *AJR* 1990; 155: 1221-6.
14. Sironi S, Livraghi T, DelMaschio A. Small hepatocellular carcinoma treated with percutaneous ethanol injection: MR imaging findings. *Radiology* 1991; 180: 333-6.

15. Livraghi T, Goldberg SN, Lazzaroni S, Meloni F, Solbiati L, Gazelle GS. Small hepatocellular carcinoma: Treatment with radio-frequency ablation *versus* ethanol injection. *Radiology* 1999; 210: 655-61.
16. Adson MA, Heerden van J, Adson MH, Wagner JS, Ilstrup DM. Resection of hepatic metastases from colorectal cancer. *Arch Surg* 1984; 119: 647-51.
17. Fong Y, Blumgart LH. Hepatic colorectal metastasis: current status of surgical therapy. *Oncology (Huntingt)* 1998; 12: 1489-98; discussion 1498-1500, 1503.
18. Hughes KS, Simon R, Songhorabodi S, et al. Resection of the liver for colorectal carcinoma metastases: A multi-institutional study of indications for resections. *Surgery* 1988; 103: 278-88.
19. Jenkins LT, Millikan KW, Bines SD, Staren ED, Doolas A. Hepatic resection for metastatic colorectal cancer. *Am Surg* 1997; 63: 605-10.
20. Harrison LE, Brennan MF, Newman E, et al. Hepatic resection for non-colorectal, non-neuroendocrine metastases: a fifteen-year experience with ninety-six patients. *Surgery* 1997; 121: 625-32.
21. Lorenz M, Waldeyer M. The resection of the liver metastases of primary colorectal tumours. The development of a scoring system to determine the individual prognosis based on an assessment of 1,568 patients. *Strahlenther Onkol* 1997; 173: 118-9.
22. Maksan SM, Lehnert T, Bastert G, Herfarth C. Curative liver resection for metastatic breast cancer. *Eur J Surg Oncol* 2000; 26: 209-12.
23. Mariette D, Fagniez PL. Hepatic metastasis of non-colorectal cancers. Results of surgical treatment. *Rev Prat* 1992; 42: 1271-5.
24. Petrelli NJ, Nambisan RN, Herrera L, Mittelman A. Hepatic resection for isolated metastasis from colorectal carcinoma. *American Journal of Surgery* 1985; 149: 205-8.
25. Scheele J, Altendorf-Hofmann A, Stangl R, Schmidt K. Surgical resection of colorectal liver metastases: Gold standard for solitary and completely resectable lesions. *Swiss Surg Suppl* 1996; 4: 4-17.
26. Yoon SS, Tanabe KK. Surgical treatment and other regional treatments for colorectal cancer liver metastases. *Oncologist* 1999; 4: 197-208.
27. Kaplan EL, Meier P. Nonparametric estimation from incomplete observation. *J Am Stat Assoc* 1958; 53: 457-81.
28. Stangl R, Altendorf Hofmann A, Charnley RM, Scheele J. Factors influencing the natural history of colorectal liver metastases. *Lancet* 1994; 343: 1405-10.
29. Finlay IG, Seifert JK, Stewart GJ, Morris DL. Resection with cryotherapy of colorectal hepatic metastases has the same survival as hepatic resection alone. *Eur J Surg Oncol* 2000; 26: 199-202.
30. Charnley RM, Doran J, Morris DL. Cryotherapy for liver metastases: a new approach. *Br J Surg* 1989; 76: 1040.
31. Seifert JK, Achenbach T, Heintz A, Bottger TC, Junginger T. Cryotherapy for liver metastases. *Int J Colorectal Dis* 2000; 15: 161-6.
32. Shapiro RS, Shafir M, Sung M, Warner R, Glajchen N. Cryotherapy of metastatic carcinoid tumours. *Abdom-Imaging* 1998; 23: 314-7.
33. Hewitt PM, Dwerryhouse SJ, Zhao J, Morris DL. Multiple bilobar liver metastases: cryotherapy for residual lesions after liver resection. *J Surg Oncol* 1998; 67: 112-6.
34. Wang SS, VanderBrink BA, Regan J, et al. Microwave radiometric thermometry and its potential applicability to ablative therapy. *J Interv Card Electrophysiol* 2000; 4: 295-300.
35. Livraghi T, Lazzaroni S, Pellicano S, Ravasi S, Torzilli G, Vettori C. Percutaneous ethanol injection of hepatic tumours: single-session therapy with general anesthesia. *Am J Roentgenol* 1993; 161: 1065-9.
36. Douillard JY, Cunningham D, Roth AD, et al. Irinotecan combined with fluorouracil compared with fluorouracil alone as first-line treatment for metastatic colorectal cancer: a multicentre randomised trial [published erratum appears in *Lancet* 2000; 355 (9212): 1372]. *Lancet* 2000; 355: 1041-7.

37. Douillard JY, Bennouna J, Vavasseur F, *et al.* Phase I trial of interleukin-2 and high-dose arginine butyrate in metastatic colorectal cancer. *Cancer Immunol Immunother* 2000; 49: 56-61.
38. Kemeny N, Huang Y, Cohen AM, *et al.* Hepatic arterial infusion of chemotherapy after resection of hepatic metastases from colorectal cancer. *N Engl J Med* 1999; 341: 2039-48.
39. Kemeny NE. Regional chemotherapy of colorectal cancer. *Eur J Cancer* 1995; 31A: 1271-6.
40. Kemeny NE, Atiq OT. Non-surgical treatment for liver metastases. *Baillieres Best Pract Res Clin Gastroenterol* 1999; 13: 593-610.
41. Lorenz M, Heinrich S, Staib-Sebler E, *et al.* Relevance of locoregional chemotherapy in patients with liver metastases from colorectal primaries. *Swiss Surg* 2000; 6: 11-22.
42. Ardalan B, Sridhar KS, Benedetto P, *et al.* A phase I, II study of high-dose 5-fluorouracil and high-dose leucovorin with low-dose phosphonacetyl-L-aspartic acid in patients with advanced malignancies. *Cancer* 1991; 68: 1242-6.
43. Rossi S, Di Stasi M, Buscarini E, *et al.* Percutaneous RF interstitial thermal ablation in the treatment of hepatic cancer. *AJR* 1996; 167: 759-68.
44. Solbiati L, Goldberg SN, Ierace T, *et al.* Hepatic metastases: Percutaneous radio-frequency ablation with cooled-tip electrodes. *Radiology* 1997; 205: 367-73.
45. Livraghi T, Goldberg SN, Monti F, *et al.* Saline-enhanced radio-frequency tissue ablation in the treatment of liver metastases. *Radiology* 1997; 202: 205-10.
46. Vogl TJ, Mack M, Straub R, *et al.* MR-guided laser-induced thermotherapy (LITT) of malignant liver and soft tissue tumours. *Med Laser Appl* 2001; 16: 91-102.
47. Vogl TJ, Mack M, Straub R, *et al.* Magentic resonance (MR)-guided percutaneous laser-induced interstitial thermotherapy (LITT) for malignant liver tumours. *Sur Technol Int* 2002; 10: 89-98.
48. Vogl TJ, Balzer J, Mack M, Bett G, Oppelt A. Hybrid MR interventional imaging system: combined MR and angiography suites with single interactive table. Feasibility study in vascular liver tumour procedures. *European Radiology* 2002; 12: 1394-400.
49. Vogl TJ, Eichler K, Mack M, Straub R. MR-guided laser-induced thermotherapy of malignant liver tumours. Experience with complications in 899 patients. *Radiology* 2002; 225: 367-77.
50. Vogl TJ, Mack M, Balzer J, *et al.* Neoadjuvant downsizing of liver metastases by transarterial chemoembolisation (TACE) before laser-induced thermotherapy (LITT). *Radiology* 2003 (in press).
51. Vogl TJ, Straub R, Eichler K, Söllner O, Mack M. Laser-induced interstitial thermotherapy (LITT) of colorectal carcinoma metastases in the liver – local tumour control and survival data. *Radiology* 2003 (in press).

V

Lower GI malignancy

Critical appraisal of staging rectal cancer

R.G.H. Beets-Tan

Department of Radiology, University Hospital Maastricht, The Netherlands

One of the concerns after rectal cancer surgery is the local recurrence rate. It is now proven through randomized trials that the best local control rate for rectal cancer patients taken together as a whole group is obtained by a short pre-operative course of radiotherapy followed by a total mesorectal excision [1, 2]. There are however subgroups of rectal cancer patients with different risks for recurrences. On one side of the spectrum there is the stage I disease who are at very low risk for local recurrence. At the other end of the spectrum is the group of patients with a locally advanced tumour who are at very high risk and who would benefit from a more extensive neo-adjuvant treatment schedule. Paramount for the selection and differentiated treatment is a reliable pre-operative test that can distinguish between these groups [1].

So far there has been no consensus on the role of diagnostic imaging tests in the management of patients with primary rectal cancer. Patients are often considered for surgery without pre-operative imaging of the pelvic area. This indirectly indicates that it has been difficult for pre-operative imaging to obtain accuracy levels that are high enough for clinical decision making. There have been many reports on rectal cancer imaging with endorectal ultrasound, CT or MRI, but most studies only focused on T and N stage determination, rather than the more relevant mesorectal fascia. Endoluminal ultrasound (EUS) is now an established modality for the evaluation of the integrity of the rectal wall layers. With accuracies for T staging varying between 67% and 93% it is at present the most accurate imaging modality for the assessment of tumour ingrowth into the rectal wall layers [3-9]. A meta-analysis of 11 studies however has shown that the sensitivity was affected by the T stage [3-10]. Endorectal ultrasound is highly accurate for staging superficial rectal cancer, but performs less well in staging advanced rectal cancer. Resolution may be improved by increasing the frequency of the ultrasound probe but at the expense of tissue penetration. Therefore the mesorectal fascia and surrounding organs are difficult to identify on endorectal sonography.

T stage determination with MRI

The introduction of magnetic resonance imaging (MRI) was a major advance in diagnostic imaging. MRI provides images in multiple planes and with a high soft tissue contrast resolution, without the need for ionizing radiation. Initial reports on magnetic resonance imaging of the pelvic region were promising, and MRI was soon evaluated for rectal diseases. The conventional MR techniques with a body coil showed a resolution that was still insufficient to differentiate the layers of the rectum. The overall accuracy reported for body coil MRI ranges from 59% to 95% [11-18] and is not better than CT.

Efforts were therefore aimed at increasing the signal to noise ratio in order to obtain small voxel sizes. With the introduction of endoluminal coils, spatial resolution improved and detailed evaluation of the layers of the rectal wall was feasible [19]. This was also reflected in the improved and more consistent accuracy figures for T staging ranging between 66% and 91% [19-28].

Although endorectal MRI is very accurate for the assessment of tumour ingrowth in the rectal wall layers and shows accuracies comparable to EUS, some problems still remain. The major shortcoming of the endoluminal technique is the sudden signal drop off at short distance from the coil which limits its field of view. Therefore the mesorectal fascia and surrounding pelvic structures are difficult to visualize [29]. Furthermore the positioning of an endoluminal device can be difficult or impossible in patients with high and/or stenosing tumours, and failure rates for the insertion as high as 40% have been reported in patients with rectal cancer.

With the introduction of dedicated surface coils, phased array coils, improvement of MRI performance was expected [30-34]. A phased array coil consists of an arrangement of multiple surface coils that result in a considerable increase of the signal to noise ratio. With this high signal to noise ratio images can be obtained with a high spatial resolution but at a large field of view. However the first MR studies that used the multiple surface coil technique reported an overall accuracy for T staging of only 55% to 65% and obviously showed no benefit as compared to the body coil MR technique or even to CT [35-36]. The low performance of MRI in these studies could have been attributed to the low spatial resolution that was used. But even when a higher spatial resolution was applied with the newer generation phased array coil MR techniques, the accuracy for T staging was not as high as anticipated with figures varying between 67% and 83% [32-37] and with a considerable interobserver variability [32]. One exception to above findings are those of Brown and colleagues who reported a 100% accuracy and complete agreement between two readers on the prediction of tumour stage with phased array MRI [33].

Most staging failures with MRI occur in the differentiation of T2 and borderline T3 lesions with overstaging as the main cause of errors. These staging difficulties apply to both the endoluminal and the phased array MR technique. Overstaging is often caused by desmoplastic reactions [27, 32, 38] and it is difficult to distinguish on MRI between speculation in the perirectal fat caused by fibrosis only (stage pT2) from speculation caused by fibrosis that contains tumour cells (stage pT3) [32].

Endoluminal MR techniques using dynamic contrast enhanced sequences have been proposed to solve this problem because it can more reliably show complete disrupture of the muscular rectal wall [27]. However the high interobserver variability reported for this technique questions its reliability [39].

How relevant is it to distinguish between the different T stages pre-operatively? Although the TNM staging system is a very reliable prognostic indicator, it does have its shortcomings. Indeed it may be valuable to pre-operatively identify those patients with small superficial (T1) tumours that can be treated with transanal resection. The majority of rectal cancer patients however have T2 or T3, both of which require complete excision. A T3 tumour that has just breached the muscular rectal wall and minimally penetrates the mesorectal fat, will have a lower risk for recurrence than a T3 tumour that invades the mesorectal fascia. Therefore there is little benefit in differentiating between tumours limited to the rectal wall (T2) and tumours that have just breached the wall (minimal T3) when it does not affect pre-operative or operative management.

Determination of the circumferential resection margin with MRI

It has been repeatedly shown that it is the distance from the tumour to the circumferential resection margin that is the most powerful predictor for the local recurrence rate [40-42] and not the T stage. It would therefore be of far more importance to be able to identify pre-operatively by imaging those tumours that will have a close resection margin so that they can be selected for a more extensive neo-adjuvant treatment and more extensive surgery. Recent editorials in the Lancet and NEJM have stressed the importance of differentiated treatment in rectal cancer and the need for an accurate tool to select patients on the basis of risk factors [43, 44].

Prediction of the circumferential resection margins has not been the subject of many imaging studies. The reason is that radiologists were not acquainted with the concept of total mesorectal excision, and were not used to evaluate the mesorectal fascia as an anatomic border. The very first report on the identification of the mesorectal fascia by imaging dated from 1983 [45], but since that time nothing has been published until only very recently [33, 34]. In one report the mesorectal fascia was visualized with a high resolution phased array MR technique, and although the authors concluded that the depth of tumour extension could be predicted, the more relevant distance between tumour and fascia was not studied [33]. With a postoperative MRI of the resected specimens Blomqvist and colleagues were able to predict the tumour-free lateral resection margin with high accuracy [34].

We reported a study on the MR evaluation of circumferential resection margins in patients with rectal cancer published in the *Lancet* early 2001 [32]. Using a high resolution phased array MR technique we found a higher accuracy for the prediction of the circumferential resection margin in 76 rectal cancer patients than for the prediction of the T stage. An important finding is the high agreement of the measurements both between and within the observers in contrast to the only moderate intra- and interobserver agreement for the T stage determination. This indicates that phased array MRI is more reliable for the assessment of the circumferential resection margin than for the assessment of the T stage. These results were confirmed in a third study on the MR determination of the circumferential resection margins in 43 patients [46]. The authors not only reported a 95% accuracy on the MR prediction of the tumour free lateral resection margin with a phased array technique, they also proved in a cadaver study that the fascia that was visualized on high resolution phased array MRI, was indeed the mesorectal fascia.

Although the value of a pre-operative MRI in patient management is presently being evaluated in larger clinical trials, these findings already suggest that the anatomical information provided by a high resolution MRI is very detailed, reliable and easy to communicate.

Assessment of local tumour extent in locally advanced and recurrent rectal cancer

Ten to twenty percent of rectal tumours are locally advanced with fixation to surrounding pelvic organs. In these cases the patient's best chance for cure is a radical en bloc resection of the tumour and the surrounding invaded structures [47]. Accurate and detailed anatomic information on tumour extent is essential not only for the selection of patients for an extensive course of chemoradiation in order to obtain tumour shrinkage but also for planning of the optimal surgical procedure. The same holds true for locally recurrent rectal cancer [48].

In imaging literature only few studies have addressed the problems of predicting tumour infiltration in neighbouring organs for primary rectal cancer [12, 37, 49, 50]. Based on the initial optimistic results for CT in staging advanced rectal cancer [11, 14, 51-54] this modality has since been used in clinical practice to evaluate the local tumour extent in patients with fixed rectal cancer or recurrent rectal cancer. The exact value of MRI has never fully been investigated. Although MRI has extensively been compared with CT for its accuracy in detecting local recurrences, only few publications exist comparing CT and MRI for the prediction of local tumour extent [55-57]. In an early study Blomqvist *et al.* found a better prediction for organ invasion with pelvic phased array MRI (6/9) than with CT (3/9) but this was based on only a limited number of patients. The same author recently published the results of a study in 16 patients with advanced rectal cancer. This study showed superior performance for MRI in the prediction of urinary bladder and uterus invasion [57]. Beets-Tan *et al.* found phased array MRI far more accurate than CT in predicting pelvic floor invasion, pyriform muscle invasion and subtle bone invasion but the large difference in outcome between the two modalities could partially be attributed to the fact that a state of the art high resolution MR technique was compared with conventional CT techniques [55].

Theoretically newer generation multi-slice spiral CT techniques with optimal bolus timing and reconstructions in multiple planes may perform better than conventional CT [58, 59]. In a study of 105 rectal cancer patients undergoing a spiral CT an improved overall accuracy for T staging (82%) was reported [58]. However this study only included four T4 lesions. Thus to date the role of multi-slice spiral CT in rectal cancer imaging has not been fully explored.

Difficulties in reading rectal cancer MRI

Despite the high accuracy of phased array MRI in the pre-operative selection of the different risk groups of rectal cancer patients, some pitfalls exist. Difficulties may arise in the prediction of the circumferential margins in distal and irradiated rectal cancer. These difficulties are discussed below.

Prediction of the circumferential resection margin in distal rectal cancer

Tumours located in the distal rectum, in specific the low and anteriorly located rectal cancer, can pose a problem for surgeons as well as for radiologists. These tumours generally show a higher rate of local recurrence [1]. Due to its tapered anatomy the mesorectum contains less mesorectal fat on the ventral and distal site. Technically it is more difficult for surgeons to obtain a complete resection of these tumours. But also from the imaging point of view many problems arise in staging low rectal cancer as a consequence of the rectal anatomy. Even the best staging method, EUS, fail in accurate staging of these tumours [6, 60]. The main message is that one need to be aware of a very close or involved resection margin on the anterior site when dealing with low rectal tumours.

Prediction of the circumferential resection margin in irradiated rectal cancer

MR images of rectal cancer patients who have had a long course of radiotherapy may be difficult to interpret. Radiation therapy can induce fibrosis, both in normal tissue and in areas of tumour necrosis. MRI cannot reliably distinguish between fibrosis with and without tumour cells [49, 55, 61]. This can pose diagnostic problems in predicting whether the cancer is close to or actually invades the mesorectal resection plane and/or surrounding organs. In order to minimize such interpretation problems the assessment of organ invasion should be made on a baseline MRI before radiotherapy [55].

Conclusions

Since the recent introduction of new treatment strategies for rectal cancer (pre-operative radiotherapy and total mesorectal excision) there is a growing need for an accurate imaging tool to select pre-operatively patients with different risk for local recurrences so that treatment can be given according to risks.

For superficial rectal cancer that can be treated with surgery only, endoluminal ultrasound (EUS) remains the most accurate staging modality for the assessment of tumour ingrowth into the muscular rectal wall. Endorectal MRI is as accurate as EUS. At present EUS remains the imaging modality of first choice for staging superficial tumours because it is more available and less expensive than MRI. Although both endoluminal techniques provide clear details of the rectal wall it is less accurate for the evaluation of the outer border of the mesorectum: the mesorectal fascia and its relation to the tumour (the circumferential resection margin).

For all remaining mobile and fixed rectal cancer a high resolution phased array coil MRI is at present the most reliable imaging tool to evaluate the mesorectal plane and the circumferential resection margins. Pre-operative identification of these margins allows pre-operative selection of patients at different risk for recurrences so that each patient can be given the most appropriate treatment.

Despite the many potentials of the multi-slice spiral CT to date its role in rectal cancer imaging has not been fully explored.

References

1. Kapiteijn E, Marijnen CA, Nagtegaal ID, *et al.* Pre-operative radiotherapy combined with total mesorectal excision for resectable rectal cancer. *N Engl J Med* 2001; 345 (9): 638-46.
2. Investigators SRCT. Improved survival with pre-operative radiotherapy in resectable rectal cancer. Swedish Rectal Cancer Trial. *N Engl J Med* 1997; 336 (14): 980-7.
3. Akasu T, Sugihara K, Moriya Y, Fujita S. Limitations and pitfalls of transrectal ultrasonography for staging of rectal cancer. *Dis Colon Rectum* 1997; 40 (Suppl. 10): S10-5.
4. Beynon J, Foy DM, Roe AM, Temple LN, Mortensen NJ. Endoluminal ultrasound in the assessment of local invasion in rectal cancer. *Br J Surg* 1986; 73 (6): 474-7.
5. Glaser F, Schlag P, Herfarth C. Endorectal ultrasonography for the assessment of invasion of rectal tumours and lymph node involvement. *Br J Surg* 1990; 77 (8): 883-7.
6. Herzog U, von Flue M, Tondelli P, Schuppisser JP. How accurate is endorectal ultrasound in the pre-operative staging of rectal cancer? *Dis Colon Rectum* 1993; 36 (2): 127-34.
7. Katsura Y, Yamada K, Ishizawa T, Yoshinaka H, Shimazu H. Endorectal ultrasonography for the assessment of wall invasion and lymph node metastasis in rectal cancer. *Dis Colon Rectum* 1992; 35 (4): 362-8.
8. Milsom JW, Graffner H. Intrarectal ultrasonography in rectal cancer staging and in the evaluation of pelvic disease. Clinical uses of intrarectal ultrasound. *Ann Surg* 1990; 212 (5): 602-6.
9. Rifkin MD, Ehrlich SM, Marks G. Staging of rectal carcinoma: prospective comparison of endorectal US and CT. *Radiology* 1989; 170 (2): 319-22.
10. Solomon MJ, McLeod RS. Endoluminal transrectal ultrasonography: accuracy, reliability, and validity. *Dis Colon Rectum* 1993; 36 (2): 200-5.
11. Butch RJ, Stark DD, Wittenberg J, *et al.* Staging rectal cancer by MR and CT. *AJR Am J Roentgenol* 1986; 146 (6): 1155-60.
12. Cova M, Frezza F, Pozzi-Mucelli RS, *et al.* Computed tomography and magnetic resonance in the pre-operative staging of the spread of rectal cancer. A correlation with the anatomicopathological aspects. *Radiol Med* (Torino) 1994; 87 (1-2): 82-9.
13. Guinet C, Buy JN, Ghossain MA, *et al.* Comparison of magnetic resonance imaging and computed tomography in the pre-operative staging of rectal cancer. *Arch Surg* 1990; 125 (3): 385-8.
14. Hodgman CG, MacCarty RL, Wolff BG, *et al.* Pre-operative staging of rectal carcinoma by computed tomography and 0.15T magnetic resonance imaging. Preliminary report. *Dis Colon Rectum* 1986; 29 (7): 446-50.
15. McNicholas MM, Joyce WP, Dolan J, Gibney RG, MacErlaine DP, Hyland J. Magnetic resonance imaging of rectal carcinoma: a prospective study. *Br J Surg* 1994; 81 (6): 911-4.
16. Okizuka H, Sugimura K, Ishida T. Pre-operative local staging of rectal carcinoma with MR imaging and a rectal balloon. *J Magn Reson Imaging* 1993; 3 (2): 329-35.
17. Starck M, Bohe M, Fork FT, Lindstrom C, Sjoberg S. Endoluminal ultrasound and low-field magnetic resonance imaging are superior to clinical examination in the pre-operative staging of rectal cancer. *Eur J Surg* 1995; 161 (11): 841-5.

18. Zerhouni EA, Rutter C, Hamilton SR, et al. CT and MR imaging in the staging of colorectal carcinoma: report of the Radiology Diagnostic Oncology Group II. *Radiology* 1996; 200 (2): 443-51.
19. Vogl TJ, Pegios W, Hunerbein M, Mack MG, Schlag PM, Felix R. Use and applications of MRI techniques in the diagnosis and staging of rectal lesions. *Recent Results Cancer Res* 1998; 146: 35-47.
20. Chan TW, Kressel HY, Milestone B, et al. Rectal carcinoma: staging at MR imaging with endorectal surface coil. Work in progress. *Radiology* 1991; 181 (2): 461-7.
21. Imai Y, Kressel HY, Saul SH, et al. Colorectal tumours: an *in vitro* study of high-resolution MR imaging. *Radiology* 1990; 177 (3): 695-701.
22. Indinnimeo M, Grasso RF, Cicchini C, et al. Endorectal magnetic resonance imaging in the pre-operative staging of rectal tumours. *Int Surg* 1996; 81 (4): 419-22.
23. Joosten FB, Jansen JB, Joosten HJ, Rosenbusch G. Staging of rectal carcinoma using MR double surface coil, MR endorectal coil, and intrarectal ultrasound: correlation with histopathologic findings. *J Comput Assist Tomogr* 1995; 19 (5): 752-8.
24. Maldjian C, Smith R, Kilger A, Schnall M, Ginsberg G, Kochman M. Endorectal surface coil MR imaging as a staging technique for rectal carcinoma: a comparison study to rectal endosonography. *Abdom Imaging* 2000; 25 (1): 75-80.
25. Pegios W, Vogl J, Mack MG, et al. MRI diagnosis and staging of rectal carcinoma. *Abdom Imaging* 1996; 21 (3): 211-8.
26. Schnall MD, Furth EE, Rosato EF, Kressel HY. Rectal tumour stage: correlation of endorectal MR imaging and pathologic findings [see comments]. *Radiology* 1994; 190 (3): 709-14.
27. Vogl TJ, Pegios W, Mack MG, et al. Accuracy of staging rectal tumours with contrast-enhanced transrectal MR imaging. *Am J Roentgenol* 1997; 168 (6): 1427-34.
28. Zagoria RJ, Wolfman NT. Magnetic resonance imaging of colorectal cancer. *Semin Roentgenol* 1996; 31 (2): 162-5.
29. DeSouza NM, Hall AS, Puni R, Gilderdale DJ, Young IR, Kmiot WA. High resolution magnetic resonance imaging of the anal sphincter using a dedicated endoanal coil. Comparison of magnetic resonance imaging with surgical findings. *Dis Colon Rectum* 1996; 39 (8): 926-34.
30. Beets-Tan RG, Beets GL, van der Hoop AG, et al. High-resolution magnetic resonance imaging of the anorectal region without an endocoil. *Abdom Imaging* 1999; 24 (6): 576-81; discussion 582-4.
31. Beets-Tan RG, Beets GL, van der Hoop AG, et al. Pre-operative MR imaging of anal fistulas: Does it really help the surgeon? *Radiology* 2001; 218 (1): 75-84.
32. Beets-Tan RG, Beets GL, Vliegen RF, et al. Accuracy of magnetic resonance imaging in prediction of tumour-free resection margin in rectal cancer surgery. *Lancet* 2001; 357 (9255): 497-504.
33. Brown G, Richards CJ, Newcombe RG, et al. Rectal carcinoma: thin-section MR imaging for staging in 28 patients. *Radiology* 1999; 211 (1): 215-22.
34. Blomqvist L, Rubio C, Holm T, Machado M, Hindmarsh T. Rectal adenocarcinoma: assessment of tumour involvement of the lateral resection margin by MRI of resected specimen. *Br J Radiol* 1999; 72 (853): 18-23.
35. Hadfield MB, Nicholson AA, MacDonald AW, et al. Pre-operative staging of rectal carcinoma by magnetic resonance imaging with a pelvic phased-array coil. *Br J Surg* 1997; 84 (4): 529-31.
36. De Lange EE, Fechner RE, Wanebo HJ. Suspected recurrent rectosigmoid carcinoma after abdomino-perineal resection: MR imaging and histopathologic findings. *Radiology* 1989; 170 (2): 323-8.
37. Blomqvist L, Holm T, Rubio C, Hindmarsh T. Rectal tumours-MR imaging with endorectal and/or phased-array coils, and histopathological staging on giant sections. A comparative study. *Acta Radiol* 1997; 38 (3): 437-44.
38. Meyenberger C, Huch Boni RA, Bertschinger P, Zala GF, Klotz HP, Krestin GP. Endoscopic ultrasound and endorectal magnetic resonance imaging: a prospective, comparative study for pre-operative staging and follow-up of rectal cancer. *Endoscopy* 1995; 27 (7): 469-79.

39. Drew PJ, Farouk R, Turnbull LW, Ward SC, Hartley JE, Monson JR. Pre-operative magnetic resonance staging of rectal cancer with an endorectal coil and dynamic gadolinium enhancement. *Br J Surg* 1999; 86 (2): 250-4.
40. Quirke P, Dixon MF. The prediction of local recurrence in rectal adenocarcinoma by histopathological examination. *Int J Colorectal Dis* 1988; 3 (2): 127-31.
41. Wibe A, Rendedal PR, Svensson E, *et al.* Prognostic significance of the circumferential resection margin following total mesorectal excision for rectal cancer. *Br J Surg* 2002; 89 (3): 327-34.
42. Nagtegaal ID, Marijnen CA, Kranenbarg EK, van De Velde CJ, van Krieken JH. Circumferential margin involvement is still an important predictor of local recurrence in rectal carcinoma: Not one millimeter but two millimeters is the limit. *Am J Surg Pathol* 2002; 26 (3): 350-7.
43. Radcliffe A, Brown G. Will MRI provide maps of lines of excision for rectal cancer? *Lancet* 2001; 357 (9255): 495-6.
44. Nelson H, Sargent DJ. Refining multimodal therapy for rectal cancer. *N Engl J Med* 2001; 345 (9): 690-2.
45. Grabbe E, Lierse W, Winkler R. The perirectal fascia: morphology and use in staging of rectal carcinoma. *Radiology* 1983; 149 (1): 241-6.
46. Bissett IP, Fernando CC, Hough DM, *et al.* Identification of the fascia propria by magnetic resonance imaging and its relevance to pre-operative assessment of rectal cancer. *Dis Colon Rectum* 2001; 44 (2): 259-65.
47. Poeze M, Houbiers JG, van de Velde CJ, Wobbes T, von Meyenfeldt MF. Radical resection of locally advanced colorectal cancer. *Br J Surg* 1995; 82 (10): 1386-90.
48. Sagar PM, Pemberton JH. Surgical management of locally recurrent rectal cancer. *Br J Surg* 1996; 83 (3): 293-304.
49. Lange de EE, Fechner RE, Wanebo HJ. Suspected recurrent rectosigmoid carcinoma after abdominoperineal resection: MR imaging and histopathologic findings. *Radiology* 1989; 170: 323-8.
50. Popovich MJ, Hricak H, Sugimura K, Stern JL. The role of MR imaging in determining surgical eligibility for pelvic exenteration. *Am J Roentgenol* 1993; 160 (3): 525-31.
51. Moss AA. Imaging of colorectal carcinoma [see comments]. *Radiology* 1989; 170 (2): 308-10.
52. Thoeni RF. Colorectal cancer. Radiologic staging. *Radiol Clin North Am* 1997; 35 (2): 457-85.
53. Thoeni RF, Moss AA, Schnyder P, Margulis AR. Detection and staging of primary rectal and rectosigmoid cancer by computed tomography. *Radiology* 1981; 141 (1): 135-8.
54. Zaunbauer W, Haertel M, Fuchs WA. Computed tomography in carcinoma of the rectum. *Gastrointest Radiol* 1981; 6 (1): 79-84.
55. Beets-Tan RG, Beets GL, Borstlap AC, *et al.* Pre-operative assessment of local tumour extent in advanced rectal cancer: CT or high-resolution MRI? *Abdom Imaging* 2000; 25 (5): 533-41.
56. Blomqvist L, Holm T, Goranson H, Jacobsson H, Ohlsen H, Larsson SA. MR imaging, CT and CEA scintigraphy in the diagnosis of local recurrence of rectal carcinoma. *Acta Radiol* 1996; 37 (5): 779-84.
57. Blomqvist L, Holm T, Nyren S, Svanstrom R, Ulvskog Y, Iselius L. MR imaging and computed tomography in patients with rectal tumours clinically judged as locally advanced. *Clin Radiol* 2002; 57 (3): 211-8.
58. Chiesura-Corona M, Muzzio PC, Giust G, Zuliani M, Pucciarelli S, Toppan P. Rectal cancer: CT local staging with histopathologic correlation. *Abdom Imaging* 2001; 26 (2): 134-8.
59. Horton KM, Abrams RA, Fishman EK. Spiral CT of colon cancer: imaging features and role in management. *Radiographics* 2000; 20 (2): 419-30.
60. Sailer M, Leppert R, Kraemer M, Fuchs KH, Thiede A. The value of endorectal ultrasound in the assessment of adenomas, T1- and T2-carcinomas. *Int J Colorectal Dis* 1997; 12 (4): 214-9.
61. Kahn H, Alexander A, Rakinic J, Nagle D, Fry R. Pre-operative staging of irradiated rectal cancers using digital rectal examination, computed tomography, endorectal ultrasound, and magnetic resonance imaging does not accurately predict T0, N0 pathology. *Dis Colon Rectum* 1997; 40 (2): 140-4.

Endoscopic management of early colorectal lesions

Brian Saunders

Wolfson Unit for Endoscopy, St. Mark's Hospital, Harrow, Middlesex, HA1 3UJ

Colonoscopy provides the best opportunity for the detection of early colorectal cancer. In endoscopic series early colorectal cancer accounts for approximately 10% of all colonic cancer and can be divided into polypoid and non-polypoid cancer [1, 2]. Polypoid lesions are usually easy to detect but flat or minimally-elevated lesions can be more subtle and require careful inspection with the use of dye (indigocarmine 0.2%) to highlight mucosal irregularities. Change in patient position, use of antispasmodic & antifoaming agents, optimising bowel cleansing and aspiration of retained fluid help to improve the quality of the examination during withdrawal. If the lesion is on a stalk then endoscopic resection using conventional snare diathermy is safe and often curative. Multiple publications testify to the conservative management of polyp cancers provided the cancer is not poorly differentiated, the resection margin is clear histologically and the endoscopist is confident of complete resection [3-7]. The importance of vessel or lymphatic involvement despite a clear resection margin is less clear but would probably sway management in favour of a segmental resection to exclude any risk lymph node metastases in a patient fit for surgery [8, 9]. Regardless of the final management strategy it is important to tattoo the polypectomy site for future endoscopic or surgical recognition. If this has not been done at the initial colonoscopy then an early repeat examination before complete healing at the polypectomy site has occurred & once the histology is known, is indicated. Commercially-available, sterile India ink solutions are available and should be injected into a submucosal bleb created by injecting saline to define the submucosal plain [10]. This two step technique avoids inadvertent spillage of Ink into the peritoneal cavity or the bowel lumen.

Endoscopic management of sessile or flat lesions is more difficult but has been greatly improved by the use of endoscopic mucosal resection (EMR). EMR has become an established procedure in colonoscopy practice and is now accepted as the optimal technique for removing large sessile or flat adenomas and flat or sessile, early colorectal cancers. EMR has gained increased importance with the advent of colorectal cancer screening by endoscopy which has allowed earlier detection of colorectal neoplasia. In experienced

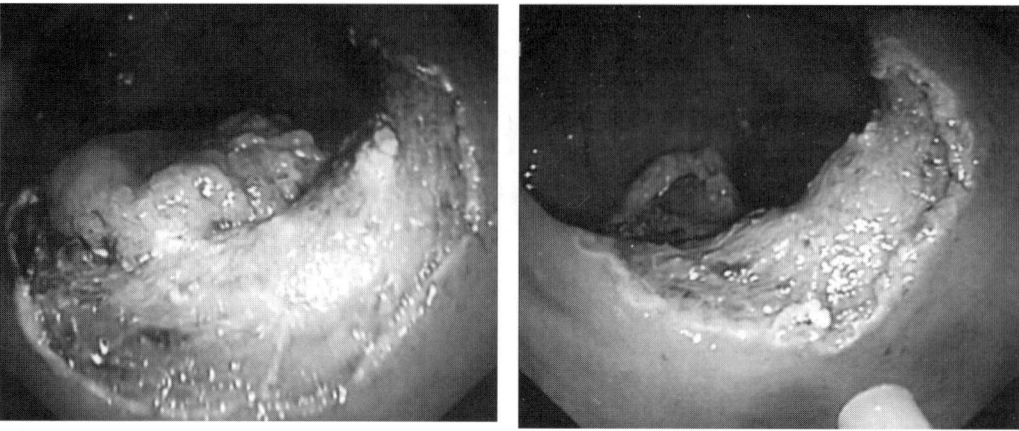

Figure 1. Large (6 cm by 6 cm) sessile colonic polyp completely resected by EMR.

hands benign lesions greater the 50% of the bowel wall circumference can be resected whilst maintaining low complication rates and high rates of neoplasia clearance. However it is important to note that most of the scientific literature relating to EMR has been anecdotal with few randomised trials analysing different techniques or comparing EMR to surgery (open or laparoscopic).

A variety of techniques for EMR have been described but all involve injection of a solution into the submucosal space to separate and lift the mucosa from the muscularis propria [11, 12, 13]. Single lesions up to approximately 2 cm can be resected in one piece but larger lesions require a piecemeal technique. There has been interest recently in improving the duration and quality of the mucosal "lift" by using different injection solutions. In the authors experience using dilute adrenaline provides benefits in terms of haemostsasis whilst addition of a few drops of methylene blue helps to stain the muscularis propria and submucosa defining tissue planes during resection. Hyaluronate has advantages in terms of duration and extent of mucosal lift but is very expensive [14]. Other solutions such as hydroxymethylcellulose, twice normal saline and 50% dextrose have also been proposed.

Most EMR in the colon can be achieved successfully with a standard, single-channel colonoscope and a diathermy snare. Variations on this theme include use of barbed or spiked snares to help grasp mucosa and facilitate removal of flat lesions and the use of the suction cap to perform aspiration mucosectomy. A twin-channel colonoscope can be employed to use a "lift and cut" technique where grasping forceps are used to retract the mucosa through the open snare.

Two key areas related to the EMR technique remain problematic:

- **Accurate *in vivo* assessment of depth of invasion** is needed to avoid inappropriate endoscopic resection. Early cancers confined to the first third of the submucosa are very unlikely to have metastasised to regional lymph nodes and are probably best treated by EMR alone; however deeper invasion usually mandates surgery to ensure lymph node

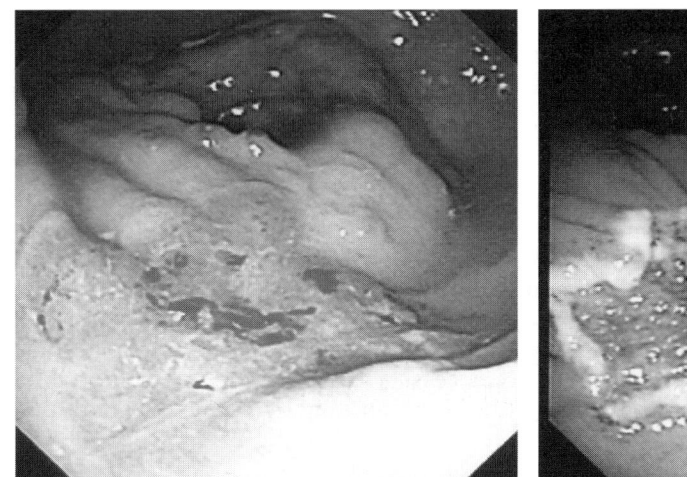
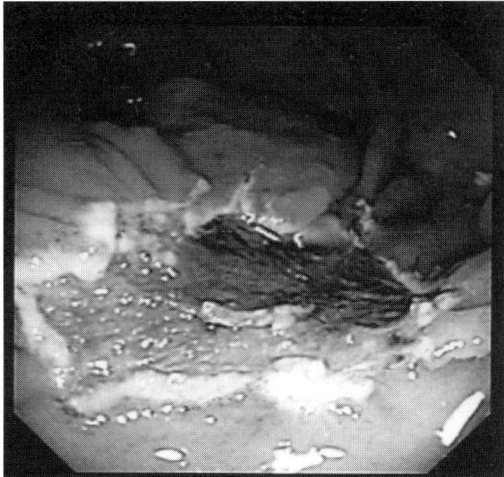

Figure 2. Flat adenoma (2 cm by 2 cm) completely resected by EMR utilising a lift and cut technique and a twin channel colonoscope.

resection & to provide the best chances of cure [15]. Inadvertent snare resection of advanced lesions may risk local complications and even possibly cancer dissemination. Methods of improving lesion differentiation include using the "non-lifting sign", EUS and magnification endoscopy. Of these techniques the assessment of the lifting characteristics of the lesion is the simplest.

- Saline is injected alongside the lesion and complete lifting suggests that invasion if present is very superficial and that EMR is safe to perform with a high probability of cure [16]. If the lesion does not lift then endoscopic resection is neither safe nor feasible. EMR may still be possible after partial lifting but this is suggestive of deeper submucosal invasion where the risk of lymph node metastases may be as high as 25%. Endoscopic ultrasound using a dedicated scope or through-the-scope high frequency mini-probes (20-30 MHz) can define the hyperechoic submucosal layer with up to 90% accuracy in determining depth of invasion [17]. An alternative and possibly complimentary approach is to use magnification endoscopy. After staining & defining the pit (crypt-opening) pattern with crystal violet, the appearance of a disrupted, pit pattern is suggestive of invasive malignancy [17]. A severely disrupted surface pattern has been associated with lymph node involvement. Perhaps the optimal approach to *in vivo* assessment would be the combination of magnification and EUS, however a more pragmatic and simpler approach is to assess the lifting characteristics of the lesion and if it lifts perform EMR and if it doesn't refer for surgery, either laparoscopic or open.

- **Endoscopic piecemeal resection** of large lesions remains technically difficult, somewhat time-consuming and often results in incomplete or difficult to interpret histology. Piecemeal resection commits the patient to at least 2 endoscopies to ensure complete healing of the polypectomy site and often results in residual polyp tissue and the necessity of further endoscopic therapy. There is also some evidence that partial resection of adenomas may accelerate the process of carcinogenesis [18, 19]. Argon plasma coagulation to treat resection margins has been shown to significantly reduce recurrence/ residual neo-plastic tissue, and the author recommends this approach routinely after piecemeal EMR [20]. En-bloc resection of large lesions is clearly advantageous and ideally would also include a margin of normal mucosa to aid interpretation of completeness of excision. Possible methods of en-bloc endoscopic resection include circumferential incision with the I-T (insulation-tipped) knife followed by a large snare resection or submucosal dissection using endoscopic scissors or diathermy devices [21, 22]. Sessile lesions invariably lie over contoured haustral folds and a dissection technique whereby the submucosal plane is established and developed gradually is likely to be the safest and most effective approach. Establishing the submucosal plane is relatively easy using diathermy knives with or without insulation tips but optimal dissection devices (scissors/knives) have yet to be developed. To enable dissection of the submucosal plane, traction on the mucosa above the line of dissection is usually necessary and this could be achieved by utilising a twin channel instrument with grasping forceps or by using two ultra-thin endoscopes in parallel. The twin-endoscope technique has been trialled successfully in an animal model [23].

In conclusion careful examination technique augmented by the appropriate use of mucosal dyes enhances detection of colonic neoplasia and early cancer. *In vivo* assessment of endoscopic respectability is made from visual assessment, the lifting characteristics of the lesion and when available EUS and magnification. New resection methods incorporating endoscopic mucosal resection allow some very early cancers and large sessile, benign lesions to be successfully & appropriately resected endoscopically, avoiding the need for surgical intervention. Although there are few good data to accurately define its role, standard EMR appears safe and effective. The main challenges to improve the technique include the accurate staging of early cancer, the development of the optimal submucosal injection solution and the integration of new equipment and techniques to allow, rapid, easy en-bloc resection.

References

1. Kudo S, Kashida H, Tamura T, *et al*. Colonoscopic diagnosis and management of nonpolypoid early colorectal cancer. *World J Surg* 2000; 24 (9): 1081-90.
2. Williams CB, Saunders BP, Talbot IC. Endoscopic management of polypoid early colon cancer. *World J Surg* 2000; 24 (9): 1047-51.
3. Netzer P, Forster C, Biral R, *et al*. Risk factor assessment of endoscopically removed malignant colorectal polyps. *Gut* 1998; 43 (5): 669-74.
4. Cooper HS, Deppisch LM, Gourley WK, *et al*. Endoscopically removed malignant colorectal polyps: clinicopathologic correlations. *Gastroenterology* 1995; 108 (6): 1657-65.
5. Volk EE, Goldblum JR, Petras RE, Carey WD, Fazio VW. Management and outcome of patients with invasive carcinoma arising in colorectal polyps. *Gastroenterology* 1995; 109 (6): 1801-7.
6. Netzer P, Binek J, Hammer B, Lange J, Schmassmann A. Significance of histologic criteria for the management of patients with malignant colorectal polyps and polypectomy. *Scand J Gastroenterol* 1997; 32 (9): 910-6.
7. Morson BC, Whiteway JE, Jones EA, Macrae FA, Williams CB. Histopathology and prognosis of malignant colorectal polyps treated by endoscopic polypectomy. *Gut* 1984; 25 (5): 437-44.

8. Geraghty JM, Williams CB, Talbot IC. Malignant colorectal polyps: venous invasion and successful treatment by endoscopic polypectomy. *Gut* 1991; 32 (7): 774-8.
9. Muller S, Chesner IM, Egan MJ, Rowlands DC, Collard MJ, Swarbrick ET, Newman J. Significance of venous and lymphatic invasion in malignant polyps of the colon and rectum. *Gut* 1989; 30 (10): 1385-91.
10. Sawaki A, Nakamura T, Suzuki T, *et al.* A two-step method for marking polypectomy sites in the colon and rectum. *Gastrointest Endosc* 2003; 57 (6): 735-7.
11. Hawes RH. Perspectives in endoscopic mucosal resection. *Gastrointest Endosc Clin N Am* 2001; 11 (3): 549-52.
12. Waye JD. Endoscopic mucosal resection of colon polyps. *Gastrointest Endosc Clin N Am* 2001; 11 (3): 537-48.
13. Kudo S, Tamegai Y, Yamano H, Imai Y, Kogure E, Kashida H. Endoscopic mucosal resection of the colon: the Japanese technique. *Gastrointest Endosc Clin N Am* 2001; 11 (3): 519-35.
14. Yamamoto H, Koiwai H, Yube T, *et al.* A successful single-step endoscopic resection of a 40 millimeter flat-elevated tumour in the rectum: endoscopic mucosal resection using sodium hyaluronate. *Gastrointest Endosc* 1999; 50 (5): 701-4.
15. Nascimbeni R, Burgart LJ, Nivatvongs S, Larson DR. Risk of lymph node metastasis in T1 carcinoma of the colon and rectum. *Dis Colon Rectum* 2002; 45 (2): 200-6.
16. Kato H, Haga S, Endo S, *et al.* Lifting of lesions during endoscopic mucosal resection (EMR) of early colorectal cancer: implications for the assessment of resectability. *Endoscopy* 2001; 33 (7): 568-73.
17. Matsumoto T, Hizawa K, Esaki M, *et al.* Comparison of EUS and magnifying colonoscopy for assessment of small colorectal cancers. *Gastrointest Endosc* 2002; 56 (3): 354-60.
18. Kunihiro M, Tanaka S, Haruma K, *et al.* Electrocautery snare resection stimulates cellular proliferation of residual colorectal tumour: an increasing gene expression related to tumour growth. *Dis Colon Rectum* 2000; 43 (8): 1107-15.
19. Matsuda K, Masaki T, Abo Y, Uchida H, Watanabe T, Muto T. Rapid growth of residual colonic tumour after incomplete mucosal resection. *J Gastroenterol* 1999; 34 (2): 260-3.
20. Brooker JC, Saunders BP, Shah SG, Thapar CJ, Suzuki N, Williams CB. Treatment with argon plasma coagulation reduces recurrence after piecemeal resection of large sessile colonic polyps: a randomized trial and recommendations. *Gastrointest Endosc* 2002; 55 (3): 371-5.
21. Gotoda T, Kondo H, Ono H, *et al.* A new endoscopic mucosal resection procedure using an insulation-tipped electrosurgical knife for rectal flat lesions: report of two cases. *Gastrointest Endosc* 1999; 50 (4): 560-3.
22. Yoshikane H, Hidano H, Sakakibara A, *et al.* Endoscopic resection of laterally spreading tumours of the large intestine using a distal attachment. *Endoscopy* 1999; 31 (6): 426-30.
23. Brooker JC, Saunders BP, Suzuki N, Sibbons P. Twin-endoscope scissors resection (T-ESR): a new minimally invasive technique for performing colonic mucosectomy. *Surg Endosc* 2001; 15 (12): 1463-6.

Multi-modality treatment in advanced rectal tumours

Lars Påhlman

Department of. Surgery, Colorectal Unit, University Hospital, Uppsala, Sweden

Introduction

Modern rectal cancer treatment has changed dramatically during the last two decades. Among several things it has been shown that the individual surgeon is one of the most important prognostic factor for a good outcome. Also the new knowledge of adjuvant and neo-adjuvant radiotherapy with or without a combination with chemotherapy has changed the outcome substantially. However, with an unselective use of chemotherapy and radiotherapy we will have a lot of overtreatment. To diminish this, it is important to have a proper pre-operative staging before the patients are scheduled for a specific treatment.

This review will summarise the modern view of the staging processes among patients with an advanced rectal cancer and the appropriate approach and use of neo-adjuvant treatment as well as proper surgery.

Staging

In rectal cancer, as in all other cancer forms, the stage of disease is of outmost importance to know pre-operatively. One of the first things is to rule out whether or not there are any signs of distant metastases. The most common places for these metastases are the liver and lungs and those areas should be screened before any decision is taken for treatment. The next step is to evaluate the local tumour stage. Before imaging techniques are used, a clinical staging is essential. With the "experienced fingers" it is obvious for most surgeons whether or not a tumour is considered an "early one" or if it is a "late one". The early tumour is a mobile tumour confined to the bowel wall and the late tumour is a tumour growing outside the bowel wall, and in some cases growing close to or into the surrounding organs, *i.e.*, tethered or fixed tumours [1].

To evaluate a small early lesion, it is essential to see whether the tumour has grown through the muscularis mucosa layer, *i.e.* a T1 tumour, or if it has grown into the *muscularis propria* layer, *i.e.*, a T2 tumour. Of course, it is also of value to know whether there is a T3 tumour indicating that the tumour has invaded the bowel wall and reached the surface. The best examination for those early lesions is endorectal ultrasound, where it is possible to disclose T1 tumours from T2 tumours. A T1 tumour could be suitable for local surgery but T2 and T3 tumours should have an abdominal procedure.

The late stage tumours, *i.e.* more than T2 tumours, MRI has become the best staging facility today [3]. With good MRI examination it is possible to classify T3 – T4 tumours in three main categories, "the good", "the bad" or "the ugly". A "good" cancer is a T3 tumour growing into the mesorectum but with a good distance to the circumferential margin. A "bad" tumour is a tumour growing very close to but not through the circumferential margin indicating a high risk of local recurrence if the patient is treated with surgery alone. Finally, the "ugly" ones are tumours growing through the circumferential margin.

Based upon this definition with ultrasound in "the early lesions" it is possible to decide which type of procedure is appropriate for that type of patient. If the tumour is a "late one" the decision making is how to use neo-adjuvant treatment.

Radiotherapy

Most data indicate that if radiotherapy should be used it should be given pre-operatively. The effect on local recurrence rate is better with pre-operative radiotherapy and also there is an effect on survival benefit. This knowledge is based on theoretical grounds [4] but also on data derived from the meta-analyses [5].

According to the T-staging based on MRI, for patients who have a tumour classified as a "good" T3 one radiotherapy is probably superfluous. If the tumour is disclosed as a "bad" one, radiotherapy should be considered. In those cases it might be enough with just radiotherapy but chemotherapy could be discussed (see below). This treatment could probably be given with the so-called Swedish model 5×5 Gy followed by surgery the next week [6]; conventional radiotherapy with 25×2 Gy could also be used. The third group of patients, those with an "ugly" tumour, should probably be given radiotherapy with a prolonged course. The issue with this type of treatment is to have a downsizing making it possible to resect those tumours, which are considered not resectable. There are very few strong supports for chemoradiotherapy but most doctors today do support a chemoradiotherapy approach to those patients [7].

According to the knowledge there is no real use for postoperative radiotherapy or chemoradiotherapy [5, 8]. However, in patients with a early lesion, where a local excision has been performed and it turns out to be a T1 tumour or a very favourable T2 tumour, one could consider postoperative chemoradiotherapy. The same situation can exist in patients with a "good" tumour based upon MRI, where surgery has been done and the pathological report indicates a very close circumferential margin. In those cases it is probably worthwhile to consider postoperative chemoradiotherapy to reduce the local recurrence rate [9].

Chemotherapy

The whole issue with local recurrences has been solved with good surgery and appropriate radiotherapy. The next issue to evaluate and improve is actually the occult distant metastases. Therefore chemotherapy must be evaluated even more aggressively. Again, the literature is very confusing and most studies indicating that the value of chemotherapy in rectal cancer patients is not that good [10]. The reason for this is very difficult to explain since we know that there is an effect on colon cancer but not on rectal cancer [11]. An interesting observation is that those patients who have the best effect of chemotherapy are those with a micro-satellite instability compared to patients with stable micro-satellites. Since the left sided part of colon has more tumours with stable micro-satellites this might be an explanation why chemotherapy does not work as well in rectal cancer patients as in colon cancer patients and especially in the right sided ones, where most of them have unstable micro-satellites. New trials are essential to try to disclose whether we should use chemotherapy in rectal cancer. However, in many protocols and routines rectal cancer patients are treated as colon cancer patients.

Sphincter preservation

Another very important option for radiotherapy is sphincter preservation. Again, the literature is very confusing. With chemoradiotherapy many authors have claimed that more sphincters can be preserved. These data come from recent institutional series compared with historical controls from the same institution. One has to realise that the historical controls are not useful in this comparison. The reason is that most of the historical controls are not valid due to the modern philosophy in sphincter-saving surgery. We do accept much lesser distant margins today and the only way to prove whether or not this is true is to do randomised trials. So far, there are very few data supporting that more sphincters can be preserved if chemoradiotherapy is used in the pre-operative setting. Actually, some data do not support this at all [12]. Therefore this is still a question which should be studied in randomised controlled trials.

Surgery

Local excision in early tumours is a valid option as long as the pre-operative examination has not disclosed a tumour with a high grade of malignancy. Whether this is done transanal or with a TEM (transanal endoscopic microsurgical) technique is optional but according to literature the best specimens are provided with the TEM technique [13]. As mentioned above, some of those patients should have postoperative chemoradiotherapy. On the other hand, there are also surgeons proposing a pre-operative chemoradiotherapy in T2 and T3 tumour lesions and then a TEM procedure should be done in selective cases with a good tumour regression [14]. This treatment option must be considered experimental and long term results are awaited.

In most patients T3-T4 tumours must be operated upon with an abdominal procedure. The gold standard today is a proper TME (total mesorectal excision) procedure [15, 16]. In patients with a T4 tumour pre-operative radiotherapy is mandatory and in many centres a shift to pre-operative chemoradiotherapy has already been done [17]. Dependent upon the tumour extension different surgical options can be considered. A more or less aggressive approach to the pelvic organs must be followed dependent upon the tumour extension. Tumours growing into a vagina should be resected with a posterior vagina wall. If the uterus is involved, the uterus should of course be taken out on block. Rarely, a total pelvic exenteration is necessary in women. In men, however, for tumours growing anteriorly into the prostate or the base of the bladder, a pelvic exenteration is often necessary. The key issue after having taken out a huge tumour in the pelvis is the reconstruction for the bowel function and the urinary function. If the tumour is high enough, a low anterior resection with a colonic pouch is possible in many of the patients. If the bladder and prostate are taken out, it is possible to do a conventional Bricker conduit or a Bricker deviation according to the Kock pouch technique. The third option is, of course, to create an orthotoptic bladder sutured to the urethra.

Tumours growing out in the bony pelvis must, if possible, be resected. To that purpose orthopaedic surgeons are necessary. Also in those cases it might be of importance to have facilities with intraoperative radiotherapy although very little evidence-based data support this approach. Again, this is something which must be considered an experimental treatment and exploratory trials are important.

Summary and conclusion

Modern rectal cancer treatment is essential to be run with a multidisciplinary team. First of all, good access to staging procedures is important. The use of radiotherapy and chemotherapy must be considered in all cases and when surgery is planned for the advanced case, again a team is necessary. Surgeons, urologists, gynaecologists and orthopaedics are specialists which must be available in such an approach.

References

1. Nicholls RJ, York Mason A, Morson BC, Dixon AK, Kelsey Fry I. The clinical staging of rectal cancer. *Br J Surg* 1982; 69: 404-9.
2. Lindmark G, Elwin A, Glimelius B, Påhlman L. The value of endosonography in pre-operative staging of rectal cancer. *Int J Colorectal Dis* 1992; 7: 162-6.
3. Blomqvist L. Preoperative staging of colorectal cancer – computed tomography and magnetic resonance imaging. *Scan J Surg* 2003; 92: 35-43.
4. Glimelius B, Påhlman L. Perioperative radiotherapy in rectal cancer. *Acta Oncol* 1999; 38: 23-32.
5. Colorectal Cancer Collaborative Group. Adjuvant radiotherapy for rectal cancer: a systematic overview of 22 trials involving 8,507 patients. *Lancet* 2001; 358: 1291-304.
6. Swedish Rectal Cancer Trial. Improved survival with pre-operative radiotherapy in resectable rectal carcinoma. *N Engl J Med* 1997; 336: 980-7.
7. Frykholm-Jansson G, Påhlman L, Glimelius B. Combined chemo- and radiotherapy *vs* radiotherapy alone in the treatment of primary, nonresectable rectal carcinoma. *Int J Radiation Oncology Biol Phys* 2001; 50: 427-34.
8. Frykholm G, Glimelius B, Påhlman L. Pre-operative or postoperative irradiation in adenocarcinoma of the rectum: Final treatment results of a randomized trial and evaluation of the late secondary effects. *Dis Colon Rectum* 1993; 36: 564-72.
9. Tveit KM, Gudvog I, Hagen S, *et al.* Randomised controlled trial of postoperative radiotherapy and short-term time-scheduled 5-fluorouracil against surgery alone in the treatment of Dukes' B and C rectal cancer. *Br J Surg* 1997; 84: 1130-5.
10. Zoetmulder FAN, Taal BG, van Tinteren H. Adjuvant 5FU plus levamisole improves survival in stage II and III colonic cancer, but not in rectal cancer. *Proc ASCO J Clin Oncol* 1999; 18: 266a.
11. IMPACT-study. Efficacy of adjuvant fluorouracil and folinic acid in colon cancer. *Lancet* 1995; 354: 939-44.
12. Francois Y, Nemoz CJ, Baulieux J, *et al.* Influence of the interval between pre-operative radiation therapy and surgery on downstaging and on the rate of sphincter-sparing surgery for rectal cancer: The Lyon R90-01 randomized trial. *J Clin Oncol* 1999; 17: 2396-402.
13. Buess G, Hutterer F, Theiss R, *et al.* Das System für die transanale, endoskopishe Rectumoperation. *Chir* 1984; 55: 677-80.
14. Lezoche E, Guerrieri M, Paganini A, *et al.* Is transanal microsurgery (TEM) a valid treatment for rectal tumours? *Surg Endosc* 1996; 10: 736-41.
15. Heald RJ, Husband EM, Ryall RDH. The mesorectum in rectal cancer surgery – the clue to pelvic recurrence? *Br J Surg* 1982; 69: 613-6.
16. Lehander Martling A, Holm T, Rutqvist L-E, *et al.* Effect of a surgical training programme on outcome of rectal cancer in the County of Stockholm. *Lancet* 2000; 356: 93-6.
17. Hatfield P, Sebag-Montefiore D. The use of radiotherapy in rectal cancer. *Scand J Surg* 2003; 92: 65-73.

The role of stenting as temporary and palliative treatment

M.C. Parker

Department of Surgery, Davent Valley Hospital Dartford, United Kingdom

Introduction

The management of malignant obstruction of the colon should aim to clarify the extent of the disease in order to determine whether therapeutic intervention is intended to be curative or palliative. It is recognised that due to the critical nature of colonic obstruction it may not be possible to determine the presence of distal metastases at the time of this intervention.

Prior to the introduction of self expanding colonic stents (SEMS) both curative and palliative surgical procedures carried significant risks to the patient. In those with localised obstructing disease the choice of surgical procedure, if the patient was suitable for surgery, was dependent on the position of the lesion. For right sided colonic lesions resection and construction of an ileo-colic anastomosis was often undertaken. The surgical management of left sided colonic lesions was more complex and often necessitated formation of an end colostomy after resection. The reversibility of this stoma was variable. Stamatakis *et al.* (1999) showed that, although 59% with a left-sided colonic obstruction had a successful one-stage surgical resection, 41% had a Hartmann procedure. Patients with advanced malignant disease are more frail and surgical management may involve either a colonic bypass procedure, resection with stoma formation, formation of a stoma alone, or no procedure at all.

Though the surgical options have varied little SEMS provide an alternative option in the management of malignant colorectal obstruction. They may assist in two ways. Firstly to provide a "bridge to surgery" where the obstruction is initially relieved and the patient may satisfactorily recover prior to definitive surgery being undertaken. This interval also allows a formal assessment of the spread of the disease if not done so already. This definitive surgery could involve a one staged colonic resection with a primary anastomosis.

The second way that SEMS may help is to provide adequate palliation for advanced colonic lesions, mainly to restore rapid recovery of colonic function. This also permits a comparatively comfortable and dignified quality of remaining life for patients with irresectable or terminal disease.

Stents

An ideal colonic stent should be able to be inserted easily transrectally, negotiate the colonic folds, be deployed comfortably, remain in position, and should allow a sufficient channel for faecal material to pass. There are numerous stents commercially available; most have a mesh design and are constructed from steel or Nitinol. Nitinol stents are constructed from a nickel and titanium alloy; they have "shape memory" reverting to a predetermined configuration after deployment, usually after two to five days. The inherent flexibility of Nitinol affords some colonic peristalsis. SEMS differ in their final expanded diameter and length after deployment. The FDA (Food and Drug Administration) in the United States have approved three stents for use in malignant colonic obstruction: the Enteral Wallstent (Microvasive Corporation, Natick, Massachusetts, USA), the BARD Memotherm stent (BARD, Billerica, Massachusetts, USA) and the colonic Z-stent (Wilson-Cook Medical, Winston-Salem, North Carolina, USA). Though the latter two have larger deployment diameters, the Enteral Wallstent has a longer and smaller diameter delivery system making it suitable for endoscopic placement, and as such it may be preferred for more proximal colonic lesions.

Stent placement

A combined approach as advocated by Soonawalla *et al.* (1998) with both a surgical endoscopist and an interventional radiologist is recommended for successful insertion of a SEMS. The nature and position of the obstructing lesion may permit non-fluoroscopically-guided SEMS placement, where the endoscope first traverses the lesion (this may require balloon dilatation of the stricture). The SEMS may then be deployed either using a stent delivered through the working channel of the endoscope or with a guide wire placed across the lesion to assist SEMS placement. Alternatively if the endoscope cannot traverse the lesion a guide wire may be placed across the lesion under fluoroscopic control. If a guide wire is used for SEMS placement the passage of a second safety wire proves useful if the initial guide wire should become displaced during stent placement. The stent position is checked fluoroscopically and endoscopically. Characteristic features of correct placement include "flaring" of the ends and the appearance of a central "waist".

Early attempts at colonic decompression with Lecluk *et al.* (1986) use of a nasogastric tube and Keen and Orsay's (1992) use of a chest tube were unsuccessful as the tubes were of small calibre and were prone to obstruction. Dohmoto (1991) first described the use of a metal stent to relieve malignant rectal obstruction. This was followed by sporadic similar reports predominately for the palliation of obstructing lesions.

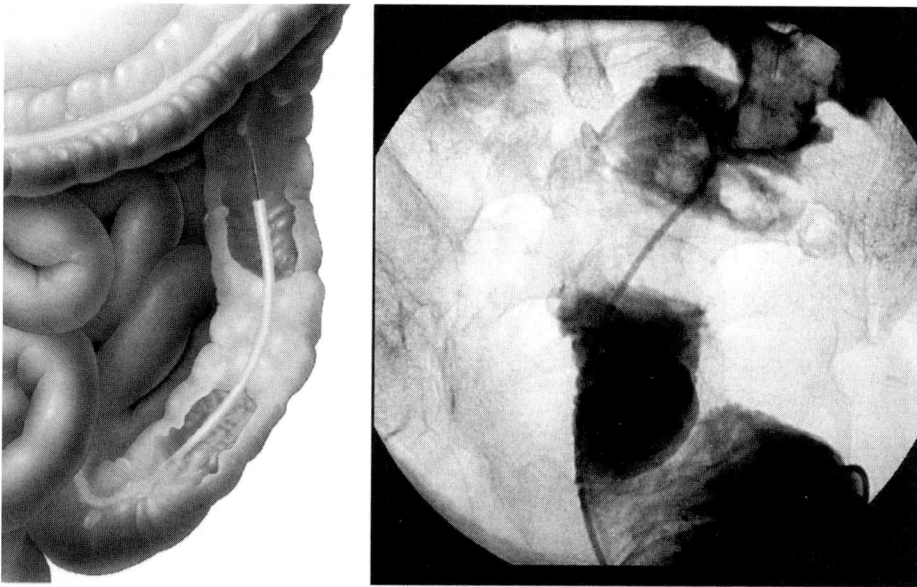

Figure 1. Insertion of guide wire through colonic stricture (by kind permission of Boston Scientific, MA, USA).

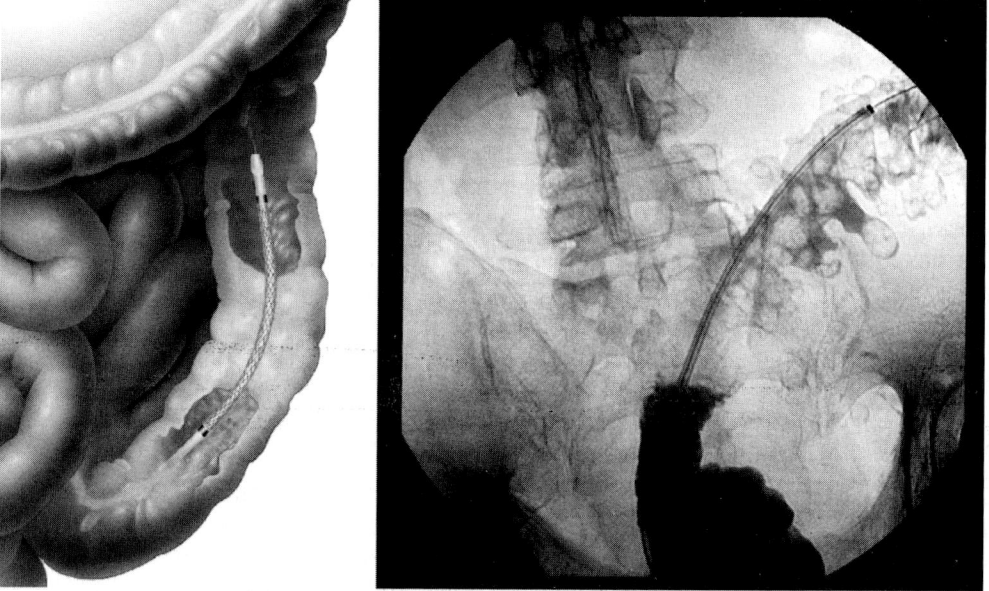

Figure 2. Insertion of stent over guide wire (by kind permission of Boston Scientific, MA, USA).

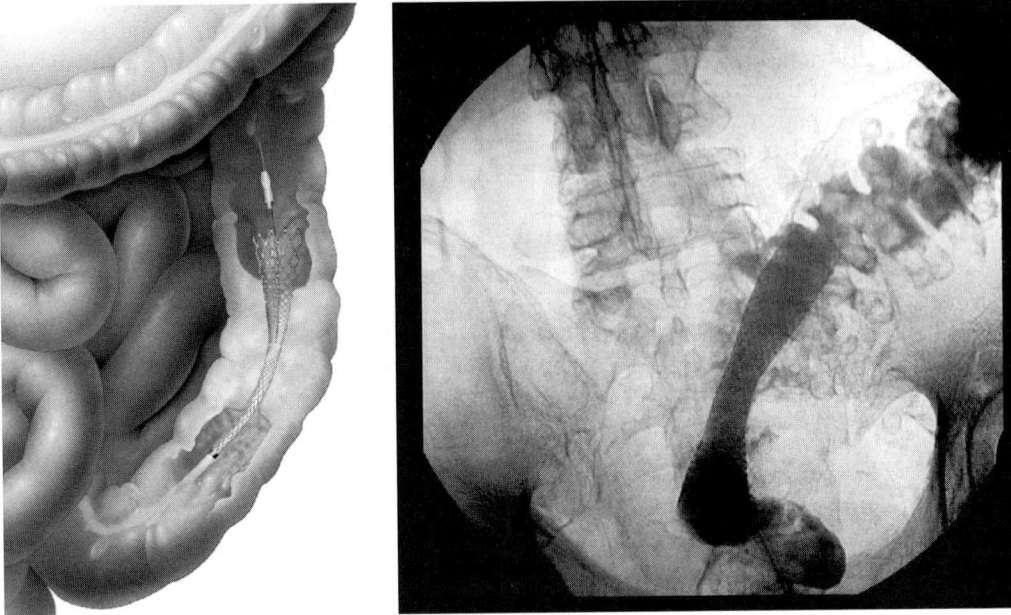

Figure 3. Deploying the stent (by kind permission of Boston Scientific, MA, USA).

"Bridge to surgery"

Tejero *et al.* (1994) outlined the following phases for the treatment of malignant obstruction of the colon:

1) stent placement to relieve the obstruction,
2) recovery of the patient and staging the disease,
3) definitive resection.

They performed this procedure successfully in two patients, demonstrating that this procedure was safe and effective and advocated this treatment as the method of choice for the management of malignant colonic obstruction. Further work from the same unit by Mainar *et al.* (1996) demonstrated successful SEMS placement in all 12 patients evaluated. Obstructive symptoms and signs were relieved in 10 (83%) within 24 hours. Ten patients underwent elective single-stage surgery, and in the remaining two SEMS placement was considered palliative due to disseminated disease. Saida *et al.* (1996) described successful SEMS placement in 12 (80%) of 15 patients. Of the remaining three patients, in one the delivery system could not reach the lesion, and in the remaining two the guide wire could not negotiate the stricture. The mean "bridging time" was 5.8 days (range 2 to 16). All but two had a primary anastomosis constructed following resection. The remaining two patients underwent a Hartmann's procedure; one patient had a low rectal lesion and was of advancing age and in the second patient the stent dislocated during the operation. Tejero *et al.* (1997) described within a series of 38 patients, 25 who had completion surgery after

SEMS placement. In 23 the obstruction was relieved after SEMS placement. In one patient the lesion was too long for the stent and in the remaining patient surgery was performed when complete radiological resolution of the obstruction was not achieved. In this last patient the end of the stent was abutting the pelvic wall, thus preventing emptying of the colon. Of the 23 patients described, one had an early laparotomy because of strangulation of the small bowel from unrelated pathology. In the remaining 22 patients surgery was undertaken with a mean interval of 10 days (range 5 to 20). One patient died after resection; this patient was deemed to have a high anaesthetic risk (ASA IV).

Choo et al. (1998) described a similar bridging interval in 12 patients with malignant colorectal obstruction. Twelve patients underwent SEMS placement prior to surgery; eight underwent elective single-stage resection with a "bridging" interval of 5-7 days. Mainar et al. (1999) reviewed a series of 71 patients and evaluated the use of SEMS for malignant obstruction before surgical resection. Seventy-two SEMS were placed within 24 hours of diagnosis, 64 (90%) of which were initially placed successfully.

In two patients the lesions could not be traversed and in five cases the SEMS was poorly placed, three of which required further stents. Sixty-six (93%) showed clinical improvement within 24 hours and the mean "bridging" interval was 8.6 days (range 6 to 16). Camunez et al. (2000) demonstrated a mean "bridging" time of 7 days (range 4-10) in 33 patients who underwent elective surgery after SEMS placement, though his series consisted of a total of 80 patients, the majority of whom SEMS were placed for palliation. Law et al. (2000) and Liberman et al. (2000) have reported successful deployment of SEMS prior to surgery, though their series involved six and nine patients respectively. Martinez-Santos et al. (2002) compared primary colonic anastomosis after SEMS placement in 43 patients and emergency surgery for left-sided colonic obstruction in 29 patients. In the SEMS group the obstruction was relieved in 41 (95%). Of the 26 who underwent surgery after SEMS placement a primary anastomosis was possible in 22. Though the anastomotic failure rate was similar in both groups, the intensive care unit stay and the number with severe complications were significantly lower in the SEMS group. These results reaffirmed the role of SEMS placement in planning appropriate therapy. The authors also suggested that after the initial relief of the obstruction pre-operative evaluation could be performed in an ambulatory setting, thus minimising hospitalisation. Young et al. (2002) reported our own unit's NHS results: of 43 patients where a SEMS was placed from April 1997 to May 2002, 11 went on to have surgery, with a median "bridging" interval of 22 days.

Palliation of malignant colorectal obstruction

The ACPGBI (Association of Coloproctology of Great Britain and Ireland) Colorectal Cancer Study (2002) have highlighted the challenges that patients with advanced malignancy pose. Surgery may be considered inappropriate in this group of patients who are often frail, and whose co-morbid conditions may not be fully optimised pre-operatively. All palliative procedures were shown to have a significantly higher mortality rate. Spinelli et al. (1993) demonstrated successful stent placement in 12 (92%) of 13 patients. At a mean follow up of seven months 10 (83%) had a patent stent lumen with no reports of discomfort. Turegano-Fuentes *et al.* (1998) reported relief of obstruction in 7 (64%) of 11 patients with advanced disease. Surgical intervention was prevented in 6 (55%), five of whom died with an unobstructed colon from 26 days to seven months after SEMS placement. Tack *et al.* (1998) described the use of a Nd:YAG laser to create a channel for SEMS placement. In their series 9 (90%) of 10 patients had successful stent placement and the patients remained free of obstruction for 103 ± 31 days. However in three the stent migrated and reobstruction from tumour ingrowth occurred in another patient.

De Gregorio *et al.*'s (1998) multi-centre study of 24 patients treated palliatively showed successful stent placement in all patients, and in 23 (96%) there was relief of obstruction within 24 hours. The mortality rate at 6 months was 24%. In Paul *et al.*'s series of 16 patients treated with SEMS, successful placement occurred in 15. In three cases the stent migrated and in three the stents occluded. The mean life span was 130 days and none of the patients had symptoms and signs of obstruction at the time of death. In a larger series by Fernandez *et al.* (1999) involving 41 patients with advanced malignancy the obstruction was relieved within 24-96 hours in 38 (93%). In Repici *et al.*'s (2000) series where 15 (93%) of 16 had successful SEMS placement there was no obstruction seen at a median follow up of 21 weeks. SEMS also has a role in patients with advanced malignancy of extra colonic aetiology. Xinopoulos *et al.*'s (2002) study consisted of 11 patients who presented with advanced malignant colonic obstruction of whom eight had colorectal adenocarcinoma; in two malignancy was ovarian and in the remaining patient the obstruction was due to an infiltrating bladder carcinoma. SEMS placement with the additional use of a Diomed laser in 5 cases to deal with late tumour ingrowth proved successful in all cases. Gandhi *et al.* (2000) described a useful technique for the palliation of right-sided colonic lesions. In this case the stent was placed in an antegrade fashion after creation of caecostomy performed through a Lanz incision under local anaesthetic.

Complications of colorectal stents

Khot *et al.* (2002) conducted a systematic review of the efficacy and safety of colorectal stents by examining the literature from January 1990 to December 2000. Of these 29 case series were included. Stent insertion was attempted in 598 cases; technical success was achieved in 551 (92%) and clinical success, defined by colonic decompression within 96 hours without endoscopic or surgical reintervention, was achieved in 525 (88%). 302 (90%) of 336 were adequately palliated and 223 (85%) of 262 went on to have a successful bridge to surgery. Technical failure was seen in 47 (8%) of 598 cases and was predominantly related to inability to place a guide wire across the lesion (36 cases). Other main causes of technical failure included stent malposition and perforation of the colonic wall. Clinical failure was mainly due to perforation, persistence of obstructive symptoms and adhesions of the colonic wall.

Stent migration occurs in approximately 10% of cases, usually after three days post deployment. Most of these cause no symptoms and are often identified on routine radiological follow up. In those stents that migrate further stents can be inserted, particularly in those patients being treated palliatively. In some cases stents that dislodge through the anal canal require manual or endoscopic removal. Factors that predispose to stent migration include laser pre-treatment, chemotherapy or the presence of benign tumours. Perforation of the colonic wall as a complication can be immediate, at the time of insertion, or post deployment. It has the disadvantage of shedding malignant cells into the peritoneal cavity. It occurs in approximately 4% of cases and prior balloon dilatation is a contributing factor. Clinical reobstruction after placement of a SEMS may be due to tumour ingrowth or overgrowth of the stent, stent migration or faecal impaction. Pain occurs in 5% of patients with SEMS placed. Simple analgesics can often help. If a SEMS is placed within 6 cm of the anal verge the patients may experience significant discomfort and tenesmus. Though bleeding is uncommon it is thought to arise in the most part from the friable tumour. Occasionally the stent may cause some mucosal damage. Transfusion is rarely required.

Conclusion

Self expanding metal stents (SEMS) have a valuable role in allowing a satisfactory quality of life, both for those patients in whom a curative single-staged operative procedure is anticipated and for those in whom surgery is either not curative or efficacious. Osman *et al.* (2000) estimated the cost of a palliative case was less than half that of a surgically decompressed case. Furthermore the cost of a "bridge to surgery" was also significantly lower than compared with a two staged surgical procedure. A multidisciplinary approach is essential and there is a learning curve to overcome. SEMS provide an additional useful option to the colorectal surgeon to deal with malignant colorectal obstruction.

References

1. Camunez F, Echenagusia A, Simo G, Turegano F, Vazquez J, Barreiro-Meiro I. Malignant colorectal obstruction treated by means of self-expanding metallic stents: effectiveness before surgery and in palliation. *Radiology* 2000; 216: 492-7.
2. Choo IW, Do YS, Suh SW, *et al.* Malignant colorectal obstruction: treatment with a flexible covered stent. *Radiology* 1998; 206: 415-21.
3. De Gregorio MA, Mainar A, Tejero E, *et al.* Acute colorectal obstruction: stent placement for palliative treatment-results of a multicenter study. *Radiology* 1998; 209: 117-20.
4. Dohmoto M. New Method – endoscopic implantation of rectal stent in palliative treatment of malignant stenosis. *Endoscopica Digestiva* 1991; 3: 1507-12.
5. Fernandez Lobato R, Pinto I, Paul L, *et al.* Self-expanding prostheses as a palliative method in treating advanced colorectal cancer. *Int Surg* 1999; 84: 159-62.
6. Gandhi P, Osman HS, Rashid HI, Sathananthan N, Parker MC. Palliative on-table antegrade stenting of proximal colon cancer. *Colorectal Disease* 2000; 2: 281-7.
7. Keen RR, Orsay CP. Rectosigmoid stent for obstructing colonic neoplasms. *Dis Colon Rectum* 1992; 35: 912-3.
8. Khot U, Wenk Lang A, Murali K, Parker M C. Systematic review of the clinical evidence on colorectal self-expanding metal stents. *Br J Surg* 2002; 89: 1096-102.
9. Law WL, Chu KW, Ho JW, Tung HM, Law SY, Chu KM. Self-expanding metallic stents in the treatment of colonic obstruction caused by advanced malignancies. *Dis Colon Rectum* 2000; 43: 1522-7.

10. Lelcuk S, et al. Endoscopic decompression of acute colonic obstruction. Avoiding staged surgery. *Ann Surg* 1986; 203: 292-4.
11. Liberman H, Adams DR, Blatchford GJ, Ternent CA, Christensen MA, Thorson AG. Clinical use of the self-expanding metallic stent in the management of colorectal cancer. *Am J Surg* 2000; 180: 407-11.
12. Mainar A, Tejero E, Maynar M, Ferral H, Castaneda-Zuniga W. Colorectal obstruction: treatment with metallic stents. *Radiology* 1996; 198: 761-4.
13. Mainar A, De Gregorio Ariza MA, Tejero E, et al. Acute colorectal obstruction: treatment with self-expandable metallic stents before scheduled surgery-results of a multicenter study. *Radiology* 1999; 210: 65-9.
14. Martinez-Santos C, Lobato RF, Fradejas JM, Pinto I, Ortega-Deballon P, Moreno-Azcoita M. Self-expandable stent before elective surgery *vs* emergency surgery for the treatment of malignant colorectal obstructions: comparison of primary anastomosis and morbidity rates. *Dis Colon Rectum* 2002; 45: 401-6.
15. Osman HS, Rashid HI, Sathananthan N, Parker MC. The cost effectiveness of self expanding metal stents in the management of malignant left-sided large bowel obstruction. *Colorectal Disease* 2000; 2: 233-7.
16. Paul DL, Pinto P, I, Fernandez LR, Montes LC. Palliative treatment of malignant colorectal strictures with metallic stents. *Cardiovasc Intervent Radiol* 1999; 22: 29-36.
17. Repici A, Reggio D, De Angelis C, et al. Covered metal stents for management of inoperable malignant colorectal strictures. *Gastrointest Endosc* 2000; 5: 735-40.
18. Saida Y, Sumiyama Y, Nagao J, Takase M. Stent endoprosthesis for obstructing colorectal cancers. *Dis Colon Rectum* 1996; 39: 552-5.
19. Soonawalla Z, et al. Use of self-expanding metallic stents in the management of obstruction of the sigmoid colon. *AJR Am J Roentgenol* 1998; 171: 633-6.
20. Spinelli P, Dal Fante M, Mancini A. Rectal metal stents for palliation of colorectal malignant stenosis. *Bildgebung* 1993: 60 (Suppl. 1); 48-50.
21. Stamatakis J, Thompson M, Chave H. *National audit of bowel obstruction due to colorectal cancer*, April 1998-March 1999. The Association of Coloproctology of Great Britain and Ireland, July 2000 edition.
22. Tack J, Gevers AM, Rutgeerts P. Self-expandable metallic stents in the palliation of rectosigmoidal carcinoma: a follow-up study. *Gastrointest Endosc* 1998; 48: 267-71.
23. Tejero E, Mainar A, Fernandez L, Tobio R, De Gregorio MA. New procedure for the treatment of colorectal neo-plastic obstructions. *Dis Colon Rectum* 1994; 37: 1158-9.
24. Tejero E, Fernandez-Lobato R, Mainar A, et al. Initial results of a new procedure for treatment of malignant obstruction of the left colon. *Dis Colon Rectum* 1997; 40: 432-6.
25. Tekkis PP, Poloniecki JD, Thompson MR, Stamatakis JD. *ACPGBI Colorectal cancer study 2002*. Part A: Unadjusted outcomes. Dendrite Clinical Systems: Oxfordshire, 2002.
26. Turegano-Fuentes F, Echenagusia-Belda A, Simo-Muerza G, et al. Transanal self-expanding metal stents as an alternative to palliative colostomy in selected patients with malignant obstruction of the left colon. *Br J Surg* 1998; 85: 232-5.
27. Xinopoulos D, Dimitroulopoulos D, Tsamakidis K, Apostolikas N, Paraskevas E. Treatment of malignant colonic obstructions with metal stents and laser. *Hepatogastroenterology* 2002; 49: 359-62.
28. Young H, Bhardwaj R, Parker MC. *Colonic stenting in palliation and as a bridge to surgery for obstructing colonic lesions*. Abstracts of the proceedings of the British Association of Surgical Oncology 2002. London.

Rationale and techniques of intra-operative hyperthermic intraperitoneal chemotherapy in peritoneal surface malignancy

A.J. Witkamp, V.J. Verwaal, S. van Ruth, E. de Bree, F.A.N. Zoetmulder

Department of Surgical Oncology, The Netherlands Cancer Institute/Antoni van Leeuwenhock Hospital, Amsterdam, The Netherlands

Introduction

Peritoneal surface malignancy has always been a major problem in cancer management. Surgery alone can never be complete at microscopic level and in gastrointestinal cancers systemic chemotherapy has only limited value. Residual or recurrent disease will occur in almost all cases and patients usually die of gastrointestinal malfunction and cachexia. In recent years it has been emphasised that peritoneal seeding can be understood as regional spread, comparable to lymph node metastases. This means that it is a poor prognostic sign, but no proof for distant metastases. This provides a rationale for regional therapy, as effective regional control will postpone death in most cases and possibly cure some of the patients. Intra-operative heated chemoperfusion of the abdominal cavity was introduced in the prevention and treatment of peritoneal surface malignancy in the early eighties. The current report reviews the literature concerning the rationale and techniques of this treatment option in the treatment of peritoneal metastases with a main emphasis on gastrointestinal tract cancers. A literature search was performed through PubMed (United States National Library of Medicine) using hyperthermia, hyperthermic, intraperitoneal, chemotherapy, colorectal cancer, gastric cancer and pseudomyxoma peritonei as keywords, using English language only.

Intraperitoneal chemotherapy

In most cases peritoneal metastases from primary gastrointestinal tract cancer are relatively resistant to intravenous cytotoxic drugs with a clear dose-effect relation, but with the effective dose exceeding the toxic dose. Intraperitoneal administration of cytotoxic drugs can increase the local exposure with less systemic toxicity compared to intravenous administration. An additional advantage is that the blood drainage of the peritoneal surface through the portal vein to the liver provides an increased exposure of potential hepatic micro metastases to intraperitoneally administered cytotoxic drugs. The concept of intraperitoneal chemotherapy is not new. Already in 1955 Weissberger *et al.* reported the treatment results of intraperitoneal nitrogen mustard in 7 patients with ovarian cancer [1]. However, most of the early reports on the clinical use of intraperitoneal chemotherapy failed to produce a clear survival benefit in patients with peritoneal surface malignancy. It lasted till 1978 when Dedrick and his co-workers took a more studied look at the pharmacokinetic favours of intraperitoneal chemotherapy [2]. They found that hydrophilic cytotoxic drugs can maintain a significant concentration gradient along the peritoneal-plasma barrier, with high intraperitoneal concentrations, when added in the abdominal cavity in large volumes [3]. However, they also emphasised that the most limiting factor in the clinical use of intraperitoneal chemotherapy is the restrictive penetration depth of the used drugs in tumour tissue (probably 1-3 mm). Dedrick's findings are confirmed by more recent studies in ovarian cancer [4-6]. It is now generally accepted that the only patients that will possibly benefit from intraperitoneal chemotherapy are patients with minimal residual disease after surgery.

Surgery

The aim of cytoreductive surgery before intraperitoneal chemotherapy is to obtain complete resection of macroscopic tumour and the complete lysis of pre-existent intra-abdominal adhesions in order to create an optimal exposure to intraperitoneal drugs. Often complete removal of all macroscopic tumours is not possible. Most groups consider intraperitoneal therapy only useful if residual tumour nodules are smaller than 3 mm, in view of recorded drug penetration depth. The importance of cytoreductive surgery on survival has already been studied in ovarian cancer [7, 8]. However, it was Sugarbaker who developed a specific surgical procedure which made it possible to perform large peritonectomy procedures with the use of electro-surgery in order to obtain maximal cytoreduction in peritoneal carcinomatosis [9]. He described 6 different peritonectomy procedures which can be performed separately or all together: greater omentectomy-splenectomy, left upper quadrant peritonectomy, right upper quadrant peritonectomy, lesser omentectomy-cholecystectomy with stripping of the omental bursa, pelvic peritonectomy with sleeve resection of the sigmoid colon and antrectomy. Using this cytoreductive technique combined with an aggressive approach towards affected intra-abdominal organs makes it possible to create an optimal situation for intraperitoneal chemotherapy in most patients. When surgical cytoreduction is performed in advance of intra-operative intraperitoneal chemotherapy, bowel reconstruction after resections is usually postponed till after the chemotherapy perfusion in order to minimise the risk of tumour cells seeding at anastomotic sites. Sugarbaker also developed an objective method to score the presence and size of macroscopic tumours in 13 different abdominal regions (Peritoneal Cancer Index) before and after cytoreductive surgery [10]. This Peritoneal Cancer Index is based on the natural route of tumour implantation and is an important help in estimating the likelihood of complete cytoreduction in peritoneal surface malignancy. The use of this scoring system should be encouraged in the surgical treatment of peritoneal carcinomatosis because it prevents unnecessary surgery in high risk patients, thus decreasing postoperative morbidity. In The Netherlands Cancer Institute a simplified version of the Peritoneal Cancer Index is used which contains 7 abdominal regions (small pelvis, ileocolic, omentum and transverse colon, small bowel and mesentery, subhepatic, subdiaphragm left and subdiaphragm right).

Hyperthermia

True clinical hyperthermia is defined as the use of temperatures of 41° C and higher. The scientific basis for the use of hyperthermia in malignancy is multifactorial. Hyperthermia itself has a direct cytotoxic effect caused by impaired DNA repair, denaturation of proteins, induction of heat-shock proteins which may serve as receptors for natural killer-cells, induction of apoptosis and inhibition of angiogenesis [11, 12]. The cytotoxic effect of hyperthermia is not only temperature dependent, but is also related to the exposure time and the time-relation to other therapies. Furthermore hyperthermia also shows a synergism with certain cytotoxic drugs *(Table I)*. Increased cell-membrane permeability at higher temperatures, can increase drug uptake by tumour tissue [13]. Pharmacokinetics of these drugs can also be affected by altered active drug transport and cell metabolism. This synergism can already occur at temperatures as low as 39 to 41° C (mild hyperthermia) in some cytotoxic drugs as cisplatinum, ifosfamide, melphalan and mitomycin C [13]. Besides this synergistic effect hyperthermia can also diminish the systemic toxicity of some drugs (*e.g.* doxorubicin and cyclophosphamide) by increasing their alkylation and/or excretion [14].

Table I. Interaction between hyperthermia and cytotoxic drugs that are used during HIPEC procedures [69]. Although enhancement of penetration depth should theoretically apply for all drugs, this has only been proved for cisplatinum

	Synergism	Non cell-cycle specific
Mitomycin C	Yes (linear ≥ 39° C)	Yes
Cisplatinum	Yes (linear ≥ 39° C)	Yes
Melphalan	Yes (linear ≥ 39° C)	Yes
Mitroxantrone	Yes (linear ≥ 39° C)	Yes
Bleomycin	Yes (threshold ≥ 42° C)	Yes
Doxorubicin	Yes (threshold ≥ 42° C)	Yes
Taxanes	No	Yes
5-FU	No	No

Hyperthermic intraperitoneal chemotherapy

In the late 1970's Spratt *et al.* began experiments in dogs in which they tried to combine hyperthermia and continuos perfusion of the abdominal cavity, in order to find a selective local treatment option for peritoneal carcinomatosis [15]. They created a model that was based on the earlier findings of the direct cytotoxic effect of hyperthermia, the synergism between hyperthermia and cytotoxic drugs and the pharmacokinetic advantage of intraperitoneal chemotherapy. Five dogs were treated with a continuous 2 hours perfusion of the abdominal cavity at 41° C without direct toxicity and a quick and homogeneous distribution of the added drug over the peritoneal cavity. This finally resulted in the first intra-operative heated intraperitoneal chemotherapy (HIPEC) perfusion in a human being with pseudomyxoma peritonei in February 1979 [16]. After surgical debulking of the macroscopic tumour mass, the abdominal cavity was perfundated with a cell cycle nonspecific agent (thiotepa) directly postoperative during $1\frac{1}{2}$ hour at 42° C. Five days postoperatively, this was followed by a cell cycle specific agent (methotrexate), which was administered during $\frac{1}{2}$ hour. No major complications or toxicity was recorded. In the following years other authors developed different clinical perfusion models for intraoperative HIPEC in respectively pseudomyxoma peritonei, colorectal- and gastric cancer.

Different perfusion techniques

Peritoneal expansion

In first reports the HIPEC procedure was performed early postoperatively, as described by Spratt. However, experiments with blue dye showed that intraperitoneal fluid distribution was not optimal, probably due to early postoperative adhesions and the development of preferential intraperitoneal pathways for perfusion fluid as soon as the abdomen is closed [17]. Therefore peritoneal expansion is applied in most centers to optimise exposure of the intra-abdominal organs and the parietal peritoneum to the perfusate. This can be achieved by different methods. Sugarbaker introduced the so called coliseum technique [18]. The skin of the abdomen is attached to a retractor ring, which is placed above the laparotomy wound. The abdominal cavity is covered with a plastic sheet with a small opening in the centre allowing entrance for the surgeon's hand to stir the abdominal contents, resulting in a better exposure of the seroperitoneal surfaces and a more uniform distribution of drug and heat. Yonemura and his co-workers were the first to introduce a "peritoneal access device" to achieve optimal peritoneal expansion [19, 20]. This expander is made of a transparent acrylic cylinder, which is fitted in the laparotomy wound. Creating peritoneal expansion according this technique makes it possible to add large volumes of perfusion fluid allowing the small bowel to float in the cavity expander. Major advantage of the two above-described techniques is that it creates a controlled distribution of fluid, heat and cytotoxic drugs. Disadvantages however are heat loss through the open laparotomy wound and more important, possible leakage of drugs thus creating a health risk for the OR personnel. Another disadvantage in the use of the peritoneal expander might be that small parts of the parietal peritoneum are not fully exposed thus creating a risk area for tumour recurrence [21]. Fujimoto and Koga both developed separately from each other a perfusion system in which the abdomen is closed during perfusion by a running suture of the skin [22, 23]. This way the whole peritoneal surface is exposed and it prevents drug spillage and heat loss. This technique also provides the possibility of increasing the abdominal pressure by adding large volumes of perfusion fluid (up to 9 litres) which might lead to increased drug penetration of macromolecular agents [24]. The latter has only been proved in a rat model using doxorubicin [25]. However, homogeneous distribution of the perfusion fluid with a closed abdomen remains very uncertain [17, 21]. Other attempts to promote the distribution of the perfusion fluid include external massage of the abdomen and an increased flow rate of perfusion fluid [26, 27].

Perfusion models

Another difference in perfusion techniques is the use of an open *versus* a closed perfusion model. Most centers use one curled Tenckhoff inflow catheter (placed centrally in the abdomen or at the site of highest risk for recurrence) and two or more outflow catheters (placed subdiaphragmaticly and in the small pelvis) to obtain a continuous flow of perfusion fluid equally distributed throughout the abdominal cavity. These catheters are inserted through separate stab incisions in the abdominal wall. When both the inflow and outflow catheters are connected to a perfusion pump, fluid filter and heat exchanger, a closed circuit is formed [26]. In an open perfusion model the outflow catheters are connected to a separate compartment, thus preventing re-use of perfusion fluid [23]. The advantage of the closed model is that it creates more control over the whole perfusion system and that it is easier to maintain adequate hyperthermia of the perfusion fluid. Disadvantage is the theoretical possibility of reintroduction of tumour cells into the abdominal cavity.

Hyperthermia control

There is no consensus yet on the optimal temperature during HIPEC procedures. As pointed out above, synergism between various cytotoxic drugs and hyperthermia starts at a temperature of $39°$ C but is stronger at higher temperatures. On the other hand, at temperatures above $43°$ C this synergism seems to decrease in most cytotoxic drugs [13] and the small bowel toxicity of heat increases above $43°$ C. Another problem in the use of hyperthermia during perfusion is the development of thermotolerance due to the activation of heat shock proteins at temperatures of around $43°$ C during short exposure time (30 minutes or less) [11]. Hyperthermia $\leq 43°$ C itself appears to have no influence on the complication rate in HIPEC procedures [28]. Most groups perfuse therefore at temperatures between 41 and $43°$ C during 60 minutes or longer. Temperature probes are attached to the in- and outflow catheters in the abdominal cavity and to the heat exchanger to control the distribution of heat. In The Netherlands Cancer Institute the intraperitoneal temperature control at multiple locations (subdiaphragmatic left and right, small pelvis and centrally in the abdominal cavity) are used as main help to register the fluid distribution. Insufficient perfusion in an area of the abdomen will very quickly result in a drop of temperature. However, manual stirring of the abdominal contents during perfusion leads to an homogeneous heat (and thus fluid) distribution. A probe in the esophagus or larynx monitors the core temperature in order to prevent malignant hyperthermia of the patient.

Choice of drug and pharmacokinetics

The pharmacokinetic advantage of intraperitoneal chemotherapy is the most important rational for HIPEC in peritoneal surface malignancy. The movement of large molecular drugs from the intraperitoneal cavity to the systemic compartment of the body is much slower than the clearance of drugs from the systemic compartment. This principle creates a concentration gradient over the peritoneal-plasma barrier, strongly in favour of the intraperitoneal concentration after intraperitoneal drug administration. Stripping of large surfaces of the peritoneum as common in peritonectomy procedures does not alter this phenomenon [29]. Rubin *et al.* showed that removal of intra-abdominal viscera also has no effect on the effectiveness of the peritoneal-plasma barrier [30]. It has to be noted that for the treatment of free intraperitoneal tumour cells high intraperitoneal drug concentrations seems of main importance. However, for invasive peritoneal tumour deposits it is more important to achieve high drug concentrations in superficial tissue bordering the peritoneal cavity. Therefore, high intraperitoneal/plasma drug concentration ratios are not automatically associated with higher efficacy, but may even be undesirable if it means that no drug has entered the target tumour residues.

Cytotoxic drugs used

For use during HIPEC procedures drugs should fulfil the following criteria: they have to be of large molecular weight and be water-soluble, they must be rapidly cleared from the systemic circulation and their effectiveness must be enhanced by (mild) hyperthermia. Non cell-cycle specific drugs are an advantage because they are cytotoxic after even a relatively short exposure time. *Table I* shows commonly used chemotherapeutical agents that meet these criteria. Although 5-fluorouracil has been widely used in postoperative intraperitoneal chemotherapy, it seems not an ideal drug for HIPEC procedures because it shows no synergism with hyperthermia and its cytotoxicity is cell-cycle dependent.

Pharmacokinetics and dosage

Both clinical and pre-clinical studies have shown the pharmacokinetic advantage of HIPEC. High intraperitoneal drug concentrations can be obtained in HIPEC procedures in combination with relatively low plasma concentrations [31-39]. This is also found when the area under the time concentrations curve (AUC) is used as a more exact measure of total drug exposure. However, comparison between the different studies regarding pharmacokinetics is difficult because of the difference in drugs, dosage and perfusion techniques used. Most clinical experience in HIPEC procedures is gained with mitomycin C (MMC) and platinum containing therapy. With MMC, peritoneal-plasma concentration ratios up to 28 are described [32], while rapid absorption leads to high tissue levels [35]. *Tables II and III* show various pharmacokinetic studies in MMC and cisplatinum in HIPEC procedures. It appears that higher abdominal temperatures lead to higher peritoneal/plasma concentration- or AUC-ratios. Although it has to be noticed that in some of the reported studies the plasma AUC is only calculated for the duration of the perfusion, while in other studies the AUC is calculated for the first 24 hours during and after perfusion. The duration of perfusion seems to have no influence on the peritoneal/plasma ratios. In most of the reported studies intraperitoneal drug half-life is 90 minutes or less. This finding pleads

Table II. MMC pharmacokinetics during HIPEC

Study	n	Dose	Abdomen	Mean i.p. temp.	Perfusion time	i.p. t$_{1/2}$ (min)	MMC]$_{max}$ pe/pl	AUC pe/pl
Loggie [56]	7	20 mg/L	Closed	40.5° C (inflow)	120 min.	97 min. (±31)	27	–
Fujimoto [32]	21	10 mg/L	Closed	45° C (outflow)	118 (±17) min.	–	28	–
Beaujard [39]	83	10 mg/L	Closed	42° C	90 min.	–	20	–
Panteix [35]	18	10 mg/L	Closed	42° C	90-120 min.	–	24	–
Fernandez-Trigo [26]	10	5-10 mg/L	Closed	41-43° C	120 min.	58 (±13) min.	–	22
Jacquet [42]	18	10 mg/L	Open	41-43° C	120 min	58 (±10) min	–	23.5
Neth. Cancer Institute	118	18 mg/L	Open	40-41° C	90 min	–	25	13

Table III. Cisplatin pharmacokinetics during HIPEC

Study	n	Dose	Abdomen	Mean i.p. temp.	Perfusion time	i.p. t$_{1/2}$ (min)	MMC]$_{max}$ pe/pl	AUC pe/pl
Stephens [70]	13	86.4 mg	Closed	40.6° C	120 min.	48 (±14)	–	6.9 (±3.6)
Van de Vaart [36]	5	108 mg	Open	41.5° C	90 min.	–	15	–
Ma [37]	9	300 mg	Closed	41° C	90 min.	30	13	21

for a perfusion time of 90 minutes or less, or a divided drug administration, in order to maintain effective intraperitoneal drug concentrations. When MMC is used, higher ratio's are reached compared to cisplatinum. DNA-adduct measurements after HIPEC procedures with cisplatinum have shown that penetration of cisplatinum in tissue is significantly improved when compared to normothermic intraperitoneal therapy [36, 40]. There are no data on the penetration depth of MMC after intraperitoneal use. However, therapeutic MMC concentrations are found in the urothelium, lamina propria and even the muscle layer of the bladder after intravesical instillation therapy, suggesting the penetration of at least a few millimetres [41]. Different dose schedules are described. Most authors dose per litre volume of perfusion fluid (mg/L) [32, 38, 42]. Other studies use a dosage based on body surface (mg/m^2) [43] or a combination of both (mg/m^2/L) [44]. The latter seems the most accurate because the total volume of perfusate used can differ significantly inter-individually. There are few reports on the maximum tolerated dose of cytotoxic drugs in HIPEC procedures [45]. In our own institution we have performed HIPEC procedures with MMC in colorectal carcinoma and pseudomyxoma peritonei at different dose levels. We used 15, 25, 35 and 40 mg/m^2. Pharmacokinetic analysis showed that the best peritoneal-plasma AUC ratio was at 35 mg/m^2. Unacceptable systemic toxicity occurred at 40 mg/m^2 (*i.e.* grade IV leucocytopenia), finally resulting in two postoperative deaths. Therefore 35 mg/m^2 MMC was chosen as standard dose in HIPEC procedures in The Netherlands Cancer Institute.

Complications

The combination of aggressive surgical cytoreduction and HIPEC is associated with a relatively high morbidity rate. Complications that occur may arise as a result from the surgical procedure, hyperthermia or the intraperitoneal chemotherapy. There is a wide variation in reported morbidity (0-39%) and mortality rates (0-20%), regardless of indication, technique and cytotoxic drug used [23, 24, 39, 46-50].

Surgical complications

The major surgical complications described include mainly bowel perforations, anastomotic leakage and fistula. Also bile leakage, pancreatitis, postoperative bleeding, wound dehiscence, deep vein thrombosis and pulmonary embolism, pneumothorax, cardiovascular arrest and ischaemic cerebral damage are reported. It is often difficult to separate complications related to surgery from those that are related to intraperitoneal chemotherapy or heat. Most of the described major complications appear to be related to the aggressive surgical procedure. Number of previous laparotomies, duration of surgery, number of peritonectomy procedures, number of visceral resections and number of suture lines are associated with major morbidity [49]. Fumagalli *et al.* found that MMC impairs the heeling of suture lines, resulting in an increased anastomotic leakage after HIPEC with MMC in rats [51]. Randomised studies in gastric cancer have shown no clinical proof for this [19, 23, 52, 53]. Bowel perforations are probably caused by surgical trauma of the bowel surfaces, maybe enhanced by thermal and chemotherapeutic damage [46, 54, 55]. However, by using a control group that was treated with intra-operative normothermic intraperitoneal chemotherapy, Shido *et al.* showed that hyperthermia itself does not cause peritoneal damage when used in HIPEC procedures.

Systemic toxicity

Systemic toxicity includes renal failure in cisplatinum perfusions and grade III and IV hematologic toxicity in MMC perfusions. Renal failure after HIPEC is generally reversible, however postoperative death due to severe renal failure has been described [56]. There is also a case report of anaphylactic reaction after intraperitoneal chemotherapy with cisplatin [57]. Bone marrow suppression resulting in leucocytopenia and thrombocytopenia is clearly a result from intraperitoneal chemotherapy and is dose and drug (MMC) related [49, 55]. Remarkable is the observation that the nadir of bone marrow suppression after HIPEC with MMC is < 2 weeks postoperatively, while the nadir after systemic MMC is 4-6 weeks after administration [38]. The haemolytic-uraemic-syndrome (HUS), which sometimes occurs after intravenous MMC or cisplatinum administration, is not described after HIPEC procedures.

Survival after HIPEC

Most clinical experience with aggressive surgical cytoreduction in combination with HIPEC has been gained in gastric cancer, pseudomyxoma peritonei and peritoneal carcinomatosis from colorectal origin *(Table IV)*. Other positive results have been reported in intraperitoneal mesothelioma, sarcomatosis and advanced ovarian cancer [37, 58-60]. An important prognostic factor in most studies reporting survival is the completeness of cytoreduction achieved during surgery. Unfortunately there are no reliable data on the influence of drug dosage on survival. Aggressive surgical cytoreduction followed by HIPEC appears to be an effective treatment in peritoneal carcinomatosis from gastric origin, resulting in an improved survival rate [61]. At this time randomised data on survival after HIPEC in gastric cancer are only available from studies in which HIPEC was used as prophylactic adjuvant treatment during primary surgery for high-risk gastric cancer [47, 62, 63]. These studies show that survival in high risk gastric cancer can be improved by using HIPEC as adjuvant treatment *(Table V)*.

Table IV. Results regarding survival after extensive surgical cytoreduction and HIPEC in patients with pseudomyxoma peritonei and peritoneal carcinomatosis of colorectal and gastric origin (* = follow-up for whole group of treated patients, not specified for colorectal carcinoma, ** = randomised study)

Study	Year	Tumour site	n	Median follow-up	Survival
Sugarbaker [65]	1999	Appendix carcinoma	161	–	2 yrs 50%, 5 yrs 30%
Schneebaum [64]	1996	colorectal carcinoma	15	10 months	NED in 1 patient, all alive
Loggie [68]	2000	colorectal carcinoma	38	27 months*	2 yrs 39%, 3 yrs 24%
Cavaliere [66]	2000	colorectal carcinoma	14	30 months*	2 yrs 64%
Witkamp [50]	2000	colorectal carcinoma	29	38 months	2 yrs 45%, 3 yrs 23%
Elias [67]	1997	colorectal carcinoma	23	12 months*	2 yrs 40%
Neth Cancer Institute	2003	colorectal carcinoma	105	21.6 months**	2 yrs 45% vs 22%
Witkamp [43]	2000	pseudomyxoma peritonei	46	12 months	3 yrs 81%
Sugarbaker [65]	1999	pseudomyxoma peritonei	224	–	5 yrs 80%
Fujimoto [61]	1997	Gastric cancer	48	–	3 yrs 42%, 5 yrs 31%
Yonemura [71]	1999	Gastric cancer	83	–	5 yrs 11%
Beaujard [39]	2000	Gastric cancer	23	–	1 yr 48%, 2 yrs 33%

Table V. Results of randomised studies regarding HIPEC as adjuvant prophylactic treatment in high risk (stage III, TNM classification) gastric cancer

Study	Year	n° of patients surgery alone	n° of patients surgery + HIPEC	5 yrs survival surgery alone	5 yrs survival surgery + HIPEC
Yu [62]	1998	81	78	18.4%	49.1%
Ikeguchi [63]	1995	39	33	44%	66%
Fujimoto [47]*	1999	70	71	49%**	62%**

* Both low-risk and high risk patients included;
** 8 years survival.

Phase II data on colorectal cancer and pseudomyxoma peritonei are promising [43, 50, 64-68]. For that reason a randomised trial was performed at the Netherlands Cancer institute. Between February 1998 and August 2001, 105 patients were randomised to receive either standard treatment consisting of systemic chemotherapy (5-FU/Leucovorin) with or without palliative surgery or experimental therapy consisting of aggressive cytoreduction with HIPEC, followed by the same systemic chemotherapy regime. The primary end-point was survival. After a median follow-up period of 21.6 months, the median survival was 12.6 months in the standard therapy arm and 22.3 months in the experimental therapy arm (log rank test: $p = 0.032$). The treatment related mortality in the aggressive therapy group was 8%, while most complications from HIPEC were related to bowel leakage. Subgroup analysis of the HIPEC group showed that patients with 0 to 5 of the 7 regions of the abdominal cavity involved by tumour at the time of the cytoreduction had a significantly better survival than patients with 6 or 7 affected regions (log rank test: $p < 0.0001$). If the cytoreduction was macroscopically complete (R-1), the median survival was also significantly better than in patients with limited (R-2a), or extensive residual disease (R-2b) (log rank: $p < 0.0001$).

Conclusions

Aggressive cytoreductive surgery followed by intra-operative HIPEC has recently been introduced in the treatment of peritoneal surface malignancy. Pharmacokinetic studies have shown a clear dose advantage for HIPEC *versus* systemic chemotherapy. The prerequisites for HIPEC are minimal residual disease after surgery and the absence of extra-abdominal metastases. During perfusion expansion of the abdominal cavity is applied to optimise drug exposure. Various drugs can be used, but most experience has been gained in MMC and cisplatinum. Local complications after HIPEC are mainly surgery related, while systemic toxicity is caused by the intraperitoneal chemotherapy. The latter is dose and drug dependent. Randomised studies have shown that HIPEC reduces the risk of peritoneal recurrence when used during primary surgery in high-risk gastric cancer. A randomised study in peritoneal carcinomatosis from colorectal origin recently performed at the Netherlands Cancer Institute showed a significant improved 2-years survival for patients treated with cytoreductive surgery and HIPEC with MMC.

References

1. Weissberger AS, Levine B and Storaasli JP. Use of nitrogen mustard in treatment of serous effusions of neo-plastic origin. *JAMA* 1955; 159: 1704-7.
2. Dedrick RL, Myers CE, Bungay PM, DeVita VT Jr. Pharmacokinetic rationale for peritoneal drug administration in the treatment of ovarian cancer. *Cancer Treat Rep* 1978; 62: 1-9.
3. Jones RB, Myers CE, Guarino AM, et al. High volume intraperitoneal chemotherapy ("belly bath") for ovarian cancer. Pharmacologic basis and early results. *Cancer Chemother Pharmacol* 1978; 1: 161-6.
4. Howell SB, Zimm S, Markman M, et al. Long-term survival of advanced refractory ovarian carcinoma patients with small-volume disease treated with intraperitoneal chemotherapy. *J Clin Oncol* 1987; 5: 1607-12.
5. Alberts DS, Liu PY, Hannigan EV, et al. Intraperitoneal cisplatin plus intravenous cyclophosphamide *versus* intravenous cisplatin plus intravenous cyclophosphamide for stage III ovarian cancer. *N Engl J Med* 1996; 335: 1950-5.
6. Ozols RF, Gore M, Tropé C, et al. Intraperitoneal treatment and dose-intense therapy in ovarian cancer. *Ann Oncol* 1999; 10: 59-64.
7. Griffiths CT, Parker LM and Fuller AF Jr. Role of cytoreductive surgical treatment in the management of advanced ovarian cancer. *Cancer Treat Rep* 1979; 63: 235-40.
8. Eisenkop SM, Friedman RL and Wang HJ. Secondary cytoreductive surgery for recurrent ovarian cancer. A prospective study. *Cancer* 1995; 76: 1606-14.
9. Sugarbaker PH. Peritonectomy procedures. *Ann Surg* 1995; 221: 29-42.
10. Sugarbaker PH, Ronnet B, Archer A, et al. Pseudomyxoma peritonei syndrome. *Adv Surg* 1996; 30: 233-80.
11. Christophi C, Winkworth A, Muralihdaran V, Evans P. The treatment of malignancy by hyperthermia. *Surg Oncol* 1999; 7: 83-90.
12. Dahl O, Dalene R, Schem BC, Mella O. Status of clinical hyperthermia. *Acta Oncol* 1999; 38: 863-73.
13. Storm FK. Clinical hyperthermia and chemotherapy. *Radiol Clin N America* 1989; 27: 621-7.
14. Bull JMC. An update on the anticancer effects of a combination of chemotherapy and hyperthermia. *Cancer Res* 1984; 44: 4853s-6s.
15. Spratt JS, Adcock RA, Sherrill W, Travathen S. Hyperthermic peritoneal perfusion system in canines. *Cancer Res* 1980; 40: 253-5.
16. Spratt JS, Adcock RA, Muskovin M, et al. Clinical delivery system for intraperitoneal hyperthermic chemotherapy. *Cancer Res* 1980; 40: 256-60.
17. Averbach AM, Sugarbaker PH. Methodologic considerations in treatment using intraperitoneal chemotherapy. *Cancer Treat Res* 1996; 82: 289-309.
18. Sugarbaker PH. Management of peritoneal-surface malignancy: the surgeon's role. *Langenbecks Arch Surg* 1999; 384: 576-87.
19. Fujimura T, Yonemura Y, Muraoka K, et al. Continuous hyperthermic peritoneal perfusion for the prevention of peritoneal recurrence of gastric cancer: randomised controlled study. *World J Surg* 1994; 18: 150-5.
20. Yonemura Y, Fujimura T, Fushida S, et al. Hyperthermo-chemotherapy combined with cytoreductive surgery for the treatment of gastric cancer with peritoneal dissemination. *World J Surg* 1991; 15: 530-6.
21. Elias D, Damia E, Puizillout J, et al. Thermic homogeneity and standardization of intraperitoneal chemohyperthermia for peritoneal carcinomatosis. *Reg Cancer Treat* 1996; 9: 54-9.
22. Fujimoto S, Shrestha R, Kokobun M, et al. Intraperitoneal hyperthermic perfusion combined with surgery effective for gastric cancer patients with peritoneal seeding. *Ann Surg* 1988: 36-40.

23. Koga S, Hamazoe R, Maeta M, et al. Prophylactic therapy for peritoneal recurrence of gastric cancer by continuous hyperthermic peritoneal perfusion with mitomycin-C. Cancer 1988; 61: 232-7.
24. Tsiftis D, de Bree E, Romanos J, et al. Peritoneal expansion by artificially produced ascites during perfusion chemotherapy. Arch Surg 1999; 134: 545-9.
25. Jacquet P, Stuart OA, Chang D, Sugarbaker PH. Effects of intra-abdominal pressure on pharmacokinetics and tissue distribution of doxorubicin after intraperitoneal administration. Anticancer Drugs 1996; 7: 596-603.
26. Fernandez-Trigo V, Stuart OA, Stephens AD, et al. Surgically directed chemotherapy: heated intraperitoneal lavage with mitomycin C. Cancer Treat Res 1996; 81: 51-61.
27. Otani S, Maeta M, Oka A, et al. Long term survival of 5 years following initial surgery for gastric cancer and simultaneous disseminated peritoneal metastasis. Surg Today 1995; 25: 959-61.
28. Shido A, Ohmura S, Yamamoto K, et al. Does hyperthermia induce peritoneal damage in continuous hyperthermic peritoneal perfusion. World J Surg 2000; 24: 507-11.
29. Jacquet P, Sugarbaker PH. Peritoneal-plasma barrier. Cancer Treat Res 1996; 82: 53-63.
30. Rubin J, Jones Q, Planch A, Bower JD. The minimal importance of hollow viscera to peritoneal transport during peritoneal dialysis in the rat. Am Soc Artif Intern Organs Transact 1988; 34: 912-5.
31. Ceelen WP, Hesse U, de Hemptinne B, Pattyn P. Hyperthermic intraperitoneal chemoperfusion in the treatment of locally advanced intraabdominal cancer. Br J Surg 2000; 87: 1006-15.
32. Fujimoto S, Shrestha RD, Kokobun M, et al. Pharmacokinetic analysis of mitomycin C for intraperitoneal hyperthermic perfusion in patients with far-advanced or recurrent gastric cancer. Reg Cancer Treat 1989; 2: 198-202.
33. Nicoletto MO, Padrini R, Galeotti F, et al. Pharmacokinetics of intraperitoneal hyperthermic perfusion with mitoxantrone in ovarian cancer. Cancer Chemother Pharmacol 2000; 45: 457-62.
34. Jacquet P, Averbach A, Stuart OA, et al. Hyperthermic intraperitoneal doxorubicin: pharmacokinetics, metabolism, and tissue distribution in a rat model. Cancer Chemother Pharmacol 1998; 41: 147-54.
35. Panteix G, Guillaumont M, Cherpin L, et al. Study of the pharmakokinetics of mitomycin C in humans during intraperitoneal chemothermia with special mention of the concentration in local tissues. Oncology 1993; 50: 366-70.
36. Van de Vaart PJM, Van der Vange N, Zoetmulder FAN, et al. Intraperitoneal cisplatin with regional hyperthermia in advanced ovarian cancer: pharmacokinetics and cisplatin-DNA adduct formation in patients and ovarian cancer cell lines. Eur J Cancer 1998; 34: 148-54.
37. Ma GY, Bartlett DL, Reed E, et al. Continuous hyperthermic peritoneal perfusion with cisplatin for the treatment of peritoneal mesothelioma. Cancer J Sci Am 1997; 3: 174-6.
38. Loggie BW, Fleming RA. Complications of heated intraperitoneal chemotherapy and strategies for prevention. 1996: 221-233.
39. Beaujard AC, Glehen O, Caillot JL, et al. Intraperitoneal chemohyperthermia with mitomycin C for digestive tract cancer patients with peritoneal carcinomatosis. Cancer 2000; 88: 2512-9.
40. Los G, van Vucht MJ, Pinedo HM. Response of peritoneal solid tumours after i.p. chemohyperthermia treatment with cisplatin or carboplatin. Br J Cancer 1994; 69: 235-41.
41. Wientjes MG, Badalament RA, Wang RC, et al. Penetration of mitomycin C in human bladder. Cancer Res 1993; 53: 3314.
42. Jacquet P, Averbach A, Stephens AD, et al. Heated intra-operative intraperitoneal mitomycin C and early postoperative intraperitoneal 5-fluorouracil: pharmacokinetic studies. Oncology 1998; 55: 130-8.
43. Witkamp AJ, de Bree E, Kaag MM, et al. Extensive surgical cytoreduction and intra-operative hyperthermic intraperitoneal chemotherapy in patients with pseudomyxoma peritonei. Br J Surg 2001; 88: 458-63.
44. Cavaliere F, Di Filippo F, Botti C, et al. Peritonectomy and hyperthermic antiblast perfusion in the treatment of peritoneal carcinomatosis. Eur J Surg Onc 2000; 26: 486-91.

45. Steller MA, Egorin MJ, Trimble EL, et al. A pilot phase I trial of continuous hyperthermic peritoneal perfusion with high-dose carboplatin as primary treatment of patients with small-volume residual ovarian cancer. *Cancer Chemother Pharmacol* 1999; 43: 106-14.
46. Jacquet P, Stephens AD, Averbach AM, et al. Analysis of morbidity and mortality in 60 patients with peritoneal carcinomatosis treated by cytoreductive surgery and heated intra-operative intraperitoneal chemotherapy. *Cancer* 1996; 77: 2622-9.
47. Ikeguchi M, Kondou A, Oka A, et al. Effects of continuous hyperthermic peritoneal perfusion on prognosis of gastric cancer with serosal invasion. *Eur J Surg* 1995; 161: 581-6.
48. Yonemura Y, Ninomiya I, Kaji M, et al. Prophylaxix with intra-operative chemohyperthermia against peritoneal recurrence of serosal invasion-positive gastric cancer. *World J Surg* 1995; 19: 450-5.
49. Stephens AD, Alderman R, Chang D, et al. Morbidity and mortality analysis of 200 treatments with cytoreductive surgery and hyperthermic intra-operative intraperitoneal chemotherapy using the coliseum technique. *Ann Surg Oncol* 1999; 6: 790-96.
50. Witkamp AJ, de Bree E, Kaag MM, et al. Extensive cytoreductive surgery followed by intra-operative hyperthermic intraperitoneal chemotherapy with mitomycin-C in patients with peritoneal carcinomatosis from colorectal origin. *Eur J Cancer* 2001.
51. Fumagalli U, Trabucchi E, Soligo M, et al. Effects of intraperitoneal chemotherapy on anastomotic healing in the rat. *J Surg Res* 1991; 50: 82-7.
52. Hamazoe R, Maeta M, Kaibara N. Intraperitoneal thermochemotherapy for prevention of peritoneal recurrence of gastric cancer. Final results of a randomised controlled study. *Cancer* 1994; 73: 2048-52.
53. Fujimoto S, Shrestha R, Kokobun M, et al. Positive results of combined therapy of surgery and intraperitoneal hyperthermic perfusion for far-advanced gastric cancer. *Ann Surg* 1990; 212: 592-6.
54. Sayag-Beuajard AC, Francois Y, Glehen O, et al. Intraperitoneal chemohyperthermia with mitomycin C for gastric cancer patients with peritoneal carcinomatosis. *Anticancer Res* 1999; 19: 1375-82.
55. Witkamp AJ, Muller SH, de Bree E, et al. Impact of mitomycin-C kinetics on surgical complications after hyperthermic intraperitoneal chemotherapy (HIPEC). *Eur J Surg Oncol* 2000; 26.
56. Loggie BW, Fleming RA. Complications of heated intraperitoneal chemotherapy and strategies for prevention. *Cancer Treat Res* 1996; 82: 221-33.
57. Özgüroglu M, Demir G, Demirelli F, Mandel NM. Anaphylaxis from intraperitoneal infusion of cisplatin; a case report. *Am J Clin Oncol* 1999; 22: 172-3.
58. De Bree E, Christodoulakis M, Tsiftis D. Malignant peritoneal mesothelioma treated by continuous hyperthermic peritoneal perfusion chemotherapy. *Ann Oncol* 2000.
59. Eilber FC, Rosen G, Forscher C, et al. Surgical resection and intraperitoneal chemotherapy for recurrent abdominal sarcomas. *Ann Surg Oncol* 1999; 6: 645-50.
60. Van der Vange N, van Goethem AR, Zoetmulder FAN, et al. Extensive cytoreductive surgery combined with intra-operative intraperitoneal perfusion with cisplatin under hyperthermic conditions (OVHIPEC) in patients with recurrent ovarian cancer; a pilot study. *Eur J Surg Onc* 2000.
61. Fujimoto S, Takahashi M, Mutou T, et al. Improved mortality rate of gastric carcinoma patients with peritoneal carcinomatosis treated with intraperitoneal hyperthermic chemoperfusion combined with surgery. *Cancer* 1997; 79: 884-91.
62. Yu W, Whang I, Suh I, et al. Prospective randomised trial of early postoperative intraperitoneal chemotherapy as an adjuvant to resectable gastric cancer. *Ann Surg* 1998; 228: 347-54.
63. Fujimoto S, Takahashi M, Mutou T, et al. Successful intraperitoneal hyperthermic chemoperfusion for the prevention of postoperative peritoneal recurrence in patients with advanced gastric carcinoma. *Cancer* 1999; 85: 529-34.
64. Schneebaum S, Arnold MW, Staubus A, et al. Intraperitoneal hyperthermic perfusion with mitomycin C for colorectal cancer with peritoneal metastases. *Ann Surg Oncol* 1996; 3: 44-50.
65. Sugarbaker PH and Chang D. Results of treatment of 385 patients with peritoneal surface spread of appendiceal malignancy. *Ann Surg Oncol* 1999; 6: 727-31.

66. Cavaliere F, Perri P, Di Filippo F, *et al.* Treatment of peritoneal carcinomatosis with intent to cure. *J Surg Oncol* 2000; 74: 41-4.
67. Elias D, Dubé P, Blot F, *et al.* Peritoneal carcinomatosis treatment with curative intent: the Institut Gustave-Roussy experience. *Eur J Surg Onc* 1997; 23: 317-21.
68. Loggie BW, Fleming RA, McQuellen RP, *et al.* Cytoreductive surgery with intraperitoneal hyperthermic chemotherapy for disseminated peritoneal cancer of gastrointestinal origin. *Am Surgeon* 2000; 66: 561-8.
69. Rietbroek RC. Hyperthermia in combination with chemotherapy: from laboratory bench to bedside. 1996: 13-37.
70. Stephens AD, Belliveau JF, Sugarbaker PH. Intra-operative hyperthermic lavage with cisplatin for peritoneal carcinomatosis and sarcomatosis. *Cancer Treat Res* 1996; 81: 15-30.
71. Yonemura Y, Fujimura T, Nishimura G, *et al.* Effects of intra-operative chemohyperthermia in patients with gastric cancer with peritoneal dissemination. *Surgery* 1996; 119: 437-44.

Achevé d'imprimer par 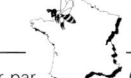 Corlet, Imprimeur, S.A.
14110 Condé-sur-Noireau
N° d'Imprimeur : 73288 - Dépôt légal : octobre 2003

Imprimé en France